AIDS,
ETHICS
&
RELIGION

p. 200

p. 153

p. 206 QUALITY CARE

p. 208 POSITIVE LIVING

p. 212 QUOTE — "VISION"

AIDS,
ETHICS
&
RELIGION

Embracing a World of Suffering

KENNETH R. OVERBERG, S.J.
Editor

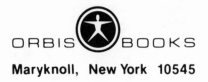

ORBIS BOOKS
Maryknoll, New York 10545

Compilation and Introduction Copyright © 1994 by Kenneth R. Overberg, S.J.

Grateful acknowledgment is made to authors and publishers who granted permission to reprint material. These permissions are acknowledged on the first page of each chapter.

Library of Congress Cataloging-in-Publication Data

Aids, ethics & religion : embracing a world of suffering / Kenneth R.
   Overberg, editor.
       p.   cm.
   Includes bibliographical references and index.
   ISBN 0-88344-949-8 (pbk.)
   1. AIDS (Disease)—Moral and ethical aspects.   2. AIDS (Disease)—
Religious aspects—Christianity.   3. AIDS (Disease)—Social
aspects.   I. Overberg, Kenneth R.   II. Title: Aids, ethics, and
religion.
RC644.A25A36   1994
174'.2—dc20   93-42176
                                                                  CIP

To
Tony and Rosie
in memory of
Joe and Jane
and
Aloysius Gonzaga, S.J.

Contents

Part III
Society and AIDS
Responses and Strategies

GREAT ARTICLE. INFORMA-TIVE

Part IV
Religion and AIDS
Compassion and Care

AIDS: A Worsening Crisis
Challenges Society and Religion

Kenneth R. Overberg

In a moving account of AIDS in one affluent town, the video "The Los Altos Story" describes three people infected with HIV, the virus that causes AIDS. One of these people, a senior citizen and a long-time resident of Los Altos,[1] has for many years played Santa Claus at Christmas. With tragic symbolism, this situation reminds us that AIDS is not somebody else's disease, somebody else's worry. AIDS touches all kinds of people, including a gentle man who played Santa Claus.

AIDS is *our* disease, a disease of the human family. For many of us, this fact may be difficult to accept fully. Because AIDS first spread in the homosexual community in the United States and also among those using drugs, some of us in the U.S. see AIDS as *their* disease. There may even be elements of prejudice in our reactions. Similar ignorance and intolerance can be found around the world. By presenting the facts about AIDS, this anthology challenges the misconceptions and focuses on the profound dilemmas confronting society and religion.

The Relationship of AIDS and HIV

We now know many basic facts about AIDS. We also know that we have much to learn as research continues. AIDS (Acquired Immune Deficiency Syndrome) is caused by HIV (Human Immunodeficiency Virus). This virus attacks certain white blood cells called T-cells, eventually destroying a per-

A revision of "AIDS: A Worsening Crisis Challenges Church and Society," *Catholic Update*, January 1993.

son's immune system. As a result, the individual can suffer from many diseases that a healthy immune system would reject. It is this stage of the disease—with its low T-cell count and eventually many infections including *pneumocystis carinii* pneumonia (PCP) and a rare form of cancer called Kaposi's sarcoma—which is technically defined as AIDS. One of these "opportunistic" infections finally kills the person.

The AIDS virus, HIV, is spread in several ways: sexual contact (including heterosexual and homosexual intercourse), exchange of blood (especially through sharing dirty needles for piercing, tattoos, steroids, or drugs), and the birth process (an infected mother can transmit the virus to her infant). HIV, then, is spread when certain body fluids are transferred from an infected person: in semen, vaginal fluids, blood, breast milk, as well as in the process of birth. HIV can also be transmitted through blood transfusions. While improved screening has almost completely eliminated this danger in the United States, such screening is not available in many countries around the world. HIV is *not* spread through casual contact: touching or hugging, sneezing or spitting, using bathroom facilities. We must note that in one sense HIV is relatively hard to spread (only several means are possible), and yet these very means are found in very ordinary activity (sexual intercourse) and in frequent, addictive behavior (intravenous drug use).

Once infected with HIV, a person is able to infect other persons, even though the infected person shows no signs of the disease. Indeed, we now know that the incubation period, the time from HIV infection to the development of full-blown AIDS, can be very long, even more than ten years. Yet throughout the incubation period, an HIV-positive person can transmit the infection to others. Just about everyone who is infected with HIV will most likely develop AIDS. (As this Introduction is being written, experts are stressing several points that must be kept in mind: 1. a cure or vaccine is not likely to be developed soon; 2. early diagnosis and treatment and new drug therapies, however, may significantly slow down the progression from infection to full-blown AIDS; 3. HIV infection is properly understood as a chronic disease, that is, an illness that lasts a long time and eventually gets worse.)

AIDS was first described in 1981. Since then scientists have done extensive research. Drugs such as AZT have been developed to slow the progression of AIDS. Blood screening in some countries has made blood transfusions much safer. Many researchers warn us, however, that no quick technological solution for AIDS will be found. HIV is a virus that mutates easily and different strains of HIV exist today. All this makes the development of a vaccine extremely difficult. Realistically, then, we must confront the reality of AIDS and the prospect of living with AIDS.

The Suffering Has Spread

The extent of AIDS is staggering and the human suffering involved overwhelming. Statistics constantly change,[2] but the following numbers give some sense of the magnitude of this global epidemic. By 1992 an estimated 12.9 million people had been infected with HIV. Forty percent of this number are women, an increase from 25 percent in 1990. More than a million children are HIV positive. Nearly 2.5 million people have died from AIDS.

Researchers stress that we have not yet seen the full impact of AIDS, which is still spreading with astounding rapidity. In the United States, AIDS is moving into the heterosexual community, especially through bisexuality and intravenous drug use. Given sexual promiscuity and the presence of other sexually transmitted diseases, the potential for widespread infection is serious. In Asia and Africa, AIDS is mainly spread heterosexually. Indeed, Dr. Jonathan Mann of the Harvard School of Public Health has said that if AIDS had been recognized first in Central Africa—as it could have been—then AIDS would be known as a heterosexually transmitted disease that also affects homosexuals. More than half of the world's HIV-infected persons live in Africa.

By 2000, however, Asia will overtake Africa with the largest proportion of HIV-infected persons. By that year, perhaps as many as 110 million people will be infected! Between 1992 and 1995, the number of people who develop AIDS will exceed the total who developed the disease during the entire history of the epidemic. In the same time the number of children orphaned by AIDS will more than double.

The numbers are staggering; the human suffering is overwhelming. People do not simply waste away from AIDS. The suffering is intense and prolonged. Many diseases, some of them unfamiliar to most of us, attack the person with AIDS. Later stages may also include explosive diarrhea, lung infections, blindness, and dementia.

If individual human suffering is extreme, so is the cost to society. In some countries in Africa, a significant percentage of the population is HIV-infected. A generation of young adults is dying before its time, leaving many children orphaned, leaving countries without new leaders in business and politics. The health-care system, already confronting poverty, civil war, malnutrition, tuberculosis, and malaria, can barely cope with AIDS. For example, the cost of treating ten AIDS patients in the United States is greater than the *entire budget* of Zaire's largest hospital.

In the United States, AIDS is spreading rapidly in Hispanic and African-American communities, which already face a host of problems including racial prejudice, poverty, crime, and drug abuse. Confronting these issues and their relationship to AIDS challenges the nation's political will and its commitment to the common good. The health-care system, under severe economic pressures, faces massive new demands on its resources as the number of persons with AIDS multiplies.

The first section of this book, "Geography and AIDS," presents an overview of this global spread of AIDS. Truly, AIDS is a pandemic—the articles affirm this fact and at the same time offer insight into the various routes of AIDS and its many regional differences. Only with an understanding of the basic facts and an appreciation of the global realities can we begin to grasp the challenges faced by society and religion.

AIDS Raises Moral Dilemmas

AIDS raises many medical, social, and political issues, both nationally and globally, all with profound ethical questions. These complex moral dilemmas cover the human life-span. The first cluster of moral questions is focused on birth and infancy. Ought HIV-infected women to become pregnant? Is contraception possible when AIDS is involved? What about abortion? (About 30 percent of children born to HIV-infected mothers are also HIV positive.) What is the proper treatment for HIV-infected infants? How can society care for AIDS orphans?

A second cluster of ethical questions relates to HIV-infected persons and their relationships. What are their moral responsibilities concerning risky behavior that could infect others? Must previous contacts be informed? How do couples decide about their sexual behavior? What about dealings with physicians: issues of privacy, confidentiality, truth-telling, using experimental drugs?

A third cluster of concerns centers on the end of life. How much pain must be endured? What kinds of life-support treatment are appropriate? Is there a limit to the resources to be used? Is euthanasia or physician-assisted suicide an option?

Society itself faces another cluster of moral dilemmas. Does the common good of society demand testing for the AIDS virus, and who will be tested: health-care personnel, those with high-risk behaviors, those who apply for marriage licenses, those convicted of crimes, everyone? (In some African countries, a policy of universal testing would, by itself, more than exhaust the entire health-care budget.) What about quarantine? How does society fund and manage research and testing? Is there a moral obligation concerning educational programs in the light of the growing epidemic?

What about the effects of prejudice against HIV-infected persons: in housing, parishes, employment, insurance, and medical treatment? Must HIV-infected physicians and dentists stop practicing their profession? What ought society do about the economic and social structures, nationally and globally, which contribute to the spread of AIDS? What about immigration policies? What does society do about scarce resources when there is not enough research, money, or people to treat every disease, to do everything for every person? In all these questions, who decides and by what values and norms do they decide?

This long list of disturbing questions leads to the next two sections of the book: "Ethics and AIDS" and "Society and AIDS." Although many of the issues overlap, we will first consider some major moral dilemmas. The articles allow us to wrestle with the particulars of complex questions facing individuals and societies. Some of the articles describe the reality involved (for example, costs or suicide), but may not explicitly raise all the ethical implications. Readers, whether alone or in groups, will have to bring their ethical perspectives to these topics in order to benefit fully from the articles.[3] Our cluster of questions and the selection of articles remind us how AIDS touches all times and dimensions of life and challenge us to remember that even the most personal decision must also be viewed in a social context.

Accordingly, the third section of this book, "Society and AIDS," considers a variety of strategies and responses, both in the United States and in other settings. This social perspective presents its own unique challenge, for issues of economics, racism, power, cultural change, and societal structures must be included when addressing the AIDS pandemic. Similarly, given the differences in societies, culturally appropriate education and prevention strategies need to be emphasized. These differences are highlighted in the articles—from U.S. concern about how to approach the epidemic (with serious implications for many of the issues in "Ethics and AIDS") to community-based prevention programs in some developing countries.

Religion's Response

AIDS also challenges religion to respond to complex ethical and societal issues and to profound, personal needs. The response has been mixed. Representatives of some religions have described AIDS as God's punishment for sexual sin. Some people have attempted to nuance their reactions, judging some actions as evil but also helping people in need. Still others have stressed the need to commit people and resources to compassionate care for all people with AIDS.

The Catholic bishops of the United States have addressed the AIDS epidemic in two major statements: *The Many Faces of AIDS: A Gospel Response*, from the U.S. Catholic Conference's Administrative Board in 1987, and *Called to Compassion and Responsibility: A Response to the HIV/ AIDS Crisis*, from the entire National Conference of Catholic Bishops in 1989.[4] These statements, of course, do not solve the crisis or respond to all of the complex ethical questions, but they do provide some of the basic building blocks of an authentically Christian response.

The Many Faces of AIDS combines a sensitive understanding of the experience of AIDS along with commitment to the Christian tradition. The statement begins by presenting four different but representative faces of AIDS: a young woman, married, successful in her career but HIV positive, infected by a previous partner; an inner-city young man who has done drugs; a young professional man, a sexually active homosexual recently fired from his work when his AIDS was discovered; an infant born with AIDS to a mother who was a drug addict. The document then turns to the gospel to find several significant messages: that the God revealed by Jesus is a compassionate and forgiving God; that every human person is of inestimable worth; that suffering, as terrible as it is, can open up new meaning and life.

After considering the facts of AIDS, the bishops draw six major conclusions.

1. AIDS is a human illness, not restricted to one group or social class. AIDS is an ominous presence, calling for the best possible response from the medical and scientific communities.

2. Members of the church have the responsibility to reach out with compassion and understanding to those suffering from AIDS.

3. The crisis demands of the church a clear presentation of its moral teaching concerning human sexuality. Throughout the document, the bishops stress that the only true response to the crisis includes behavior rooted in the fully integrated understanding of human sexuality that grounds the church's teaching.

4. Discrimination against persons with AIDS is unjust and immoral.

5. Society needs to develop appropriate programs, especially educational ones, to prevent the spread of AIDS. A long appendix to the document gives many specific suggestions concerning these programs.

6. Those who are HIV positive ought to live in a way that does not expose others to the disease.

In coming to these conclusions, *The Many Faces of AIDS* addresses five personal and social dilemmas: prejudice, personal responsibility, testing, treatment, and insurance. Briefly, this is what the document says about each.

The statement strongly rejects all forms of *prejudice*. Because all human life is sacred, the bishops call for the elimination of stereotyping, isolation, and condemnation of persons with AIDS. Instead, the epidemic challenges followers of Jesus (and all people of goodwill) to express courage and compassion, to walk with those who are suffering.

To persons with AIDS, the statement speaks both comforting and challenging words. They are encouraged to continue leading productive lives in their community and work, and their right to decent housing is reaffirmed. They are also reminded of their grave moral *responsibility* not to expose others to the virus. Even those who are simply "at risk" ought to be tested and, if engaging in intimate sexual contact or in other risky behavior, act so that others will not be harmed.

The Many Faces of AIDS recognizes the need for some *testing* for the AIDS virus—of persons engaging in high-risk behavior, for example. Widespread mandatory testing is rejected as inappropriate and ineffective at this time. The document supports voluntary testing, however, as long as certain safeguards are met: sufficient counseling, confidentiality, avoiding discriminatory uses of the results. Related to screening is the issue of quarantining people who are infected with the virus. The bishops oppose such action, reaffirming the nation's civic heritage of extreme restraint in restricting human rights.

The document expresses concern that some health-care professionals are refusing to provide medical or dental care to persons with AIDS. So the bishops urge the professionals to respect the moral obligation to provide *treatment* for all persons.

Although they recognize the conflict of interests in the *insurance* issue, the bishops advocate strongly for those who are excluded from health insurance coverage. They call on the government to provide additional funding for these people. They also encourage collaborative efforts by a variety of government and church agencies to provide adequate funding and care for all persons with AIDS. The bishops find in this dilemma the fundamental weakness of the nation's health-care system and so repeat their call for the development of adequate and accessible health care for all people.

The Many Faces of AIDS also acknowledges fundamental societal problems that must be addressed if AIDS prevention is to be effective. Such realities as poverty, oppression, and alienation make it difficult for many to live life fully and drive people to drugs or short-term physical intimacy as a means of escape. Recalling their pastoral letter *Economic Justice for All*, the bishops remind church and society of their responsibilities to eradicate those realities that destroy the quality of life.

The publication of *The Many Faces of AIDS* caused quite a stir within the Catholic community. Recognizing that not all people live according to Catholic morality and that the fatal possibilities of the epidemic are so great, the document stated that public educational programs, if grounded in a broader moral vision that presented a fully integrated understanding of human sexuality, could include accurate information about condoms (which some medical experts have recommended as a means of preventing AIDS). The document in no way endorsed the use of condoms, although this is what a number of critics stated. In fact, the document criticized "safe sex" practices as misleading, ultimately ineffective, and contributing to the trivialization of sexuality.

To continue to address the issue of AIDS and to stress their rejection of "safe sex" attitudes, the National Conference of Catholic Bishops issued *Called to Compassion and Responsibility: A Response to the HIV/AIDS Crisis* in 1989. This statement especially emphasizes authentic chastity and abstinence from intravenous drug use as the only adequate means to prevent the spread of the HIV epidemic. (This emphasis caused its own stir among some people working with AIDS, for they felt that such emphasis created obstacles for collaboration with government and international AIDS programs that advocate condom use.)

Called to Compassion and Responsibility stresses five calls: to compassion, to integrity, to responsibility, to social justice, to prayer and conversion. These five calls clearly summarize the bishops' guidance concerning the AIDS crisis and suggest directions for answering the pressing ethical questions. The life and teachings of Jesus shape the Christian's response to the epidemic. Faith helps us to appreciate and value the unique dignity of every person, for all are created in God's image. The experience of death and resurrection gives us a perspective on the meaning of suffering. The Christian tradition's rich understanding of the full meaning of personhood challenges our culture's trivialization of sexuality—and calls instead for respect and responsibility.

Prayer urges us to conversion, turning away from ignorance and intolerance, and to caring action for those in need. This action must be embodied in many ways: in research and health care; in just public policy concerning testing, confidentiality, discrimination; in appropriate care and counseling for persons with AIDS and for their families as they confront pain, anger, and isolation; in changing social and economic structures that foster the spread of AIDS.

The fourth section of this book, "Religion and AIDS," presents several articles from a variety of Christian perspectives, including Methodist, Orthodox, and Lutheran. These articles also offer a theological foundation for a response of compassion and a ministry of care for people with AIDS. Such compassion and care can also be critical—challenging people to acknowledge the implications of their free choices. The section begins with an enlightening sociological study of religion's impact on people's attitudes about AIDS.

The Future

Many AIDS researchers warn us that there will be no quick technological fix for this global epidemic. Moreover, we have not yet seen the full impact of the disease; things will get worse. We can read this text and become informed concerning the overwhelming facts and figures. We can wrestle with the complex ethical questions and discuss the proper responses from society and religion. But is this all we can do? How can we move from study to committed action? First, we must recognize the reality of AIDS, not yielding to the temptations of denial or lack of interest or intolerance. This first step is possible for all of us, as individuals and as local communities. Church and civic programs can help us search out the facts about AIDS, discuss the ethical issues, and examine our consciences about prejudices in our thoughts, conversations, and actions.

Second, we must compassionately care for persons with AIDS. Such care is not limited only to physicians and nurses. We must ask ourselves: How can I respond to this worsening crisis now? Again, there are many opportunities for ourselves and our communities to get involved. We can volunteer with a local AIDS agency, visiting persons with AIDS, perhaps running errands or providing some basic supplies like food. Or at least support those who can do this. Communities can organize different kinds of support systems for persons with AIDS and for those who love them: transportation, childcare, meal programs, counseling and bereavement groups. Such ordinary but real human care provides significant help and mirrors God's faithful love.

Third, as members of society and perhaps of a religion, we must develop ways to prevent the spread of AIDS, especially through education and behavior modification. Simple to state, extremely difficult to achieve. Both educators and those encouraging new behavior must recognize the great variety of values, cultures, and pressures that shape and limit people's choices. What possibility, for example, do many women in Africa have of changing oppressive cultural expectations regarding sexuality? Or in the United States, what real freedom does a person hooked on drugs have? And what influence comes from the culture of oppression and despair in which that person lives? Globally, the worsening state of economics increases the spread of AIDS, as poor families in desperate need of income sell their children into the "sex-tourism industry" or as women avoid starvation for themselves and their families through prostitution. As a result of all this, programs will have to be creatively and sensitively targeted for vastly different audiences.

For the indefinite future, we will be living with AIDS. As the crisis worsens, we indeed have an urgent need for understanding, justice, reason, and deep faith. It is fitting, then, to conclude this text with "The Way of the Cross." This brief meditation recalls the reality of suffering and the human face of AIDS. It gently yet powerfully reminds societies and religions of the need for compassion and care.[5]

Notes

1. "The Los Altos Story," a 30-minute video offering good insights into the personal dimensions of AIDS and suitable for general audiences, can be purchased from The Los Altos Rotary Club, P.O. Box 794, Los Altos, CA 94022.

2. Necessarily, time passes from research to publication to gathering in an anthology. Although the numbers are constantly changing, fundamental issues and directions are now quite clear and consistent. The articles in this book, most of them recently published, have been chosen because they accurately describe these issues and directions.

3. The choice of a method of making moral decisions is itself a most significant decision. In my book, *Conscience in Conflict*, I have presented a method rooted in the Christian tradition and sensitive to contemporary concerns. It is a method that can be applied to the variety of ethical dilemmas described in the section "Ethics and AIDS."

4. Copies of these two statements can be purchased from the USCC Publishing Services, 3211 Fourth Street, NE, Washington, DC 20017.

5. Special thanks to Linda Loomis and Susan Ernsberger for their work in preparing the manuscript and Sister Mary Annel, M.M., M.D., who suggested a number of articles on AIDS as it affects third-world countries and women.

1

GEOGRAPHY AND AIDS

Suffering's Spread

Chapter 1

The Sobering Geography of AIDS

Joseph Palca

Whenever molecular biologists are feeling cocky about the tremendous strides they have made in unraveling the mysteries of AIDS, Michael H. Merson has a way of bringing them down to earth. Merson is the director of the global program on AIDS for the World Health Organization (WHO), and when he showed up last month at a scientific meeting with his frequently updated slide show depicting the devastating spread of AIDS around the world, his audience of some of the top AIDS researchers in the United States listened with rapt attention. True, biologists have come a long way in a short time, but as Merson's slides show, they will have to pick up the pace if they are going to help alter the course of the AIDS pandemic.

The official numbers are horrifying, and they tell only part of the story. To date, Merson's office at WHO headquarters in Geneva has recorded 340,000 cases of AIDS worldwide. But those are just the documented numbers: WHO officials know that some countries in the developing world are reporting only 5 percent to 10 percent of the actual number of AIDS cases. The true figure is closer to one million. And that's just for starters — another eight to ten million are estimated to have been infected by HIV. Until recently, it took scenes from sub-Saharan Africa, where WHO figures there are now more than 700,000 AIDS cases and another six million adults harboring the virus, to make front page news in the United States. Lately, though, health officials including Merson have begun to express alarm about new data from Asia and Latin America, where the population densities could quickly create an Africa-scale debacle. Indeed, if the virus takes hold in India, the experience in sub-Saharan Africa could pale by comparison.

"The Sobering Geography of AIDS," *Science*, April 19, 1991, pp. 372-373. Joseph Palca is a member of the news staff of *Science*. Copyright © AAAS. Reprinted with permission.

Which is why WHO officials, though bound by national sensitivities not to release infection rates for any individual country, are trumpeting the alarm to the nations most at risk.

Asia and Southeast Asia

Although the number of AIDS cases in India, Thailand, and southern China is extremely small for the present, James Curran, director of the Division of HIV/AIDS at the Centers for Disease Control (CDC) in Atlanta, calls estimates of the number of people infected with HIV there "very frightening." According to James Chin, Merson's deputy who tracks the AIDS numbers, there are now approximately 500,000 people infected with HIV in Asia and Southeast Asia — mostly in India and Thailand. Making matters worse, these countries have historically high rates of sexually transmitted diseases, which can accelerate the spread of AIDS.

But even these WHO estimates may be conservative. Peter O. Way, chief of the health studies branch at the Center for International Research in the Bureau of the Census, has been collaborating with the Thai government on tracking the epidemic there. He says Thai health officials place the number of infections between 200,000 and 300,000 in their country alone. Despite difficulties getting comprehensive figures from India, there are clear warning signs that an epidemic is looming. In large cities such as Bombay and Madras, the virus is increasingly common among prostitutes, with some prevalence estimates as high as 20 percent. The fear, according to U.S. health officials who recently attended an AIDS meeting in Bombay, is that the virus will be transmitted to rural areas by migrant workers. Should this happen, it would completely overload Indian medical services.

Latin America and the Caribbean

Then there are the forgotten islands in the Western Hemisphere. Some of the highest rates of HIV infection in the world are now found in the Caribbean. In Haiti, one study found one in ten pregnant women — not prostitutes, just ordinary citizens — infected with the AIDS virus. On a grander scale, the Pan American Health Organization, which gathers statistics for WHO in the Western Hemisphere, puts the number of people infected with the virus in all of Latin America at close to one million. Some may have felt relief that the rate of new infections in North America has slowed — a conclusion CDC reached more than a year ago — but the rate of infection in the southern part of the hemisphere has continued its steep rise.

William Blattner, chief of the viral epidemiology branch at the National Cancer Institute, finds it especially worrisome that, despite what Blattner calls "very informed and appropriate" approaches to education and intervention, infection rates in countries like Jamaica and Trinidad are showing signs of shooting up after having been well below the average for the region. "It's like any other intervention against a possible threat," he says, "it's not a threat that leads to sustained behavior change. One is faced with the reality to my mind that we can't hold this problem in check with just prevention campaigns. There's an urgent need for an effective vaccine, and we're not there yet."

Not everyone is as discouraged about the possibility of behavioral approaches slowing the epidemic's spread. Jeff Harris, AIDS coordinator for the U.S. Agency for International Development (AID), says the kind of behavioral interventions that could make a difference just haven't been tried, even in the Caribbean. Harris is encouraged by campaigns like the one in Kinshasa, Zaire, where condom use has now reached 8 percent to 10 percent of the adult male population—the kind of usage figures that models of the epidemic suggest will slow its spread. But he readily admits that the $80 million AID will spend on prevention campaigns this year is only a drop in the bucket compared to what would be needed to have a major impact on the way HIV infection is spreading.

Sub-Saharan Africa

In Africa, AIDS has reached tragic proportions. WHO's Merson says of the AIDS problem, "There is no other disease on the African continent with anywhere near this impact." In addition to the nearly six million infected adults there are an estimated 500,000 infected infants. The social and cultural impact of the disease is staggering. Merson reckons as much as 15 percent to 20 percent of the workforce in Africa could die from AIDS, and there could be as many as ten million orphans in the next decade.

And even these estimates may be low because AIDS deaths may be masked by another disease that is paralleling HIV infection rates: tuberculosis. "We have seen in sub-Saharan Africa in general tuberculosis rates shooting up, starting around the mid-1980s," says Chin. Nearly half of AIDS patients in Africa also have active tuberculosis infections, which can be the direct cause of death. This has caused a morbid statistical question: "You can't kill a person twice," says Chin. "That's been the problem— whether to count this as a TB death or an HIV death with tuberculosis or a TB death with HIV. My recommendation is we keep double books."

Some of the most alarming numbers for Africa come from a computer model of the epidemic developed for the U.S. State Department's interagency working group (IWG) on AIDS. Designed by a team from the Census Bureau, Los Alamos National Laboratory, and the University of Illinois, the model uses demographic, behavioral, and epidemiologic data to project infection rates in the future. Using this model, overall infection rates in urban areas could be as high as 16 percent by the year 2015, and infection rates could be as high as 40 percent for adults in their 30s. Expected population for the whole of sub-Saharan Africa by 2015 could be reduced by as much as fifty million by the AIDS epidemic, compared with estimates without AIDS.

Like all AIDS models, IWG's rests on some risky assumptions. Population mobility, sexual activity, rates of sexually transmitted disease, prevalence of use of condoms, the prevalence of HIV infection in the population, and the likelihood of transmitting the infection from a single sexual contact are all variables that are often not well known but can affect the accuracy of the model. "It's a little bit like holding a fishing pole at the thin end," says Way. "If you have a very new epidemic, or no epidemic like China, it would be like holding the fishing pole at the tip and trying to tell where the handle is going." For Africa, Way says, researchers are still at the thin end of the pole, but now they have a better grip.

WHO makes no predictions about how infection rates will change. Chin says that with all the uncertainties about the way the virus is transmitted, predicting more than five years into the future is an extremely risky business. Still, the IWG AIDS model is serving a useful social function: It is providing a tool for countries that are interested in using it for making predictions about what intervention campaigns might work in slowing the epidemic. Last November, U.S. health officials and Ugandan scientists using the model created a scenario that convinced Ugandan President Yoweri Museveni to reverse his policy on condoms and start encouraging their use.

The Rest of the World

There are a few shreds of good news in WHO's numbers. So far the virus does not appear to have taken hold in any significant way in Eastern Europe, and the patterns of infection for North Africa and the Middle East also indicate that those areas should be relatively unaffected, for now. In Western Europe and the United States the epidemic seems to be spreading primarily in certain sub-populations. But even in developed countries the absolute number of AIDS cases will severely tax health care systems.

For the foreseeable future Merson will continue updating his slides and bringing his gloomy message to scientists and politicians. Today the critical problem is to alert health officials in Asia and Southeast Asia that a major epidemic is looming, but "it's important not just for the Indians and the Thais and the Chinese to know this," says CDC's Curran. "It's important for the whole world to know this."

Just three years ago, WHO asked epidemiologists studying AIDS to make predictions about where the epidemic would be by the year 2000. These expert guesstimates, which WHO dubbed the Delphi projections, indicated that there would be fifteen million to twenty million infected individuals by the end of this century. "The Delphi projections may be too conservative," says Chin. "We think that the Delphi numbers may be reached by mid- to slightly after mid-1990s." Whether or not Chin is right, there's no arguing with Curran's conclusion: "Things are going to get much, much worse before they get better."

Chapter 2

Panoramic View of Pandemic

Marsha F. Goldsmith

From 13 of the 133 countries that now have AIDS, physicians who care for patients with acquired immunodeficiency syndrome or human immunodeficiency virus (HIV) infection gathered to share the facts of their successes and frustrations at the American Medical Association's all-day news briefing in Amsterdam, the Netherlands.

Participation by a wide variety of nations was invited. The speakers who were able to appear at the briefing, nominated by the health authorities of their countries as experts on HIV/AIDS, represented Brazil, Canada, China, France, Great Britain, Greece, Italy, Japan, Kenya, the Netherlands, Spain, Turkey, and the United States. A physician from Poland, who could not attend, sent a detailed report.

Held immediately before the Eighth International Conference on AIDS under the title "Physicians Battling the AIDS Epidemic," the forum gave print and broadcast reporters a chance to hear the way the war is being waged around the world, as well as affording the medical soldiers themselves an opportunity to compare strategies.

These range from a comprehensive medical and social welfare program in the host country that the Dutch participant characterized as "an embarrassment of riches" to the desperate picture painted by speakers from Kenya and Brazil.

Because the pandemic is not under control anywhere, physicians from everywhere urge the need to do the only thing guaranteed to stop transmission — get people to change their sexual and drug-injecting behavior. No one anywhere knows how to accomplish this on a broad scale and for all

"Physicians at AMA Amsterdam News Seminar Offer Panoramic View of Their Varied Roles in Pandemic," *JAMA*, September 9, 1992, pp. 1237-1246. Marsha F. Goldsmith writes for *JAMA*.

time — or at least until science finds a truly vulnerable point in the virus's so far impenetrable armor. Consequently, using the best means their own cultures provide, all of the physicians who spoke at the AMA seminar continue primarily to treat the sick and comfort the dying.

However, their focus often moves beyond these traditional imperatives. The nature of HIV disease — striking disproportionately young sexually active persons, disrupting their lives, curtailing their strength in the labor force, and creating a host of sick and orphaned children — multiplies old problems and adds new ones. All present agreed when the Canadian participant said, "AIDS is the clinical entity which will really expose your health care system and how well or how poorly it works."

Prodded by their own consciences and emboldened by the example of AIDS activists, many physicians who care for people with HIV disease are calling not only for remedies for whatever deficiencies they perceive in their country's medical care system, but for betterment of the entire social infrastructure that underlies public health and well-being.

The theme of the Eighth International Conference was "a world united against AIDS." Speaking from the podium and informally with each other, the physicians at the AMA meeting embodied this global view.

In his welcoming remarks, Jerod Loeb, Ph.D., AMA assistant vice-president for science and technology, cited the ten million people worldwide estimated to be infected with HIV and the two million with AIDS. "The world medical community is justifiably proud of advances in the treatment and improved levels of care for those infected with HIV," he said; "however, we are mindful that access to advanced and even basic care varies between and within countries." Following are some illustrative points from each presentation.

Brazil

"The main point I want to make is that the potential for HIV to spread in my country is deeply linked to the existing economic crisis," says Maria Eugenia Hernandez, M.D., resident advisor for Family Health International in AIDS Control and Prevention Programs in São Paulo. Each year, $12 billion goes to service Brazil's $120 billion external debt, the minimum monthly salary is $60, and 10 percent of the population earns 47 percent of the gross national product.

"Poverty is everywhere," says Hernandez, along with illiteracy, leading to hordes of migrant workers, "legions of street kids" (of whom 9 percent were HIV-positive in 1987), and an estimated 2 million girls 10 to 15 years of age who are commercial sex workers. Traffic in and use of injectable drugs is rising, as is the rate of male-to-female transmission of HIV — from 10:1 in 1987 to 5:1 in 1992.

Brazil is the sixth most populous country in the world and fourth in the absolute number of cases of AIDS. As of May [1992], 25,000 cases had been reported to the Ministry of Health (65 percent of them from Rio de Janeiro and São Paulo) and an estimated 425,000 people are infected with HIV. If this trend continues, by 1995 there will be 87,000 deaths from the disease. Meanwhile, tuberculosis, malaria, and other endemic diseases continue to take their toll.

The Ministry of Health allocates 4.4 percent of the GNP to health care, or $60 per capita annually. The government expects to spend $88 million this year to treat AIDS patients. "Over time," says Hernandez, "I am sure we will not be able to maintain this program."

She observes: "Since the end of last year, the government is providing free AZT [zidovudine] to patients. Some of the patients get the AZT and sell it to buy food to eat."

Hernandez says, "Despite all the efforts performed by federal, state, and municipal governments, the AIDS epidemic is showing us in a tragic way the fragility of our health care system." As is true in almost every country, better care for HIV/AIDS patients is concentrated in urban centers. Still, she cites even in Rio and São Paulo a lack of hospital beds, equipment, and trained personnel and of laboratory facilities for diagnosing and monitoring patients.

Although "studies reveal people have a very good level of information on AIDS, there is not relevant behavior change." The government has planned massive prevention campaigns for the next three years, to include face-to-face intervention and control of sexually transmitted diseases. "Through effective AIDS prevention programs we will be able to slow down the spread of HIV infection," Hernandez says, "and for that, resources must be urgently committed."

Canada

As different as the Yukon from the Amazon was the report from David J. Walters, M.D., director, Department of Health Care and Promotion, Canadian Medical Association. Walters, who was director of the AIDS Education and Awareness Program for the Canadian Public Health Association, says, "Our system's strength is universal access to treatment services, with few if any cost barriers to people with HIV and AIDS."

Free access to the newest approved and investigational drugs—with few exceptions—is a major factor in reducing the case fatality rate due to opportunistic infections. The rate of *Pneumocystis carinii* pneumonia (PCP), for example, fell from 75 percent before the routine use of aerosolized pentamidine to 15 percent now. More than 2,000 patients are enrolled in drug trials at twenty treatment sites coordinated by the Canadian HIV Trials Network.

Canada has some 6,100 reported cases of AIDS, including 315 women and 70 children.

At least 80 percent of the cases are due to sexual transmission among male homosexuals. The prevalence of HIV infection is estimated to be some 30,000 to 50,000. There is a small but growing number of cases among injecting drug users and heterosexuals, particularly teenagers. Walters says a network of street centers that offer counseling, primary care, and needle exchange for injecting drug users has been set up "after quite a political battle." Each center may see up to 3,000 users.

In Montreal, Quebec, where two thirds of the HIV-infected women live, a network of family centers integrates gynecologic care and counseling and home care for partners and children. Efforts to diagnose the disease sooner in women and newborns are resulting in earlier treatment with AZT and less central nervous system disease in children.

Primary care physicians, many of whom practice in small communities dotted across the country's vast expanse, are encouraged to attend an intensive 4-day clinical traineeship in Toronto, Ontario. There they update their knowledge and practice hands-on skills needed for treating HIV/AIDS patients. Even so, problems remain in services for aboriginal peoples in remote areas. A clinical "buddy system" has been started to link community physicians with experienced colleagues who are recompensed for taking time to advise others.

Although he identified the need for more research, therapy options, and trained staff, Walters says, "We don't have to fight on an individual basis for treatment, referral, or support services for our patients in Canada. This makes life a great deal easier. You can concentrate on the social and psychological issues and help patients with HIV/AIDS achieve their goal, which is to be independent in the community and continue with their lives and their jobs."

China

The virus arrived so recently in China that at the end of last year [1991] there were only eight reported cases of AIDS and 700 cases of HIV infection, according to Yiming Shao, M.D., Ph.D., associate professor, vice director in the Department of AIDS and Department of Tumor Viruses at the Institute of Virology, Chinese Academy of Preventive Medicine, Beijing. China distinguishes between "foreigners" and Chinese citizens with the disease; three of the persons with AIDS and 115 with HIV are foreign.

Breaking out in 146 Chinese injecting drug users in the province of Yunan in 1989, the epidemic has so far affected mostly men. Of the 585 known HIV-infected Chinese, at first 91.8 percent were drug users, Shao says, "but there is a steady increase in sexually transmitted cases—from 0.7 percent in 1989 to 3.1 percent in 1980 to 19.6 percent in 1991. Unlike the drug cases, which are concentrated near the border with Burma [now called Myanmar], sexually transmitted cases are widespread in the country—in nine provinces. Sexual transmission will most likely increase in the future."

A member of the National Expert Committee on AIDS, Shao says that "Chinese physicians have very limited experience in caring for AIDS patients. In addition, the lack of specific diagnostic means and therapeutic drugs for opportunistic infections will be a great challenge to the physicians." The Ministry of Public Health has started clinical training programs, and special wards for patients in hospitals for infectious diseases are ready or under construction.

China's widespread network of local epidemic prevention stations is being put into play. A three-level management plan is under way in the epidemic area of Yunan province. Most HIV-infected persons will be cared for at the family and village level, with the help of professionals from the epidemic prevention networks and local hospitals. The second level is for those who have been rejected by the family and village because of continuous drug use. This group will be cared for in the local drug user treatment center, at the township level. The third level is for those who fall ill and progress to AIDS. They will be treated in the county AIDS prevention, control, and research center, which is under construction.

"But with the increasing number of HIV infections and the surely coming AIDS crisis, funding will become a problem, especially for those who are not covered by the public health insurance system," Shao says.

Shao pleads for including traditional medicine in the modern armamentarium. The Bureau of Chinese Traditional Medicine has been working with the Ministry of Health and Physicians in Tanzania to treat persons with AIDS in that African nation. Without elaboration, Shao says that "clinical symptoms and immune function have been improved in the related group compared with a control group. An extended treatment program with a stricter control group and close follow-up of laboratory markers is being conducted now."

Several laboratories in China are screening medicinal herbs for their effect on HIV, he says, because "we wish the Chinese and other traditional medicine could contribute to the worldwide efforts in fighting against AIDS."

France

"New research in the battle" was the subject of the address by Jean-Claude Chermann, Ph.D., research director of the National Research Institute (INSERM), Marseilles. To counteract a view that continues to surface, especially in Europe, that something else may cause AIDS, he states, "I repeat again that HIV is the only cause of AIDS. As soon as CD4 decreases in an AIDS patient or asymptomatic carrier, we isolate the virus in 100 percent of the cases."

Chermann's main research has resulted in the discovery (working with Luc Montagnier, M.D., at the Pasteur Institute) and characterization of HIV. He says that this "one virus causes five diseases"—that is, not only does HIV deplete CD4 lymphocytes, but it directly attacks several other types of cells; the diseases that result are specific to the target. It may even do so for a while leaving the CD4 cells unattacked, which explains why a person may begin to suffer from AIDS before the virus can be isolated.

Chermann explains that he and his colleagues have learned about the actions of HIV in the following order, which is not necessarily the way AIDS progresses:

The first thing known is that HIV targets CD4 lymphocytes and kills them, resulting in AIDS.

The second target is the macrophage. When HIV-infected macrophages are moving in the brain, the result is dementia; in the lung, pneumonia; in the kidney, renal insufficiency; in the synovial fluid, polyarthritis; and so on.

The third target is the bone marrow precursor. By blocking the maturation and differentiation of the red blood cell lineage, HIV causes anemia. By killing megakaryocytes, it causes thrombocytopenia.

The fourth target is the intestinal cell. When HIV replicates in the intestinal cells they become hypersecretory, resulting in so-called clean diarrhea, where no causative agent can be found. When HIV latently infects the intestinal cells, an internalization of the intestinal villi results in malabsorption of nutrients and "wasting." Moreover, Chermann says that when intestinal cells are infected with HIV, the virus's transactivator gene, *tat*, may activate human papilloma virus lurking in nearby cells, thereby causing anorectal carcinoma.

The fifth target is the lymphoid tissue. Knowing that HIV in one cell can act indirectly in another cell to cause malignancy, Chermann's group is now attempting to determine why lymphoma develops in so many persons who live with AIDS for a long time.

All of this means that HIV disease is not easy to cure, says Chermann. Among other reasons, the immune system must be reconstituted in persons without a thymus. Researchers in his laboratory are combining antiretroviral agents with soluble thymic factor. This work, which unexpectedly showed that renewing the cytotoxic CD8 cells that kill infected CD4 cells is as important as increasing the number of CD4 cells, appears very promising, he says.

Great Britain

Agreeing with Chermann that "we have to work with data," Anthony J. Pinching, D.Phil., professor of immunology, Department of Immunology,

Medical College of St. Bartholomew's Hospital, London, says that people who, ten years into the epidemic, reject scientific data in favor of fantasy and denial about the cause of AIDS are "stuck in a pathological mode." He urges physicians to talk with their patients about the reality of HIV and what they can do to avoid encountering the virus.

"I think it actually is unrealistic to imagine that public information campaigns or media campaigns are going to change behavior," says Pinching, allowing that they are vital in increasing awareness, and that his own country "has been surprisingly effective in transmitting consistent—even if not adventurous—messages over some time." The fact that the disease is no longer particularly newsworthy in countries such as England may keep people who don't want to change their behavior from talking about it with a physician, he says, but physicians must persevere.

The shape of the epidemic is changing as treatments for medical problems that are easier to manage improve, "while the more difficult areas are now haunting us more prominently." Regarding the advent of a cure for AIDS, he says, "I think that is just fantasyland. We shouldn't be asking that question. We don't have a cure for most of the diseases that occur in either the developed or the developing world. We have some very good treatments, though, and we are making progress. People with AIDS are living at least double what they were living in the early 1980s."

Whereas everyone in the United Kingdom receives medical care, paid for by taxation, that is free at the point of delivery, Pinching says, everyone need not be approached the same way. In such a multicultural society, where people have different expectations of the health care system depending on their background, "we shouldn't necessarily impose a unique model of what AIDS or death or disease is about on people whose cultural backgrounds tell them something very different. We have to be flexible."

Pinching concludes: "One of the great things of the last ten years of this tragic epidemic has been to see how many people have come out of it and shone like stars to illuminate what otherwise would be a fairly gloomy night. Those are the people with HIV and AIDS who didn't deny or blame but adapted and got on with the job of dealing with a new threat to their lives. It is they who inspire and maintain the efficacy of the health care system that we provide."

Greece

Having come a long way from its angry rejection of the country's initial AIDS patients in 1984, the Greek medical community, "through education, conviction, and belief in the Hippocratic oath," has become "very good health care providers" to those who carry the virus, according to Theodore Kordossis, M.D., assistant professor in pathologic physiology in the School of Medicine at the National University of Athens.

"During the eight years of the epidemic many things have changed," he says. "The state has introduced quite a lot of measures to alleviate the pain of the sufferers, and the press and television have become more understanding. There is still a long way to go, but physicians, nurses, and HIV-positive individuals hand in hand have won the battle" to change public attitudes.

A total of 636 cases of AIDS have been reported, 71 percent of them in Athens. Although no overall rate of seroprevalence was given, Kordossis says 52 percent of the persons infected with HIV are homosexuals or bisexuals, 6 percent are persons with hemophilia or transfusion recipients, and only 4.6 percent are intravenous drug users. "The bad news is the heterosexual group is going up—it's nearly 20 percent now." So far, twelve pediatric AIDS cases have been reported.

Serologic testing is free. Those who are HIV-seropositive and covered by the health care system are cared for as outpatients or inpatients in special infectious disease units in fifteen designated hospitals. They receive antiretroviral and antineoplastic drugs free and pay one-fourth the cost of other drugs.

People who are "penniless and uninsured" register with the local Department of Health, Welfare, and Social Security and receive care, including therapeutic drugs, only in state hospitals They may also receive a monthly social security benefit equal to US $95.

The Greeks are sensitive to issues of confidentiality and discrimination. Serologic testing is compulsory for military conscripts. Those who test positive are excluded from service, but "the exclusion certificate does not mention HIV disease as the reason for the exclusion, so the individual is not stigmatized." Also, people may not lose a job or be prevented from applying for one on the basis of HIV seropositivity. Regarding private insurance, "past contracts are honored according to the agreement signed. New contracts [since 1991] exclude remuneration for HIV disease."

Since 1988, the University of Athens has included in its curriculum a 26-hour elective course on retroviruses and AIDS, and HIV disease is included in the curricula of internal medicine and of nursing schools. "I don't say that Greece is paradise for HIV-infected individuals," concludes Kordossis, "but I think we are doing a good job."

Italy

"With Italy we are back in a country where the AIDS situation is quite dramatic," says Stefano Vella, M.D., research director in the Laboratory of Virology at the Italian National Institute of Health, Rome. "We have reported more than 14,000 AIDS cases since 1982, and we estimate that we have more than 100,000 HIV-infected patients.

"The pressing issues in our country are related to the particular epidemiology of HIV infection," because around 80 percent of the disease in Italy is related to intravenous drug use, which is also responsible for the presence of a great number of women and children with HIV infection. Approximately 3,000 cases of AIDS have been reported in women and 300 in children, with an estimated 1,500 babies born HIV-seropositive. Some of the women are themselves drug users and an increasing number are becoming infected through sexual contact with male users. In Italy, the curve of the number of intravenous (IV) drug-use-related cases is still rapidly rising and has not leveled off as it has in other industrialized countries, Vella says.

Tuberculosis, one of the underlying diseases common in IV drug users, poses another problem. Existing therapies must be individualized to fit each person's circumstances, Vella says. "The clinical care in Italy of individuals with HIV infection cannot be separated from the social care of these people, who are already discriminated against."

Various measures have been introduced to deal with the situation. The Italian parliament has passed a specific "AIDS law" that addresses issues of confidentiality in the care of persons with HIV/AIDS and prohibits discrimination against them in the course of medical care and in the work place. Efforts are also being made to inform people that care is possible for those with HIV infection. It is not a question of cost — all HIV testing and other medical care and drugs are free in Italy. But many people see a physician for the first time only after they already have AIDS, because coping with other problems in their life comes before seeking medical care.

An effort is being made to include community organizations and volunteers in reaching HIV-positive people. "We have to consider the approach to our patients with HIV as a real multidisciplinary approach," says Vella, "not only medical but social and psychological as well."

Japan

Unique in all the world, in this country 80 percent of those infected with HIV are persons with hemophilia. The next largest group is homosexual men, one of whom had the first case of AIDS reported in Japan in March 1985. For a developed country of 120 million, the total numbers of 473 AIDS cases and 2,077 HIV-infected people are surprisingly low, according to Yuichi Shiokawa, M.D., professor emeritus, Juntendo University, and chair, AIDS Expert Committee and AIDS Surveillance Committee, Tokyo.

The AIDS Surveillance Committee warned in November that the spread of HIV infection had risen sharply, and the epidemic reached a critical point this year, says Shiokawa, "mainly due to increased international traveling as well as increased immigration from Asian countries to Japan." Specifically, the committee says, the increase is seen among heterosexuals because of transmission from non-Japanese women 20 to 29 years of age who came to Japan as sex workers from Southeast Asian countries, in particular from Thailand.

A national AIDS Prevention Law that requires anonymous reporting of all HIV/AIDS cases went into effect in 1989. The National AIDS Control Program includes information and education, blood testing, counseling, and medical care. The national medical insurance system pays for all care. The limited number of persons with the disease has so far been taken care of in a limited number of institutions, and the medical care of pregnant women with HIV infection and their infants is not a problem because there are so few of them.

Shiokawa dismisses some suggestions of underreporting of HIV in Japan, saying that even if the number of "carriers" were four times as great, "that's also a very small number." The factors he considers significant are Japanese people's traditional sexual conservatism, the widespread use of condoms for contraception (by 75 percent of men in a recent survey), very few IV drug users, and the fact that "in Japan, homosexuals are still small in number, and their sexual behavior is not so active as that of western people." Also, informed through television, newspapers, magazines, and government pamphlets, 90 percent of the people are said to recognize that "AIDS is a hazardous disease" and this fact may also help prevent its spread.

However, says Shiokawa, "since liberation and diversification of sexual life are going on among young people in this country, under the influence of western countries ... Japan will have more and more to combat the spread of AIDS among its population in the future."

Kenya

Information has gone out through the mass media, public campaigns, and sex education in the school curriculum to even the remotest parts of Kenya, and there even the youngest child knows that HIV is a sexually transmitted disease, says Ruth W. Nduati, M.D., a pediatrician and lecturer in the Department of Pediatrics at the University of Nairobi. "What I'd like to know from my colleagues," she asks, "is how do you then change behavior? I think that continues to be the challenge."

Because AIDS in Africa is mainly a heterosexual disease, its impact is strongest on young families. At Kenyatta National Hospital, the major referral center in Nairobi, the prevalence of HIV infection in children five years of age or less rose from less than 1 percent in 1986 to 12.7 percent now. The prevalence among pregnant women has gone from less than 1 percent to 8 percent.

Lack of facilities for diagnosis—just one among many lacks in the developing world, especially Africa, says Nduati—means that pregnant women are not routinely screened for HIV. They are diagnosed only if the presence of TB or herpes zoster, for example, signals a problem. The presenting infection is treated and the woman is offered termination of pregnancy, but when told that the chance of having an uninfected child is 70 percent, most prefer to have the baby. Then, because the lack of clean water makes formula feeding unrealistic, the mothers are advised to nurse their children despite the proven chance of HIV transmission through breast milk. "We have not been able to make a major inroad in counseling about continued fertility," says Nduati.

It's difficult to diagnose HIV infection in children because the illnesses with which they present—diarrhea, failure to thrive, malnutrition, respiratory infections—are so common in Africa. Once diagnosed, "anticipatory management" is impossible—antiretroviral and prophylactic drugs for opportunistic infections are either unavailable or prohibitively expensive, so treatment is given only when patients again present with TB or pneumonia or candidiasis.

Social problems are proliferating. Nduati says, "We have seen major marital breakups occur in hospitals because of a diagnosis of HIV infection made on a child who is the index case for the family." Ill, desperate young mothers increasingly abandon their children, and the institutions that would normally care for the children won't take those with HIV infection. They are placed in hospitals, where they languish.

Even in intact families, when a mother is admitted to the hospital older children may have to take over her role. Then their education and their lives are disrupted.

Kenya has had some success in assuring a safe blood supply. A recent survey of children who have had multiple blood transfusions showed that they had no more HIV infection than children who were not transfused.

In Africa, Nduati says, unlike some other areas, "AIDS is not a disease of the poor. It is a disease of you and I and everybody else who is there . . . The average patient with HIV infection does not benefit from the major advances made in the management of HIV."

The Netherlands

"The Embarrassment of Riches is the title of a book on Dutch culture in the Golden Age. It is also what I experience when I address the care of HIV-infected patients in Holland, when I compare the position of patients and doctors alike with those in less affluent countries," says Pieter L. Meenhorst, M.D., Ph.D., head of the AIDS Unit in the Slotervaart Medical Center, Amsterdam.

All legal inhabitants of Holland benefit from the highly organized health care and social welfare system, whose critics say ironically that "the Dutch state takes care of its citizens from cradle to grave." Meenhorst tried to erase misunderstanding about the proceedings that may lead to the grave—

care of the terminally ill and euthanasia, or physician-assisted death—by explaining them in great detail.

A recent report of a Dutch commission estimates that up to 20 percent of all AIDS patients die as a result of euthanasia, he says. After spelling out all the lengthy, sober, obligatory steps that must be taken before a patient is helped to die, Meenhorst said, "Helping the patient under these circumstances is in my opinion, in contrast to what others believe, an example of good medical care."

During their lifetime, people with HIV/AIDS generally get state-of-the-art treatment from specially trained general practitioners and in eleven hospitals throughout the country. The hospitals receive an additional budget for this care. Physicians with more than ten AIDS patients get a complementary fee from the largest insurance company, ZAO, "in order to enable these doctors to work together with a colleague to relieve them." Some shortage of nursing home and domiciliary care facilities is anticipated, and it takes time for the newest antiretroviral drugs to be licensed and offered free, but AIDS specialists are working on these problems.

Although only 4.6 percent of the Dutch population lives in Amsterdam, 60 percent of about 2,200 persons diagnosed with AIDS in the country are in that city. In toto, about 80 percent are infected through male homosexual contact, 7 percent through heterosexual contact, 8 percent through injecting drugs, and 3.6 percent through blood and blood products. Only nineteen children less than 13 years of age have been diagnosed with AIDS, of whom ten were infected by the mother, but 7.6 percent of AIDS patients are women and the number is increasing each year.

The cumulative AIDS incidence in the country by the year 2000 is expected to be 8,000 and the cumulative HIV incidence 16,000.

In Amsterdam there are an estimated 6,000 to 8,000 drug addicts. Last summer, the estimated cumulative incidence of HIV infection among the IV drug users was about 1,050 (with 500 elsewhere in Holland). An extensive network of organizations exists to assist addicts with various problems of living, including HIV infection, and 70 percent of them are said to accept this help. "The central focus of aid to drug users has changed through the years from detoxification to harm reduction," says Meenhorst. By providing primary health care, methadone, clean needles and syringes, and condoms, it is believed that "one can stimulate a positive attitude among the IV drug users and reduce the incidence of HIV infection."

Poland

Intravenous drug use accounts for HIV infection in 1,639 (72 percent) of persons in this country, according to a written report sent by Wládysláwa Zielinska, M.D., Ph.D., head of the Infectious Diseases Department in the Institute of Internal Medicine at the Medical Academy, Gdansk. The users inject so-called Polish heroin (*kompot*), a substance they make themselves from poppy straw and often mix with benzodiazepines.

Diagnostic tests for HIV began in Poland in 1985 and have been popularized among those at risk of infection: IV drug addicts, prostitutes, sailors, and other people who travel or work abroad. In all, 2,281 people have been found HIV positive and 108 diagnosed with AIDS, of whom 50 have died.

Persons with HIV/AIDS are cared for in ambulatory clinics and special hospital wards. The first ward, in the Clinic for Infectious Diseases at the Medical Academy in Warsaw, began in 1986 and for two years admitted AIDS patients from the entire country. In 1988, the Gdansk Medical Academy established the Diagnostic-Clinical HIV/AIDS Center, whose plan of organization has been copied by other large cities. It includes a 32-bed ward and an outpatient consulting department, a detoxification ward, and three rehabilitation centers for drug addicts, and a multispecialty treatment center in the Gdansk Prison.

Laboratories perform most of the routine diagnostic procedures, although Western blotting is available only in Warsaw and the assessment of CD4/CD8 ratios is not possible at present.

Zielinska says urgent needs in Poland are (1) setting up more good educational programs about HIV/AIDS for various social and age groups "to dispel fear and popularize prevention," (2) creating foundations and allocating funds for organizing an advisory network for people at risk of the disease, and (3) increasing diagnostic capabilities throughout the country "in order to establish the basis for a rational therapeutic approach to HIV-infected persons in earlier than AIDS stages of the disease."

Spain

With the greatest rate per total inhabitants of AIDS cases in Europe — 15,000 — and 100,000 HIV-infected people, Spain attributes the infection in 60 percent of seropositive persons to IV drug use. About one-fifth of users have antibodies to HIV, says Bonaventura Clotet, M.D., Ph.D., chief of the AIDS Day Care Unit and associate professor of medicine at the University Autonoma of Barcelona. About 25 percent of HIV-infected people are male homosexuals and 7 percent are heterosexuals, although the latter category has had the greatest percent of growth in the last year.

The special day care units, sited in the major cities, are the preferred treatment venues for HIV-infected persons. Not only do patients refuse to be cared for in primary care units, saying they find trained specialists only in the main hospitals, they move from small cities in the middle of Spain to Madrid, Barcelona, and so on in order to be treated, according to Clotet. There they find AZT, didanosine (DDI), and dideoxycytidine (DDC) available. Although no combination therapy is done officially, many patients initiate combinations of the drugs on their own, ask their physicians to do so, or enroll in trials of AZT combined with thymic hormone, interferon, or other substances. Activists in Barcelona and other cities have helped all patients gain access to new drugs, and Clotet says physicians should fight to make therapies available rapidly.

Tuberculosis is the third AIDS-defining infection in Spain, after PCP and *Candida* esophagitis. It is usually extrapulmonary and sensitive to classic therapy, although some emerging resistance to isoniazid and rifampin is seen.

"We need to fight all together to make available efficacious therapy for these infections in order to prolong survival," Clotet says. "The mean survival in our center since four years ago has stretched from fourteen to twenty-two months. But of course this is still too short."

Turkey

In January, the AIDS Prevention Society of Turkey started educational programs on HIV infection in seven major cities, according to its president, Enver Tali Çetin, M.D., professor in the Department of Microbiology, Division of Virology, Faculty of Medicine, Istanbul. The timing was fortuitous; a Ministry of Health document dated February 29 states that 67 people had by then been diagnosed with AIDS. At least 200 more have been registered as HIV positive with the two major university hospitals that care for such patients, and there are thought to be others, especially in major cities and tourist centers.

Most of the original 30 patients diagnosed at Hacettepe Medical Faculty, Ankara, and Istanbul Faculty of Medicine had clinical symptoms and secondary infections. Their HIV seropositivity was detected after admission. The usual opportunistic infections were observed. There were 22 men and eight women, mainly from 30 to 49 years of age. The largest number (17) were infected through intercourse—heterosexual, homosexual, or bisexual.

With the aim of preventing unsafe sexual intercourse, the AIDS Prevention Society has prepared an "Education Program on AIDS" and presented a report to the government. "Now," says Çetin, "we are awaiting the decision of the Minister of Health."

United States

In San Francisco, California, "the city that is pointed to as a model of the most effective AIDS education in the United States," says Marcus Conant, M.D., a physician in private practice and clinical professor at the University of California Medical Center at San Francisco, "three men a day are dying of AIDS and three men a day are becoming infected with

HIV. We still have a 4 percent seroconversion rate. The epidemiology throughout the rest of the United States is even more daunting."

There are an estimated one million HIV-infected people in the country. New York City has 250,000 IV drug users, of whom 12 percent are infected. Conant says, "The difficulty that is not understood is the ongoing magnitude of the epidemic."

The AIDS epidemic has unmasked a number of failings in the U.S. health-care delivery system, he says along with many others, and points out not only that some forty million people lack any access to care but that the system was not designed for the ongoing care of people with a chronic illness like HIV disease. It was designed primarily, he says, for the elderly individual who had acute illness that required hospitalization and short-term care.

"What do you do," Conant asks, "with a 36-year-old man, living alone, who has no one with him during the day, cannot prepare his meals, has no emotional support, and clinic visits — even if he could get back and forth to them — are not included in his medical insurance plan?"

Speaking with all the accumulated anguish of the eleven years he and his colleagues have cared for a practice that now numbers some 3,000 HIV-infected men, Conant castigated many American institutions for not doing more to stop the epidemic sooner: the Republican administration, blood banks, organized medicine, the Food and Drug Administration, insurance companies, and churches. He says, "The churches stressed family values, forgetting that every person who is afflicted with HIV is some mother's son, some sister's brother, a member of the greater family of our country."

Even so, he admits that the United States has come a long way in the past decade, raising the average life expectancy from diagnosis of AIDS to death from six months to more than three and one-half years. Now he wants the nation to "put aside the bias, the denial and homophobia, that has kept us from addressing this epidemic properly so that we as physicians can be allowed to do the things we want to do to stop the dying, to alleviate the suffering, and to provide appropriate health care for all of our people."

AIDS: "Virtually Intransigent"

At a session following the physicians' presentation, George D. Lundberg, M.D., editor of the *Journal of the American Medical Association*, added his own perspective. He said, "Among the strongest drives experienced by humans are the drives to have sex and to take psychoactive drugs. While sex may not be an addiction, it certainly is basic and becomes habitual. Some psychoactive drugs produce addiction and when they do they often become a lifetime habit central to the lives of the addicts. The fact that a lethal infectious disease is transmitted primarily through satisfaction of these two basic human drives, sex and injectional drug use, renders that disease virtually intransigent."

Speaking to the assembled media representatives, Lundberg reminded them that "AIDS has been the biggest medical news story of the latter part of the century," and that some estimates suggest that the ten million people infected with HIV today may become forty million by the year 2000. Still, he said, "in many countries we seem numb to these numbers. I predict that at the end of the *next* century AIDS will still be a serious endemic disease throughout the world. No successful method of treatment or prevention will have been fully implemented."

Considering the diversity of responses to this disease epitomized by the presentations at the seminar, and the continuing nature of its threat to all the countries and peoples of the world, one can only hope that physicians meeting and sharing their knowledge and experience will be able to blunt the thrust of this prediction.

Chapter 3

Spread of Pandemic in Asia

Marsha F. Goldsmith

Asia is getting acquainted with AIDS. While most of the rest of the world has been forced to be concerned about the pandemic of acquired immunodeficiency syndrome for a decade, the conservative societies that people the largest continent have generally denied the reality of impending catastrophe.

That's the opinion of many Asian biological and social scientists, who say that the governments of their nations, which were initially bypassed by the human immunodeficiency virus (HIV), ignored the lurking threat. When HIV infection began to appear within the last five years, only Thailand responded.

In immensely populous India and in smaller nations, health authorities largely failed to seize the opportunity to teach prevention or mobilize against the inevitable assault. Now it is too late. Speaking at the Seventh International Conference on AIDS, James Chin, M.D., M.P.H., chief, Surveillance, Forecasting, and Impact Assessment Unit, Global Programme on AIDS, World Health Organization (WHO), said, "Several countries in south and southeast Asia reported large increases in HIV infections beginning in 1988; as of mid-1991, over one million infections may have occurred in this region of the world . . . because of the very large populations involved . . . infections are expected to reach a cumulative total of over 2.6 million by the mid-1990s."

Despite the lack of government support and a culture that favors denial of difficult social problems over confrontation, some Asian health authorities have learned about AIDS, and 125 of them attended the meeting in

"Rapid Spread of Pandemic in Asia Dismays Experts, Spurs Efforts To Fight Transmission," *JAMA*, August 28, 1991, pp. 1048-1049, 1053. Marsha F. Goldsmith writes for *JAMA*.

Florence. However, I. S. Gilada, M.D., secretary-general of the Indian Health Organization, pointed out, "Asia, with 60 percent of the world's population, is represented by only 1 percent of the delegates."

Two Groups Formed

Even so, the Asian health experts met and formed not just one but two new organizations dedicated to fighting the spread of HIV in their countries. Both have support from the Geneva, Switzerland-based WHO and stress the necessity for cooperation, but their goals are somewhat different.

The AIDS Society for Asia and the Pacific will attempt to influence official government policy. Its physician members plan to use their authority and prestige to get national leaders to establish or expand AIDS programs that are specifically attuned to the multicultural Asian milieu. One organizer said that while the group can learn from what has been done in Europe, the United States, and Africa, many of the interventions adopted in those areas are not applicable to an Asian setting.

Asian Solidarity Against AIDS will be a coordinating agency for the nongovernmental organizations, known as NGOs, which have long worked to ameliorate the multiple social problems that are prevalent in the developing world. It will address such issues, according to Gilada, a prime mover of the group, as traditional rather than "high tech" care of patients, human rights, women's issues, and a safe blood supply.

Asian Solidarity Against AIDS will be chaired by Takashi Kurimura, M.D., who is a professor of biology at Osaka University and technical advisor to the Japanese Foundation for AIDS Prevention. About half of the Asian contingent in Florence came from Japan, a country that in many ways is more "Western" than Asian, even to the extent of becoming aware of AIDS from the beginning, when Japanese hemophiliacs contracted HIV infection from tainted blood products produced elsewhere. Various social factors, including cultural proscription of homosexuality, little intravenous drug use, and the highest rate of condom use for contraception in the world, have so far kept the disease from spreading widely in Japan.

Now, says Kurimura, concern about the spread of HIV is growing because "several million Japanese people go abroad every year, and maybe what is happening in Thailand and India will happen in Japan."

What is happening in impoverished India and in Thailand with its commercial sex tours and to a lesser extent in Malaysia, Singapore, Indonesia, and Myanmar (formerly Burma) is a rapid expansion in the heterosexual acquisition and transmission of HIV.

Sex on the Subcontinent

India's Gilada spells it out: "In 1986 in Bombay we began screening for HIV among prostitutes, blood donors, and patients with sexually transmitted diseases [STDs]. We found only three of 600 prostitutes who were HIV-positive 0.5 percent. We tested each year, and each year the number increased, so that in mid-1991 it is 30 percent, and 35 percent in some areas. In 1986, not a single STD patient was positive — now we see 12 percent are.

"In Bombay, we have an estimated 100,000 prostitutes. On an average day, each has four or five clients, so say there are 400,000 clients every day. If 30 percent of the prostitutes are infected, then about 150,000 people in Bombay are at risk every day with the HIV-positive prostitutes. Those are big numbers."

Gilada said, "We have been warning our government for four years that we shouldn't allow Bombay to become Nairobi [Kenya, where HIV-sero-positivity among prostitutes, or sex workers in the preferred terminology, went from 5 percent in 1985 to 80 percent in 1989]. But nobody listened."

In the general population, Gilada says, a study done for the last two years of blood donors in four major Indian cities revealed that eight donors per one thousand are HIV-positive. The number of infected people among those who would not be considered at high risk of HIV in those four cities could be 70,000 in Bombay, 58,000 in New Delhi, 79,000 in Calcutta, and 39,000 in Madras.

A recent article in *Lancet* (1991;337:1534) mentions another ominous situation. It seems that India has become a center for kidney transplants from living donors who sell their organs.

A Bombay physician is quoted saying that "a number of HIV-positive patients are now trying to sell a kidney to earn a living. For every kidney donor identified as HIV positive, five slip through the net, putting many lives at risk."

The article says that "it is estimated that more than two thousand kidneys are taken from live donors and sold each year." Illegal trade in live corneas for transplantation, it adds, is also thriving.

Drugs and Brothels in Thailand

Thailand was the first of the "developing" Asian nations to tackle AIDS, which first appeared a few years ago among intravenous drug users. It is estimated that 400,000 Thais are now infected with HIV.

As the only Asian country with both a serious HIV problem and a government program aimed at controlling it, Thailand sent 32 delegates to Florence to describe its own efforts to nations with similar problems and to learn from others. Kumnuan Ungchusak, M.D., Ministry of Public Health, related the results of sentinel surveys conducted biannually since June 1989 to assess the extent of HIV spread and monitor transmission.

The prevalence of HIV infection among intravenous drug users has remained steady since surveillance began, at a median rate of approximately

30 percent. In Bangkok, 70 percent of the drug injectors are employed in legitimate occupations—the figure, cited by U.S. drug abuse expert Don C. Des Jarlais, Ph.D., does not include anybody in Thailand's sex industry. Among female sex workers, the median rate of infection is rising steadily every six months, from 3.5 percent to 6.3 percent to 9.3 percent among those in brothels, and from 0 percent to 1 percent to 1.2 percent among those of a higher class.

Seropositivity remains low among pregnant women at antenatal clinics. But it is rising slowly among blood donors and more rapidly among male patients at STD clinics.

Ungchusak said that Thai "decision makers have now been alerted to the three major HIV epidemics—intravenous drug users, female sex workers, and male STD patients. The Ministry of Public Health is also aware of and prepared for," he added, "the next HIV epidemic—housewives and newborns."

With the help of the WHO and Family Health International and other NGOs, Thailand is making diverse efforts to stem the epidemic in different groups. One study in Bangkok showed that counseling and testing intravenous drug users for HIV resulted in their using condoms more often.

A study among sex workers tried to promote use of the female condom. Provided with instructions and a two-week supply of the devices, 15 percent of the women who worked in brothels and less than 10 percent of those who worked in bars reported that they were "very satisfied users." The organizers of the trial say they expect usage to increase with time because "there is evidence that the experience of the initial innovators does spread through an establishment" and there is peer pressure to conform with safer sex practices.

Strenuous efforts are being made to promote safer sex in the numerous and flourishing brothels, which owe their existence to cultural mores as well as to general poverty and the low status of women. Since abolishing these well-recognized sites of HIV transmission doesn't appear to be an option, the emphasis is on protection for both workers and customers.

Several presentations in Florence dealt with the need to persuade the managers of all brothels in one locality to adopt a condom-only policy in their establishments. The conclusion of a study done in Khon Kaen City (and similar ones are ongoing in Chiang Mai) was that "a condom-only policy can succeed if managers and brothel workers show solidarity in rejecting all noncondom using clients." Laws may not be needed, it is said, if the establishments are given the opportunity to use "their own resourcefulness and determination."

Smaller Countries, Similar Concerns

Suriyani Gunawan, M.D., a member of the National AIDS Council in Indonesia—another country in which "greedy people" (as he said) promote sex tours among European and Asian businessmen—said that a recent survey revealed that "even the lowest paid prostitutes earn much more money than the average government official. The elite prostitutes, who cater to the wealthy people, are very rich."

Gunawan said, "We don't know the incidence of AIDS exactly," adding that so far only forty HIV-seropositive persons have been detected in Indonesia, including twenty who had AIDS. However, the number represented a doubling between January and June of this year.

Most of the cases were found by physicians, and a government-sponsored screening found "only three or four positives." Gunawan said most of the HIV-infected persons "caught it abroad or through sex with foreigners." Another delegate said that "some Indonesians who were working in the Middle East picked up AIDS there."

While intravenous drug use is very low in Indonesia, Gunawan said, the country's situation between the Asian mainland and Australia means its "sex tourists" come from both worlds. "The government is still reluctant to have a campaign against HIV," he said, "but there is some awareness that they have to do something, so we plan an AIDS meeting for NGOs in Jakarta."

In Singapore also, there is little intravenous drug use, "so the HIV problem is not as bad as in Thailand or Malaysia," said Roy Chan, M.D., one of the founding members of Asian Solidarity Against AIDS. However, Singapore, with 2.5 million people, has about 5 million tourists each year. Consequently, said Chan, "certainly I would expect that the number of HIV infections as well as AIDS would continue to rise for the next five to ten years before they start to come down a bit."

Chan pointed out that sex tourism—the main route of HIV transmission in his country—is popular among Southeast Asian nationals as well as Europeans, "so that has to be tackled and that takes a lot of political will, which will have to come from the government, with a bit of prodding."

A physician who is now a permanent resident of the United States but maintains close ties with his native China shed the only glimmer of light on what is happening there. Qingcai Zhang, M.D., who is now in Los Angeles, where he cares for many HIV-positive Asian-Americans, said that a symposium on AIDS and hepatitis B was held in April in Beijing. "At this symposium," he said with obvious skepticism, "they officially announced 470 HIV infections and five cases of AIDS, out of one billion people in China."

Sitting on a Volcano

At the opening session of the international conference, Vulimiri Ramalingaswami, M.D., professor emeritus at the All India Institute of Medical

Sciences in New Delhi, said, "I've come here to plead for a global response to this emergency."

Speaking passionately, he depicted his own country—the second largest in the world—as a society of some 850 million people that has survived for ages despite social and medical problems of staggering complexity. The scourge of HIV, striking a population that has been living with "a false sense of security," believing this is one plague that might pass over it, provides, he said, "an unprecedented opportunity for disaster."

"The picture that is emerging in the developing world is most disturbing," the physician concluded. "I believe we are sitting on the top of a volcano and we do not know yet just when it will erupt."

Chapter 4

AIDS in Africa

David Sanders
Abdulrahman Sambo

Introduction

The AIDS epidemic was first recognized in Africa in 1983 when clinicians in Europe reported the first cases among African patients.[1] Of the world total of 263,051 cases reported to the World Health Organization (WHO) as of June 1990, 64,404 or nearly 25 percent were from 47 African countries.[2] This contrasted sharply with the figures reported to the organization in June 1989 when 24,686 or 16 percent of the cumulative total were from these African countries.[3] The current estimated total number of cases of AIDS in Africa is 375,000 while the total number of people estimated to be infected is 3,500,000.[4] The different epidemiological profile of AIDS in Africa supports the hypothesis that heterosexual intercourse is the major mechanism of transmission. It is generally estimated that heterosexual intercourse and vertical (mother-to-child) transmission account for 80 percent of cases in Africa.[5]

Epidemiological Factors in Transmission

Biological and Behavioral Factors

Bidirectional heterosexual transmission is the major mode of infection in Africa. In addition, HIV infections in Africa are also more frequently

"AIDS in Africa: The Implications of Economic Recession and Structural Adjustment," *Health Policy and Planning* 6 (2) 1991, pp. 157-165. David Sanders, M.D., is associate professor of community medicine at the Medical School in Harare, Zimbabwe and Abdulrahman Sambo, M.D., is program officer for medical sciences at the National Universities Commission, Lagos, Nigeria. By permission of Oxford University Press.

spread congenitally and by blood transfusions than in the West. Case control studies in Africa have also shown that infected individuals report both a higher number of heterosexual partners than controls as well as frequent sexual contact with prostitutes. Most analysts argue that female prostitutes probably play a major role in the spread of HIV in many parts of Africa and they consistently show the highest HIV seroprevalence rates.[6] Genital ulcers, especially chancroid, syphilis and herpes may explain the rapid spread of HIV infection in Africa due to increased risk of infection with each exposure.

In Rwanda, 44 percent of 25 patients with AIDS had serological evidence of syphilis,[7] and in Zambia,[8] the Ivory Coast,[9] Kenya[10] and Zimbabwe[11] an increased prevalence of HIV-1 antibody was found among attendees of clinics for sexually transmitted diseases than was found in patients attending other hospital clinics. There may also be more rapid progression of the disease due to more frequent infections and decreased nutritional (and therefore immunological) status of patients in Africa.

We intend to critically examine statements such as Anderson's: "Infection is assumed to flow from a core group of highly sexually active female prostitutes, to males (assumed all to be moderately promiscuous) and then to the child-bearing women (assumed all to be relatively monogamous)."[12] While this view is generally accepted, we regard it as superficial and inadequate to the immense challenge of controlling this epidemic. Failure to identify and address the social and economic factors underlying the spread of HIV infection in Africa has, we believe, led to an overwhelming concentration on sexual behaviors — and certain assumptions about them — with an almost exclusive focus on modifying these, without concomitant concern for influencing their structural determinants. Although the area of sexual behavior is notoriously difficult to study and there are problems of comparability of studies, it is nonetheless revealing that there appears to be very little empirical evidence to support the popular view regarding Africans' sexuality.

Comparison with sexual activity among both HIV infected and non-infected heterosexual men in the US shows that there is little evidence that African males are, as has been frequently suggested, more promiscuous. In a survey of sexual behaviors of American adults, more than one-third of unmarried men, a significant proportion of married men and one-fifth of unmarried women between the ages of 18 and 24 reported having three or more sexual partners in the previous year.[13]

In another study to determine the association between HIV-1 seropositivity and prostitute contact in New York City, 14 percent of the 671 males enrolled in the study reported more than 50 contacts with prostitutes within a ten-year period.[14] In one of the few published studies in Africa, in Zimbabwe, 67 HIV positive heterosexual male factory workers reported an average of 16 lifetime sexual partners against 10 partners by the 119 controls (non-HIV group).[15] Assuming their mean age to be 30 years and that each had 10 years of sexual activity, the annual number of sexual partners for these HIV positive men per year would have been only 1.6. From these studies there appears to be little difference between Zimbabwean and American men in terms of the number of partners, although there is a suggestion — and this has been noted elsewhere — that a fairly high percentage of Zimbabwean men have more than one, and sometimes several sexual partners. Further, because of the predominance of men in the urban population, several men may have a sexual relationship with one woman.

Thus higher rates of HIV transmission in Africa may be more a function of the greater risk of infection with each sexual encounter than the total number of partners. Biological factors responsible for this, as suggested above, include genital ulcer disease and other sexually transmitted diseases (STDs). However, underlying the above biological and behavioral factors are women's weak position in society, the migrant labor system with its disruption of families, inadequate health services and, more recently, the economic crisis which has greatly aggravated these social and economic factors. Indeed it is predominantly these factors rather than aberrant behavior (a presumed African propensity for promiscuity) that require modification if the high risk of transmission is to be reduced.

Social and Economic Factors

Hrdy suggested that population movements in Africa contribute to the "sexual mixing" of various African groups which may be related to the spread of AIDS.[16] The long-term movement of rural populations into urban areas in most of southern and east Africa contribute to family separation and the spread of disease (including AIDS), from urban to rural areas as well as in the opposite direction. The colonization of Africa brought about large-scale economically motivated, and in some cases forced, migration of people mostly from the rural to the urban areas. In the early years of colonial rule, a degree of compulsion was required to secure an adequate supply of labor for colonial industries and mines, often achieved in collaboration with local chiefs. The construction of the Congo-Ocean Railway in the Congo in the period 1923-1934 led to large-scale flight to adjacent countries by local residents seeking to escape conscription to work on the line.

The British used forced labor, called the "Kasanvu system," in trying to get manpower in Uganda. In southern Africa, British and Belgian companies handled recruitment for the mines of South Africa and the Belgian Congo (now Zaire). Rwandans and Malawians were also actively recruited to work in colonial plantations in Uganda. In some cases camps were provided for migrant workers along the main roads.[17] This forced migration led to the formation of a permanent workforce in the towns, with the concentration of large-scale agricultural and industrial production in the hands of a few.

In order to ensure a constant supply of labor and a market in which manufactured goods could be sold, the colonialists introduced transformations in land administration and head cattle and hut taxes to force people into wage labor.[18] Such taxes provided an enormous impetus to migration and the formation of a reserve workforce. When recruitment involved movement from one country to another, efforts were made to control it by local agreements operated between the supplying country on one hand, and employing country and the industry concerned on the other, to ensure a continuing supply of workers and remittance of earnings. This arrangement pertained especially with respect to migrant labor to South Africa. This system of migrant labor, which is widespread in southern and eastern Africa and formally institutionalized in South Africa, has enforced separation of men from their wives for long periods and disrupted familial and stable sexual relationships. It has resulted in a significant predominance of men in urban, plantation and mining centers and has inevitably resulted in extramarital sexual relationships becoming the norm, often with several men frequenting a small number of women. Indeed, the previously cited study of male factory workers in Zimbabwe showed that HIV positive men were both more likely to live apart from their wives and more often reported girlfriends and more lifetime partners.[15]

Women in Africa are portrayed as the principal vectors of the AIDS epidemic. In epidemiologic investigations this has meant an emphasis on the study of female prostitutes to the exclusion of other women. Because there are few studies on the men who use prostitutes, we do not know the extent of HIV infection among this group of men. Studies linking STDs and increased susceptibility to HIV infection may be confounded however, by the association of poverty with STDs and overall ill health.[19]

In a study of 418 prostitutes in Nairobi, 62 percent of them were found to be HIV positive.[20] Of the HIV positive women, 62 percent were from Tanzania and no difference was found in the estimated daily number of sex partners between HIV positive and HIV negative women. There were, however, substantial differences in HIV seroprevalence rates between prostitutes of higher and lower socioeconomic status. Kreiss et al., in their study of Nairobi prostitutes, noted higher infection rates (66 percent) among lower socioeconomic-level prostitutes than among prostitutes of higher socioeconomic class (8 percent).[21] This has been shown in some studies to be because women of lower socioeconomic status are more susceptible to economic incentives to have unprotected sex and also their social status may limit their ability to set the terms of the sexual encounter, particularly with regard to condom use.[22]

In contrast to the Western world where the focus has been on "professional" prostitutes or Asia where economic factors and temporary migration are associated with professional prostitution, studies in Africa reveal the difficulty in labelling prostitutes and distinguishing them from "wives" or "friends." The prostitute has been shown to be both part of her community and to engage in a variety of jobs.[22,23] The majority of "prostitutes" in Africa cannot be categorized clearly and the term "prostitute" is not generally appropriate to the exchange of sexual services for money. In Kenya for example, the term "Malaya" is used to describe some form of prostitution and other informal unions that involve not only exchange of sex for money but also provision of food and lodging.[23] Day points out that accounts of slum life show prostitution to be one of the most rational choices for urban dwellers who certainly gain greater independence through prostitution than they would through alternative options as wives or other workers.[23]

Prior to the colonial period traditional African societies were patrilineal and women returned to their natal families only if divorced. Marriage was (and is) accompanied by the payment of brideprice as token compensation to the wife's family and as a sign of affection from one family to another. In post-colonial Africa however, brideprice and marriage have taken on new meaning in a market economy, with substantial payments which may take years to complete.[5] Furthermore, the colonial system introduced its own patriarchal values to Africa where colonial laws institutionalized the reduction of women to perpetual minority status under the guardianship of fathers and husbands with severely limited rights to property. A husband's commitment in marriage is not primarily sexual fidelity but financial support of the wife and children. Social and economic factors have increased family separation in Africa leading to an increase in sexual relationships outside marriage. Urban development in Africa has drained resources from the rural areas, including girls and women who came to the towns and cities in search of employment. The rural woman is at a particular disadvantage. Her husband goes away to work in the urban centers (leaving her to care for the children, the elderly and infirm) and commonly establishes new sexual liaisons; some men even form new families, marginalizing the rural household altogether. This freedom of mobility and access to many sexual partners in the urban areas increases the possibility that men will spread the virus to their wives in the rural areas.

The multiple social, economic and cultural burdens carried by the African woman of child-bearing age, much more than her choice of sexual behaviors, may pose the major risk of her acquiring HIV infection. Women in Africa generally have considerably limited control in determining their own lives and this places them at a special disadvantage with regard to their ability to protect themselves from the risk of HIV infection. Furthermore, they may have to use sex as a means of earning a living for themselves and their children. As a locus for change in the AIDS epidemic, women have the most limited options. Attempts to control HIV spread must take into account these constraints and recognize the crucial importance of increasing women's economic options through income-generating projects and political initiatives that will strengthen their position and status in society.

Impact of Economic Recession on HIV Transmission and Control

The economic recession and debt crisis in Africa, which peaked in the 1980s, forced many governments, at the behest of the International Monetary Fund (IMF), to introduce Structural Adjustment Programs (SAPs) to control the situation. Such programs essentially include trade liberalization, removal of government subsidies (on basic foodstuffs and other items), reductions in social spending, commercialization of government-owned companies and currency devaluation. These austerity measures have resulted in sharp declines in standards of living as a result of rising inflation, declining real wages, increasing unemployment and accelerated rural-urban drift. "IMF riots" have become a familiar response to these pressures in many African countries.

Violent protest has occurred in Liberia (1979), Sudan and Tunisia (1985, 1986), Zambia (1987, 1990), Algeria (1988), Nigeria (1988, 1989) and Ivory Coast (1990).[24] Twenty-four countries in sub-Saharan Africa with a total population of over 400 million were worse off in terms of average income per capita at the end of the 1980s than at the beginning of the decade.[25] Among the remaining fourteen countries populated by 63 million people, only the small countries were noticeably better off (Cape Verde, Botswana and Mauritius). For some of the countries the growth rate in investments was negative, jeopardizing the prospects for future growth.

Budgetary cuts by governments have reduced public capital investment in health, education, transportation, and other social infrastructures. Decreased investment in education has contributed to an unprecedented decline in the gross primary school enrollment rate from 80 percent in 1980 to 75 percent in 1987.[25] Declines in formal sector employment and real wages have increased householders' dependence on informal sector income. This is evidenced by an increase in urban unemployment rates in the formal sector from about 10 percent in the 1970s to about 30 percent in the mid-1980s while informal sector employment increased by 6.7 percent.[25] An increase in the informal sector labor force of females between the ages of 15 and 64 years (from 56 percent of total females in the age group in 1985 to 66 percent in 1990) has occurred in many African countries.[25] Income generation through informal sector activities (for example, food vending, beer brewing, firewood and kerosene selling) is especially important for women in Africa.

Contraction of cash incomes in the rural areas as a result of landlessness and inflation and the attraction of an urban wage has increased so that more people migrated to the urban areas in the mid 1980s. During this period African cities grew at 6 percent per year as opposed to 2 percent for rural areas. Females form a larger proportion of urban migrants than in the past, and in the absence of other employment opportunities, some turn to prostitution.[25]

In 1980, thirty countries in sub-Saharan Africa allocated on average 5 percent of central government expenditure to health, a full 1 percent less than in 1975.[25] Studies in east, west, central, and southern Africa reveal that 80 percent of the drug requirements of these countries are imported.[24] With decreased allocations to the health sector, currency devaluation, and shortages of foreign exchange, severe drug unavailability is being experienced in many countries. Cuts in drug spending have already occurred in Uganda from 1987 to 1988, and in Zambia where the 1986 allocation for drug purchase was only 25 percent of its 1983 value and only 10 percent was actually spent due to lack of foreign exchange.[25] In Gambia between 1983 and 1987 the share of the health budget going to drugs was reduced by 20 percent.[25]

In summary, economic recession and SAPs further aggravate the transmission, spread and control of HIV infection in Africa in two major ways: directly, by increasing the population at risk through increased urban migration, poverty, women's powerlessness and prostitution; and indirectly through a decrease in health care provision. The latter entails not only reduced facilities to care for patients with AIDS but also less effective treatment of genital ulcers and other STDs as well as decreased spending on health programs like health education.

Measures being taken to control the spread of HIV infection in Africa include mainly increasing the safety of blood transfusion and the promotion of condom use through health education. Ensuring condom use is a more complicated process than simply teaching how to use them. There are well-recognized cultural and social barriers to the use of condoms in Africa. A recent national survey of Zimbabwean men found that only 35 percent said they had ever used condoms and most viewed condom use as appropriate only for sexual encounters with prostitutes.[5] Although condoms cost only a few cents, providing them in adequate numbers to the sexually active population of Africa would be financially daunting, to say the least. The total number available, and their distribution, are only some of the problems being faced by many African countries. In Zimbabwe, for example, if one assumes (conservatively) that sexually active males between the ages of 15 and 50 years comprise 15 percent of the population and need two condoms each per week, the total number of condoms required for this group per year would be about 130 million. But the Zimbabwe program distributes only 26 million condoms per annum, all of them imported.[4] The foreign exchange implications of such estimates for an already depressed economy are great. In Zaire, too, it has been estimated that to provide a condom for every episode of sexual intercourse, about 700 million would be needed annually. Sales figures in Kinshasa for 1990 were, however, only 10 million.[26]

Impact of HIV and AIDS

The estimated impact of HIV and AIDS in Africa, both present and future, is based on the current number of cases reported to the WHO from the continent and projections of future prevalence rates. There are, however, major limitations to such projections. Underreporting, which is common, is due mainly to lack of reliable data and government sensitivity — due to concern for the presumed negative effects on tourism and investment as well as sensationalized (and often racist) reporting of the epidemic.[27]

Other limitations include uncertainty as to the proportions of persons infected with HIV who will develop AIDS and the fact that most seroprevalence surveys in Africa have been conducted among prostitutes, patients attending clinics for sexually transmitted diseases and blood donors — who are predominantly drawn from the sexually active age groups.

Impact on Morbidity

The infectious manifestations of HIV and AIDS vary in different populations according to the frequency of other endemic diseases. In Africa, patients commonly present with the endemic gastrointestinal, respiratory and dermatologic infections. The most commonly observed opportunistic infections in African AIDS patients include tuberculosis, fungal, parasitic and cytomegalovirus infections.[28] Because of the widespread prevalence of latent tuberculosis infection before the HIV epidemic, tuberculosis has become one of the major manifestations of AIDS in Africa. The annual number of confirmed cases of tuberculosis in Uganda doubled between 1984 and 1987.[29]

In Zaire, 33 percent of 159 confirmed pulmonary tuberculosis patients at a sanitarium were HIV positive.[30] Similarly, in Zimbabwe, between 1988 and 1989, 49 percent of TB patients aged 15-34 years and 39 percent of these aged 35-54 years were HIV positive compared to 8 percent in non-tuberculosis patients.[31] What is generally referred to as "slim disease" in Uganda is essentially enteropathic AIDS with the major symptoms of weight loss and diarrhea occurring in 99 percent and 80 percent of cases respectively.[30] In Zaire, incidence of pneumonia, diarrhea and ear infections were higher in HIV positive children who acquired the infection vertically.[32] The few studies so far done on pediatric HIV infection in Africa indicate the difficulty in distinguishing HIV associated disease on clinical grounds, where malnutrition and pulmonary infections are common pediatric problems. The impact on morbidity is further aggravated by the fact that ill health may last for many years in many patients before severe debility and death.

Demographic Impact

Anderson states: "AIDS has greater potential to depress significantly population growth rates than smallpox or bubonic plague."[12] This is mainly due to its long latent period during which HIV infection is transmissible, its ability to be transmitted both horizontally and vertically (congenitally)

and its eventual high mortality; however, it is also the case that HIV transmission is rendered less efficient than smallpox or bubonic plague by its
lower infectivity. The sex ratio among patients with AIDS and seropositive
persons is almost equal in Africa, being 1.7:1 (male:female) in contrast to
the United States where the ratio is 7:1.[28]

Seropositivity for women peaks in the third decade and for men in the
fourth. The epidemic is notably restricted to young adults and pre-school
children. About half of all known infected adults are women in the reproductive age group and this will have consequences for reproduction and
eventual population structure. Studies in Kinshasa show a bimodal age
distribution curve with peak prevalences under one year and between 16
and 29 years of age.[30] With an HIV prevalence of between 7 and 22 percent
among women attending antenatal clinics in many African countries, the
number of reproducing women can be expected to decline slowly to a point
where births will become inadequate to replace losses due to deaths.
Another contributing factor will be a reduction in reproduction by choice,
as women learn the hazards to pregnancy and the newborn infant associated
with HIV.

It has been projected that AIDS will kill a total of between 1.5 and 2.9
million women of reproductive age in Africa by the year 2000.[33] The same
study projected the number of deaths in children under five from AIDS in
ten east and central African countries to be between one quarter and half
a million annually by the year 2000. In Zimbabwe, for example, since 1989
AIDS has been reported to be the major cause in urban hospitals of childhood death.[34] The United Nations projected that in 1990, the under-five
mortality rate (U5MR) in east and central Africa would have declined from
158 per 1,000 live births to 132 by the year 1999 without the impact of
AIDS.[35] The U5MR, however, is already between 165 and 167 in 1990 as
a result of the additional impact of AIDS and is predicted to rise to 189
by the year 2000.[36] Assuming a slow decline in the transmission of AIDS
in Africa, life expectancy at birth is expected to be lowered by four years
by the year 2000.[37] The projected net demographic effect of the AIDS
epidemic in Africa is a marked and very selective decrease in population
among the young and sexually active age groups. This level of impact will
more than offset any progress made through improvements in health care.

Economic Impact

Kahn proposed two models for assessing the economic impact of HIV
infection: direct costs to the individual and cost to the community, government and the support system.[38] The costs of all financial resources used in
the course of treatment in developing countries has been estimated to range
between US$132 and US$1585 per patient.[39] But this computation is of
course largely theoretical since many patients already do not and increasingly will not receive treatment. The direct cost of AIDS to South Africa

by mid-1990 has been estimated to be about R5.25 million (about US$2 million).[40] Malawi has recently reported a loss of R70 million (approximately US$27.3m) a year after Malawian miners were prevented from going to South Africa by their government, because of the threat of their being tested for AIDS in South Africa, given the high rates of HIV infection among these migrant workers.[41] Indirect costs based on foregone earnings of the individual range from US$890 to US$5093 per person.[19] Considering the relative youth of people with AIDS, the indirect costs may be much higher than these estimates when income losses due to illness and disability and present values of future earnings lost through death are considered.

The economic impact on households will be particularly severe where dependency rates are very high. As a result of AIDS there will be fewer caring adults while the number of people needing care will increase. A study carried out in Uganda shows that the proportion of orphaned children in Rakai district (which reports 6 percent of all Ugandan AIDS cases) ranges from 10 to 17 percent of all children.[42] The corresponding range in Hoima district with 0.1 percent of all AIDS cases is 2 to 7 percent. Similarly, in Rakai 31 percent of the orphaned children are under the care of their grandparents while in Hoima the figure is 18 percent. This reflects differences in the prevalence of AIDS and its impact on the age structure of community.

At the community level, commercial and subsistence farming will be greatly affected as a result of premature deaths from AIDS. In countries where economic viability centers on food production, governments will have to consider policy options that take declining agricultural production into account. The impact will be further aggravated by the effect of the epidemic on the functioning of infrastructure and services which are dependent on the limited numbers of available skilled personnel. Carswell predicts that there will be a substantial loss of human potential for creativity and a differential loss of decision-makers and managers from some societies.[28] Prevalence of HIV in the army in countries where studies have been carried out has been found to be very high. It has been asserted that 60 percent of the military personnel in Zimbabwe are infected with HIV, although this claim has been refuted by officials.[43]

Health Sector Impact

The most visible impact of HIV and AIDS on the health system involves the direct cost of medical care. In a cost analysis undertaken in Zaire it has been determined that the total treatment costs per AIDS patient are approximately US$150 within the public health system and US$1700 within the private health care system.[37] If all persons presently infected in Zaire sought care through the public health system, annual treatment costs would total about US$75 million. Against this background is the overall downward trend of per capita government health expenditure for most countries in sub-Saharan Africa. Increasing numbers of AIDS patients will almost certainly divert resources (human, material and financial) away from the treatment of other major diseases.

Furthermore, already existing drug shortages are being aggravated because the more frequent and severe infections in patients with AIDS require repeated courses of antibiotics in higher dosages. It is reported that in a major hospital in Kampala, 40 to 45 percent of hospital beds are currently occupied by AIDS patients.[37] In Kinshasa, 50 percent of the medical and surgical patients are HIV positive and 25 percent of the deaths are AIDS related.[37] The substantial amounts of money that may be required for national AIDS programs will divert scarce resources away from other public health programs like immunization. Blood transfusion services are likely also to be adversely affected as some potential donors are rejected and others may decide not to donate for fear of learning that they are seropositive.

Conclusion

We have argued that the current AIDS epidemic in Africa is inextricably linked to socioeconomic and political factors, both current and historical, on the continent. The colonization of Africa brought about large-scale economically motivated migration of people from rural to urban areas. The current economic crisis and SAPs introduced by many African governments have aggravated both urban drift, mainly as a result of increasing landlessness, and urban poverty as a result of contraction of cash incomes and inflation. Accompanying declines in formal sector employment in most of Africa have led to increased dependence on informal income, which for women has often meant resorting to prostitution.

We have also argued that there is little evidence that African males are more promiscuous than other males, but rather that the rapid rate of increase in the HIV prevalence in Africa may be more a function of the greater risk of infection with each sexual encounter than the total number of partners. Biological factors responsible for this are genital ulcer disease and other sexually transmitted diseases which are themselves promoted by the same underlying social and economic factors. We propose, therefore, that it is primarily these social and economic factors rather than aberrant behavior that require modification if the high risk of transmission is to be reduced. Any government initiative that seriously aims to control the AIDS epidemic in Africa will, therefore, have not only to promote "safe sex" but also to address the related problems of increasing landlessness, mounting unemployment, accelerating urbanization and prostitution as well as the rapid decline in health services needed to treat those affected by HIV infection and to control its spread. It is clear that the success of such initiatives will be perilously limited if they fail to confront such fundamental structural issues as the migrant labor system, women's position in society and the current economic recession with its attendant structural adjustment programs.

Notes

1. Clumeck N, Mascart-Lemone F, de Maulbeuge J, et al. 1983. Acquired Immune Deficiency Syndrome in Black Africans, *Lancet* i; 642.
2. Statistics from WHO 1990. *AIDS* 4:703-7.
3. Mann JM. 1989. Global AIDS in the 1990's. V International Conference on AIDS, Montreal, Canada, June.
4. Hooper Ed. 1990. *New Scientist*. 7 July.
5. Bassett MT, Mhloyi M. 1991. Women and AIDS in Zimbabwe: the making of an epidemic. *International Journal of Health Services*. 21; 143-156.
6. Bigger RJ. 1986. The AIDS problem in Africa. *Lancet*. 11 January.
7. Van de Parre P, Le-Page P, Kestelyn P, et al. 1984. Acquired immunodeficiency syndrome in Rwanda. *Lancet* ii:67-69.
8. Melbye M, Bayley A, Manuwele JK, et al. 1986. Evidence of heterosexual transmission and clinical manifestations of acquired immunodeficiency virus infection and related conditions in Lusaka, Zambia. *Lancet* ii:1113-15.
9. Denis F, Barin F, Gershey-Damet GM, et al. 1987. Prevalence of human T-lymphotropic retrovirus type III (HIV) and type IV in Ivory Coast. *Lancet* i:408-11.
10. Piot P, Plummer FA, Rey AM, et al. 1987. Retrospective seroepidemiology of AIDS virus infection in Nairobi populations. *Journal of Infectious Diseases*. 155:1108-12.
11. Latif AS, Katzenstein DA, Bassett M, et al. 1989. Genital ulcers and transmission of HIV among couples in Zimbabwe. *AIDS* 3:519-23.
12. Anderson RM, May RM, McLean AR. 1988. Possible demographic consequences of AIDS in developing countries. *Nature* 332.
13. Turner CF, Miller HG. 1988. Sexual behaviors, condom use and perceptions of personal risks of HIV infection reported in a national survey of American adults. IV International Conference on AIDS, Stockholm, Sweden. June. Abstract H 8104.
14. Chiasson MA, Stoneburner RL, Lifson AR, et al. 1988. No association between HIV-1 seropositivity and prostitute contact in New York City. IV International Conference on AIDS, Stockholm, Sweden. June. Abstract D 4053.
15. Bassett MT, Emmanuel JC, Katzenstein DA, et al. 1990. HIV infection in urban men in Zimbabwe. VI International Conference on AIDS, San Francisco, California. Abstract Th C 581.
16. Hrdy DB. 1987. Cultural practices contributing to transmission of human immunodeficiency virus in Africa. *Review of Infectious Diseases* 9:6. Nov/Dec.
17. Hance WA. 1970. *Population, migration and urbanization in Africa*. Columbia University Press. New York, 134.
18. Sanders D. 1985. *The struggle for health: medicine and the politics of underdevelopment*. Macmillan, London. Page 61.
19. Padian NS. 1988. Prostitute women and AIDS: epidemiology. *AIDS* 2:413-19.
20. Simonsen JN, Plummer FA, Ngugi EN, et al. 1990. HIV infection among

lower socio-economic strata prostitutes in Nairobi. *AIDS* 4:139-44.

21. Kreiss JK, Koech D, Plummer FA, et al. 1986. AIDS virus infection in Nairobi prostitutes: spread of the epidemic to East Africa. *New England Journal of Medicine.* 314:414-18.

22. Wilson D, Sibanda B, Mboyi L, et al. 1990. A pilot study for an HIV prevention program among commercial sex workers in Bulawayo, Zimbabwe. *Social Science and Medicine* 31:609-18.

23. Day S. 1988. Prostitute women and AIDS: anthropology. *AIDS* 2:421-28.

24. Alubo SO. 1990. Debt crisis, health and health services in Africa. *Social Science and Medicine* 31:639-48.

25. Jespersen E. 1990. Household responses to the economic crisis and its impact on social services in the 1980s. UNICEF. May. (Unpublished)

26. *AIDS NEWSLETTER* 5:15. 1990. 29 October. Page 12.

27. Chirimuuta RC, Chirimuuta RJ. 1989. *AIDS, Africa, and Racism.* Free Association Books. London.

28. Carswell JW. 1988. Impact of AIDS in the developing world. *British Medical Bulletin* 44:183-202.

29. WHO Global Statistics. 1989. *Current AIDS Literature* 2:567.

30. Quinn TC, Mann JM, Curran JW, et al. 1986. AIDS in Africa: an epidemiologic paradigm. *Science* 234:955-63. 21 November.

31. Mahari M, Legg W, Houston S, et al. 1990. Association of tuberculosis and HIV infection in Zimbabwe. VI International Conference on AIDS, San Francisco, California, June. Abstract Th B 494.

32. Manzila T, Nsa W, Kabagabo U, et al. 1990. Morbidity and mortality in the first 30 months of life in 477 infants born to seropositive mothers in Zaire. VI International Conference on AIDS, San Francisco, California, June. Abstract THC 657.

33. Piot P, Carael M. 1988. Epidemiological and sociological aspects of HIV-infection in developing countries. *British Medical Bulletin* 44:68-88.

34. Sanders D. Personal observation.

35. United National Department of International Economic and Social Affairs. 1989. World population prospects 1988. *Population Studies* No. 106. New York.

36. Preble EA. 1990. Impact of HIV/AIDS on African children. *Social Science and Medicine* 31:671-80.

37. Acquired Immunodeficiency Syndrome (AIDS) in Africa: A proposed World Bank agenda for action. (Undated and unpublished.)

38. Kahn J. 1989. Socio-economic models to assess the economic impact of HIV infection. V International Conference on AIDS, Montreal, June. Abstract WHP9.

39. Nabarro D, McConnell C. 1989. The impact of AIDS on socio-economic development. *AIDS* 3 (suppl 1); S265-72.

40. Whiteside A. 1990. "AIDS in Southern Africa." Economic Research Unit. University of Natal/Development Bank of South Africa. As reported in *AIDS Newsletter* 5:15. 29 October.

41. Sunday Times (South Africa), 10.6.90. As reported in *AIDS Newsletter.* 23 July.

42. Hunter SS. 1990. Orphans as a window on the AIDS epidemic in sub-Saharan Africa; initial results and implications of a study in Uganda. *Social Science and Medicine* 31:681-90.

43. Knight VC. 1990. The numbers game. *Africa South.* July/August.

Chapter 5

A Catholic Doctor Looks at AIDS in the U.S.A.

Robert J. Barnet

In the United States, AIDS is still perceived primarily as a scourge intimately linked, not just to sexual activity, but to aberrant sexual behavior, especially homosexuality. This is in spite of the fact that there is a significant transformation taking place in the pattern and incidence of AIDS and HIV infection. As with abortion, the issue remains politicized.

The first confirmed case of AIDS in the United States was reported in California on June 5, 1981. AIDS initially was centered in five American metropolitan localities among a relatively affluent, predominantly white, gay/bisexual population. A second phase has involved large numbers of poor minorities, especially African-American and Hispanic, with the transmission frequently occurring by the sharing of contaminated needles during intravenous drug use. Currently, about a third of those infected are gay men, and a third, drug abusers.

We are now, however, in transition with a rising rate of infection transmitted through heterosexual contact involving a broader segment of the population. The problem is moving from a few metropolitan areas and the inner cities and expanding into smaller communities and rural areas.

It took eight years (from 1981 to 1989) for the first 100,000 cases of AIDS to be reported. It took only 26 months for the second 100,000. AIDS is now the sixth leading cause of premature death in the United States.

"A Catholic Doctor Looks at AIDS in the U.S.A.," *America,* February 6, 1993, pp. 6-12. Robert J. Barnet, M.D., addressed the 10th Congress of the Asian Federation of Catholic Medical Associations in Bangkok on November 9, 1992. This article is an adaptation of that address. Reprinted with the permission of Robert J. Barnet and America Press, Inc., 106 West 56th Street, New York, New York 10019. Copyright © 1993. All rights reserved.

The greatest rate of increase in new HIV cases is occurring among hetero-sexual females and adolescents. In addition, up to 2,000 infants are born infected each year. AIDS is now the ninth leading cause of death among children one to four years of age.

The incidence of HIV infection in North America continues to grow. The following figures reflect cumulative totals between 1981 and 1992: All adults infected with HIV — 1,167,000; total projected to be infected with HIV by 1995 — 1,495,000. All adults with AIDS — 257,500; total projected to have AIDS by 1995 — 534,000. Forty thousand to eighty thousand Amer-icans were projected to have become infected with the HIV virus in 1992, and at least 45,000 will die of AIDS. Related medical complications, includ-ing resistant tuberculosis and an increase in sexually transmitted disease, not just HIV alone, are now part of the problem.

Health Care Costs

Although federal funding of research has been significant and currently is in the range of $1.7 billion annually, the high cost of treatment is becom-ing an ever greater burden. Total direct and indirect annual federal spend-ing on AIDS, including funds for research, prevention, education and patient care, is estimated to be in the range of four to five billion dollars. There has been criticism of the relatively limited share of National Institute of Health funds that have been allocated to the problems of women, chil-dren and minorities.

The effect of the additional burden on private health insurance, includ-ing increased premiums, is substantial. Continuing attempts are made to reduce private insurance coverage for AIDS to a level that would make it an almost meaningless benefit. A challenge to prevent this effort has been rejected by the U.S. Supreme Court.

The financial burden is currently concentrated in a few major population centers, not the country as a whole. In 1991, five percent of the nation's hospitals cared for 50 percent of the nation's AIDS population. With the change in the pattern of the epidemic it can be anticipated that the burden of the costs will be felt over a larger segment of society. This will undoubt-edly be a major concern in what is already a broader crisis in American health care.

The United States is currently one of the few developed countries in the world that does not have a national health program. We have extremely high health care costs that currently consume in the range of 13.2 percent of our GNP. The pressure of increased costs due to AIDS will undoubtedly make it even more imperative that there be universal access to basic health services with an affordable, long-range, coherent national health policy. How the AIDS issue will be dealt with in the debate is uncertain, but it cannot be ignored.

Prejudice, Testing, Under-reporting

There is an additional concern that makes it imperative that the church continue to be in the forefront in caring for patients with AIDS. The frustration of dealing with the overwhelming burden of being ill with AIDS and the prejudice that accompanies it have resulted in significant support for euthanasia initiatives from AIDS activist groups.

A major issue that has evoked considerable debate is the mandatory testing for HIV, among health professionals on one hand and among the general population on the other. Options suggested have included universal testing, or testing of groups with high risk activities, such as physicians and health care professionals. HIV testing is frequently required to obtain life, health and disability insurance and frequently for employment — private, not governmental — decisions.

The debate on such testing has been clouded by the fact that the risk of a physician contracting the virus from a patient is far greater than the reverse. The infections contracted from a dentist in Florida are the only documented instance of transmission to patients. Some fifty American health care professionals, according to the Centers for Disease Control (CDC) in Atlanta, have contracted the virus through patient contact.

The CDC estimates that the probability of an infected surgeon transmitting HIV to a patient is approximately one in 400,000. Because the possibility of patients becoming infected is so remote, there has been a resistance to requiring infected physicians to notify their patients of the fact. The responsibility for such action lies with the individual states. Legislation has been introduced and some passed, but overall the situation is still evolving, with no firm national pattern. The most common resolution has been to require infected physicians to notify the state licensing board. This approach anticipates that there will be monitoring of the physician's activities in much the same way as is done with alcohol and drug abuse. Although there is reticence to discuss it openly, some argue that a strong policy would unjustly deprive infected physicians of their usual level of income.

There is a legitimate concern, from both a scientific and a cost standpoint, about mandatory universal testing. If the testing is done in a population group with a low incidence, there will be an unacceptable number of false positives, and the cost per case will be prohibitive. A second major objection has been that people will attempt to avoid the testing because they fear discrimination in employment, insurance and housing. And there is a related concern about preserving confidentiality.

Quarantine of infected individuals, a traditional method of control, has been rejected as an option. The way we deal with the question in the United States is strongly influenced by the American emphasis on individual freedom. It is inconceivable that the Cuban solution of the physical restriction of those with HIV would be tolerated here.

In most American hospitals relatively strict isolation procedures, often including the use of private rooms, are followed for patients with HIV infection. There is some inconsistency, however. Much less stringent precautions are often recommended for the same patients on discharge from the hospital, even though their physical contacts at home will be much closer.

A major problem, with an ethical aspect, is the reluctance of certain health care professionals, including physicians, medical students and nurses, to treat AIDS patients. In part, the problem is related to the fact that most Americans in health care who are under the age of 60 have not had an experience in which their lives were significantly threatened by exposure to infectious disease. The last time this occurred was during the polio epidemics of the early 1950s. In addition, here as well as in Europe, altruism has too often been replaced by entrepreneurship. How much the outlook of health care professionals is influenced by attitudes on sexuality is uncertain. The issue is complex but needs to be more fully addressed.

AIDS is under-reported for a number of reasons, including social stigma and family, institutional and community pressures. Federal statisticians estimate that 18 percent of AIDS cases go unreported. There is no legal requirement to report HIV infections to public health authorities. There is, however, a requirement to report AIDS and deaths due to HIV, but the mandate is delegated to the individual states. Individual physicians, typically, and not public health authorities, are the ones who certify the cause of death, contributing to the under-reporting.

Prevention Measures and Public Attitudes

Discussion of education about condoms and programs for the distribution of free needles for IV drug abusers have also evoked controversy. The public policy debate typically centers on whether programs promoting the distribution of condoms will increase promiscuity and whether the distribution of needles will encourage more IV drug abuse. The discussion about condoms, especially in Catholic circles, has often focused primarily on whether their use under all circumstances is illicit. Therefore, the data on their unreliability in vaginal and especially anal intercourse is often not fully appreciated. The fact that condoms will not make unsafe sex safe but only less risky is obscured.

The major public health response to the epidemic has involved attempts to change behavior. The results have been mixed. According to one study, only 31 percent of those who say they are using preventive methods use condoms. The most prevalent behavioral response to the epidemic has been to limit the number of sexual partners. Although this may seem reassuring, there apparently has not been a realization that if an individual has one new sex partner per year and each partner has a similar pattern, in five years many more potentially dangerous contacts will have been made, given that approximately one of every 250 Americans is infected with HIV.

Societal hostility toward those infected with HIV has probably declined. It certainly has not disappeared. Some, such as former San Francisco orthopedic surgeon Lorraine Day, assume an alarmist position. In her book *AIDS, What the Government Isn't Telling You,* she casts doubt on the fragility of the HIV virus. Part of her emphasis is on the theoretical possibility of infection through kissing or mosquitoes or through intact skin. Dr. Day takes a strong position asserting the right of physicians to avoid contact with HIV-infected patients.

The current social attitude has, on the other hand, been favorably influenced by a series of national personalities identified as having HIV infection. Some of these have been sport celebrities such as Magic Johnson and Arthur Ashe. Others include Ryan White, the young hemophiliac, and Alison Gertz, a young woman who contracted HIV during a single sexual encounter at age 16.

Reflecting the changing pattern, an important testimonial came from Mary Fisher at the Republican convention last August. With others, she has helped blunt prejudice by putting a human face on tragedy. Neither Ryan White nor Mary Fisher is the typical American with HIV. These "special victims" are often, not always, treated with compassion and have more resources available. They are perceived as "innocent victims." In the United States the typical person infected with HIV is still a member of a minority group, or gay or a drug user.

Happily, national attitudes are changing. Mary Fisher, to her credit, when asked how her former husband had acquired the virus, had the wisdom and courage to reply: "It makes no difference. It's outrageous you would ask the question. That's how the world gets divided into bad victims and innocent victims."

Continuing Ravages

Disease of any kind, for much of society, remains full of mystery. AIDS, above all, remains mysterious for too many, especially the young. The denial of vulnerability among the young, a situation not unique to AIDS, remains a problem. Approximately 20 percent of AIDS patients are now between 20 and 29 years of age. Many acquired the infection as teen-agers. From 1989 to 1992 the cumulative number of 13- to 24-year-old victims diagnosed with AIDS increased 77 percent. By June 30, 1992, almost 9,800 teen-agers and young adults between the ages of 13 through 24 had been diagnosed with AIDS. It is the seventh leading cause of death in young people ages 15 to 24. How many already have HIV is only a matter of speculation.

Studies in San Francisco indicate that in the 1980s public health measures, especially education, reduced the incidence of new cases in the gay population. However, there has been a recent increase of HIV infections in San Francisco among gay young men in their late teens and early 20s.

There is only limited appreciation in the United States that heterosexual transmission is a major and growing problem. Most data suggest only a slightly higher risk of infection for women, although one study done at the University of California indicated that females may be up to 17 times more likely to acquire the virus through sexual contact than to transmit it. From 1987 to 1991, the ratio of adolescent females to males with AIDS increased dramatically. In 1987, 17 out of every 100 adolescents who were HIV-positive were female; in 1991, 39 out of every 100 were female.

Certain social issues, including the devastating impact of HIV on the arts and other aspects of American society, have been partially documented. The obituaries of those in the arts announce part of the first wave of deaths among the gay, educated and relatively affluent. Members of this community have mobilized and supported their agenda and have had a strong influence on both guidelines and federal approval for experimental drugs. They have also, through political action committees, supported candidates sympathetic to their concerns. The gay community has shown a strong sense of social solidarity through various support groups providing comfort and counseling.

Others, less noted, are dying in larger numbers. In my own state, those with AIDS are less notable, often food and beverage workers, waiters and bartenders. A surge of deaths is occurring among the marginalized, especially drug users.

We can anticipate there will soon be a number of deaths, no cause given, recorded in the local newspapers. These deaths in the third wave will be our neighbors, friends and their children and relatives, most infected through heterosexual activity. The social impact will be just as great, only different. The financial burden will probably be greater.

U.S. Catholic Response

The attitude of the Catholic church in the United States has been a mix of compassion and doctrinal firmness. The American church has continued to struggle with the issue of human sexuality. This has had a strong influence on how it has dealt with the AIDS issue.

In 1987 the Administrative Board of the United States Catholic Conference issued a moderate statement, *The Many Faces of AIDS: A Gospel Response*. It contained the following sentences: "In such a situation, educational efforts, if grounded in the broader moral vision outlined above, could include accurate information about prophylactic devices or other practices proposed by some medical experts as potential means of preventing AIDS. We are not promoting the use of prophylactics, but merely providing information that is part of the factual picture."

There was controversy and concern, on the part of some, including U.S. bishops, that the 1987 statement condoned the use of condoms and would encourage illicit sex. A careful reading of the entire document, in my judgment, makes it clear that its moral position and vision were unambiguous and strongly affirmed the traditional Catholic position. The authors of the document felt that, in the area of education, the facts should be forthcoming and accurate. As a physician, I could not agree more with their position.

In November 1989 the U.S. Catholic Conference issued *Called to Compassion and Responsibility: A Response to the HIV/AIDS Crisis.* This document, in part responding to the objections raised over the initial statement, held that advocating prophylactics is "morally unacceptable."

The battle over stressing prevention through the use of condoms, as contrasted with abstinence, continues. The absolutism of *Humanae Vitae* prevails in the debate at the institutional church level. There has been only limited discussion of the use of condoms for prevention of HIV when one spouse is infected, even when the woman is beyond childbearing age. In such instances, when a mature, sincere and committed couple approaches the sexual act, the primary intention is mutual love and affection. It is contrary to human experience that physical procreation is the prime motive in each and every sexual act. That is also true during the early years of a marriage and certainly true during later years. The mutual surrender of sexual union can nourish and strengthen a marriage symbolically, psychologically and spiritually. The consolation and intimacy of sex may be crucial when one spouse is infected with HIV.

The AIDS crisis gives us a special opportunity to reexamine issues of sexual morality. There are distinct differences in the United States and Europe between how these issues are dealt with at the pastoral level and what is contained in magisterial pronouncements. Love, compassion and example seem a better recipe for virtue than moral interdicts. How issues of sexual morality and conduct are eventually resolved will have an important, perhaps critical, impact on the future of the U.S. Catholic church.

On the issue of care and compassion the leadership of the U.S. Catholic church has been commendable. In New York, where there has been conflict between the Cardinal Archbishop and the activist gay community, the dedication to the care of persons with AIDS has been exceptional. Hospice and outpatient programs at St. Vincent's and St. Clare's Hospitals have involved a major church commitment. In Chicago the Alexian Brothers have established a special AIDS facility. Throughout the country individual parishes and dioceses have taken a leadership role. San Francisco and New Orleans are among the many other outstanding examples.

Toward a Gospel Response

Topics certainly pertinent to the AIDS issue include pastoral care, health care delivery, homosexuality and the use of condoms. But the perception of the problem remains clouded. I recently asked a good friend, an open, enlightened priest studying at a prominent Catholic university, to send me any material he might be able to locate on the topic of AIDS and the church. What I received was a series of articles on the church's attitude on homosexuality. This incident underlines the fact that there continues to be a muddling of our approach to AIDS as a disease with questions of sexual morality. The two are not altogether separable, but they are not the same.

What is an appropriate attitude on AIDS for the Catholic church and Catholic health care community? It should be based on Catholic tradition and social and moral teaching, of course, but what should that be in practice?

There is something we can learn from the mother of Ryan White, the young hemophiliac: "I think Christianity is having a really hard part in AIDS. We are all caught up in homosexuality and whether it's right or wrong. But of all the people I know who are such good Christians and have AIDS, the ones who are gay believe in their religion even more. I almost see more spirituality, reaching out and helping more. There is no one doing more for this disease than the gay community."

Because of the manner in which the epidemic was identified here, the homophobic bias is more of a problem in North America and Europe than in Africa and Asia. But AIDS is a worldwide modern pandemic often involving especially the poorest of the poor. In his book *A Life of Jesus,* Shusaku Endo, the Japanese writer, describes the wretched people, including prostitutes and lepers, living around the shores of Lake Galilee. He notes that "towns were full of sick and crippled ones neglected by their neighbors and even by their own families." He continues: "The New Testament provides a picture of Jesus with His loving predilection for drawing close to men and women who were otherwise forsaken or held in contempt."

I would like to associate this passage with a personal story, the outcome of which I learned only years afterward. In 1961 and 1962 I was at St. Francis Mission in what is now northwest Zambia. I was initially told there was no leprosy there. Vincent worked in the bishop's house some twenty miles away. He was brought to the mission clinic with open sores on his hands. Vincent told me that he had leprosy. We spent a few *kwacha* and built him a mud house. The mission gave him more than that, however. It gave him acceptance, care, compassion. It gave him the means to sustain himself, a garden plot, some seeds and community.

But there was a problem. There was a primary school at the mission and the Sisters had a homecraft school there in the bush, primarily for better-educated young women from the cities. Some, primarily the Europeans, were worried about the stigma of a leprosy settlement and how it would affect the mission. Does that sound familiar? Is there a contemporary parallel between that story and what has happened with AIDS among many health care institutions and professionals, Catholics included?

How was the issue resolved at St. Francis? Father Joseph, a Franciscan from Palermo, Sicily, who has now been at the mission for almost forty years, said quite simply: "We must care for Vincent. He is why we are here."

That decision involved risks. Nevertheless, the leprosy settlement survives, and the schools at St. Francis thrive. If they had not, it still should not have mattered.

What is the lesson for today? Our goal, our focus, as health professionals and institutions, as lay and religious, should be to treat all persons, regardless of their illness and their life pattern, with respect and dignity. Why? Quite simply, because, by virtue of the Incarnation, they are the image of God. That is true of the least among us. That is as true of each person with AIDS as it was of Vincent, regardless of who they are and how they have become infected.

It is even more true for those with AIDS than for many others with different needs. They are the outcasts on the shores of today's Lake Galilees. We can see those infected with HIV either as problems or as mysteries. Problems can be isolated, solved and removed. Mysteries we should try to understand, accept and embrace. We need to see those with HIV as mysteries, not problems.

That is why we are here.

Chapter 6

Latin America Confronts AIDS

D. Paul Jeffrey

The infant lay naked, alone in a large room in a Brazilian hospital. On a tag stuck to the end of her crib, in the place for her name, someone had written "AIDS and syphilis."

Abandoned by her mother, a poor woman, probably a drug addict, the newborn had been given a diagnosis for a name and set aside in isolation by the overworked hospital staff. After a few days, a pastoral worker found the infant and removed her from the hospital to a Franciscan convent. There she received a name: Carolina.

Soon cured of syphilis, Carolina was adopted by a family who offered her acceptance and love. After several months her HIV-positive status converted. She is today HIV-negative. Now six years old, Carolina has a name, a family and a future.

Carolina symbolizes people living with AIDS in Latin America, a region where systemic poverty, ignorance and religious prejudice conspire to deny wholeness to a rapidly increasing population of people struggling with the disease. Yet it's also a region where people of faith are fighting back, resisting death in all its forms, turning the epidemic's ravages into an opportunity for conversion to life in all its fullness.

At a time when the most optimistic reports suggest that AIDS is peaking in North America, in the countries to the South—and within ethnic minority neighborhoods in the North—the disease is beginning to hit with a vengeance. Today about two-thirds of the AIDS cases in the Americas are in the North—mostly the U.S.A.—and one-third are in the South. By the end

"Latin America Confronts AIDS," *America,* February 13, 1993, pp. 10-12. The Reverend D. Paul Jeffrey is a Methodist missionary based in Nicaragua. Reprinted with the permission of Paul Jeffrey and America Press, Inc., 106 West 56th Street, New York, New York 10019. Copyright © 1993. All rights reserved.

of the decade, however, that proportion will be reversed. And within the United States the vast majority of people with AIDS will be black, Hispanic or Asian.

The surge of AIDS in Latin America and poor communities in the United States is part of a global acceleration of the disease. By the year 2000, reports the World Health Organization (WHO), 40 million men, women and children will be infected with the HIV virus throughout the world. The number of AIDS orphans—uninfected children whose parents have died of the disease—will number some 10 million worldwide. Other reports put the numbers even higher. A Harvard University study released in June claims the total number of infections worldwide could reach 110 million by the end of the century.

The epidemic's challenge to Latin America has moved health workers, theologians and pastoral workers to insist that AIDS cannot be seen as a medical problem alone. Poverty and AIDS are intrinsically linked, and the global spread of the disease will not be stopped or even slowed until the world rethinks its understanding of economic development.

Brazil presents a prime example of this relationship. It boasts the fourth highest number of AIDS cases in the world (behind the United States, Uganda and Tanzania). In the world today, the acute poverty of Brazil's teeming slums is a characteristic breeding ground for the HIV virus that causes AIDS. In Brazil and throughout the region, banks and multilateral lending institutions from the North are forcing debt-ridden governments to reduce spending; already inadequate health care budgets are among the first to be slashed. Public health workers face appalling choices. Do they devote dwindling resources to combat cholera, tuberculosis, diarrhea or AIDS?

With access to physicians often a luxury for the region's poor majority, many die of AIDS without knowing it. The symptoms of AIDS-related diseases are often confused with other health problems of the poor, such as tuberculosis. When people are diagnosed correctly, they frequently suffer discrimination. In often illiterate populations that have not benefitted from years of AIDS education, misunderstanding and fear are rampant. "Preconceptions kill more people than AIDS," declares Neli Lou Eqewarth, a Franciscan sister in São Paulo, Brazil, who helps poor people with AIDS who have been pushed onto the streets by families unwilling to care for them any longer.

Projects such as Sister Eqewarth's are few and far between. Throughout the region, except in Cuba (where every HIV-positive person detected in a massive screening program has to move into a government-run sanatorium), no significant government safety net exists to catch people who are poor and HIV-positive. In the South, a person with AIDS lives an average of six months after diagnosis. In the North, that period is usually several years. Costly prescription drugs that slow the progress of the disease, manufactured by U.S. and European companies more interested in profits and patents than helping the sick, are simply unavailable for the majority of HIV-infected Latin Americans. And even drugs, when available, offer cruel choices to the poor. According to Rosa Maria Dantas, a sociologist with a Catholic AIDS project in Recife, Brazil, some recipients of AZT sell their pills to buy food for their hungry families.

If the spread of the AIDS epidemic is left unchecked, Latin America's poverty will only grow worse. Medical services will grow increasingly burdened. Otherwise productive persons in the prime of life will fall victim to the disease. Without their income, however meager it was, their families will experience greater starvation and misery.

AIDS and Women

During the early years of the epidemic, the majority of victims were men. That is changing rapidly, both North and South. According to WHO, new cases of HIV infection are about evenly divided between men and women. By the turn of the century, the majority of new infections will occur among women. Perhaps a third of the babies born to these women will die during childhood from AIDS-related causes, and millions of others will be orphaned when their infected mothers fail to survive.

In Latin America, the fastest-growing and least-noted class of people now becoming infected with the HIV virus are monogamous heterosexual women, whose only "high risk" behavior is having sex with their husbands. These men usually become infected while engaging in sex with prostitutes, although a small number have caught it from bisexual activity. The wives will usually die before their husbands, given their already undernourished state of health.

The region's prevalent value system of male domination, known as *machismo,* provides the foundation for such exploitation. *Machismo* is so inbred that many parents, afraid their sons will be homosexuals, take them to prostitutes at age 13 or 14 in order to "make a man" of them.

Many programs to combat AIDS in Latin America have targeted prostitutes as disease carriers, conveniently blaming the women for the spread of the epidemic. Such prevention programs are designed to protect others from them, not them from others. The words condom and prostitute are often closely associated. Yet the women often don't have the freedom to demand that all clients use condoms; economic reality forces them literally to commit suicide in order to feed their families. It's frequently the only way to survive.

According to Dr. Tatiana Ortiz, an evangelical physician who treats poor women in Guayaquil, Ecuador, the AIDS epidemic is just another manifestation of a system that has "taken away from women our right to feel, do and say what we want." Not much will change, she argues, until the factors that impoverish women, that silence and render them invisible, are corrected.

AIDS and the Church

From the time the first priests arrived on the boats of the military conquerors, the Roman Catholic church has retained tremendous cultural and political authority throughout the region. Most AIDS activists believe the church's teachings on sexual morality hurt efforts to slow the spread of the epidemic. The Vatican officially opposes all artificial contraception measures, including condoms, even as a method to prevent AIDS. So governments, not wanting to inflame the ire of powerful bishops who, according to Dantas, are "stuck on condoms," have backed off from aggressive educational campaigns that might promote condom use and even from scientific sex education courses in public schools.

Protestants and evangelicals in the region often preach passivity in the face of the epidemic. Convinced that AIDS is just another in a string of disasters that must be withstood in preparation for the Second Coming, when humanity will be freed from the travails of this world, some have proclaimed AIDS a part of God's plan. Others offer moral condemnation, declaring people with AIDS to be evildoers rightfully punished by God for their sins.

Chilean Joel Gajardo, a Presbyterian, challenges the church's right to condemn. "So often we in the church have focused on the question of sin, asking, 'Who sinned? What's the appropriate punishment?' If we take seriously the Gospel accounts of Jesus' ministry," he says, "we discover that those are not the correct questions. What we should be asking is, 'How can we use this opportunity to express the grace of God?' "

Many Christians in the region are breaking away from traditional thinking and asking that very question.

• Rosa Farias is a nurse in a large Buenos Aires hospital with over one hundred patients suffering from AIDS. She also gives AIDS talks in public schools. Farias says several of her colleagues at first refused to work with people with AIDS, but after attending church-sponsored seminars on the subject, most changed their mind. Others quit rather than deal with AIDS. Farias, a member of the Methodist church, says many of her patients have been abandoned by their families. "They've been told that their disease is a punishment from God for their sins. It's a hard job at times to convince them that God is not bad, that God wants to help them."

• Neli Lou Eqewarth's Alliance for Life administers a series of self-help homes in poor São Paulo neighborhoods where people with AIDS live together, caring for each other. After the Catholic-sponsored group opened its first house in 1989, neighbors threatened and stoned those who arrived.

After five days of harassment, a police escort was needed to get the people with AIDS out alive.

When the Alliance received funds to build its own homes in Mairipora, a forested area north of the city, wealthy nearby residents, worried about land values, campaigned to have the church-sponsored project — christened "The Promised Land" — evicted, and Mairipora's mayor tried unsuccessfully in the courts to stop the Alliance. But it held on, and today some forty people live in the pleasant complex.

Lazaro Bozolan is one of them. When he told his wife he was HIV positive, she washed his dishes and laundry separately and started sleeping apart. Soon he was living under a bridge, where church workers found him. Today he lives in The Promised Land.

• A retired physician in Santa Clara, Cuba, Elena Iglesias started volunteering at the local AIDS sanatorium shortly after it opened three years ago. It's her ministry today. An evangelical, Iglesias spends most days at the sanatorium practicing medicine, counseling, reading the Bible and praying with patients. "The church has stayed too long inside our four walls," she argues. "We've got to leave the building, taking the Gospel's hope to those who need it but who would never come to the church."

• Cristina Gutiérrez got involved in AIDS education when the disease touched some of her friends. She helped form Popular Pastoral Action on AIDS, an ecumenical group that assists members of street gangs in Santiago, Chile, in designing their own AIDS education programs.

Gutiérrez claims most government programs against AIDS "don't respect the vision, values and organization" of target groups. "The government can spend a lot of money, but it just won't work," she says. Instead, successful programs "must be planned and carried out by the people who benefit from them." Gutiérrez trains young promoters who work with their peers on street corners and in video halls. "We don't show up with a prescription for how to do things," she states, "but rather with information and a challenge: We're poor, but what can we do with the resources we have?"

AIDS and Solidarity

Gutiérrez admits the church is one of the hardest places to mobilize people to work against AIDS. "We don't want to talk about AIDS," she laments, "because it means talking about sexuality, homosexuality, death — themes that make many in the church uncomfortable."

Cesar Parra, a Baptist chaplain in a church-run hospital in Quito, Ecuador, admits he had to struggle with prejudice when he first came into contact with someone with AIDS. "He wasn't a homosexual or a drug addict, but rather someone just like me," he remembers. "Since I couldn't label him, I was forced to respond to him as a human being, the way Jesus would have responded."

Parra hopes the AIDS epidemic can help the church "lay bare our pastoral crisis, our failure to reach out to people in need, people who are hurting but for whom we've traditionally had only judgment, not compassion or solidarity."

Gutiérrez argues that the AIDS crisis offers the church in Latin America an opportunity for conversion. "The real challenge of AIDS," she says, "is that the church will convert itself to life, that we will let go of old dogmas in order to find ourselves in new contact with real life—where people suffer, cry and are forgotten."

II

ETHICS AND AIDS

Moral Issues

Chapter 7

The Ethics of Caring for Patients with HIV or AIDS

Ruth Ann Hansen

The instant headline status of AIDS and HIV infection in both the professional and the public press reflects the universal fears and concerns regarding the containment and control of this deadly disease. The U.S. Public Health Service currently estimates that between 1 million and 1.5 million people in the United States are infected with HIV, and the Centers for Disease Control has projected that the annual incidence of AIDS will increase to 60,000 by 1990 and to 365,000 by 1992 (Heyward & Curran, 1988). The present article discusses some of the ethical dilemmas that health care professionals must face when making decisions about the identification and treatment of persons with HIV infection or AIDS. Some concerns specific to occupational therapy are also addressed.

Milliken and Greenblatt (1987) stated, "The ethical issues surrounding the acquired immunodeficiency syndrome (AIDS) epidemic have been prominent since the initial description of AIDS in homosexuals during 1981. ... As in times of previous epidemics, conflicts between individual rights and societal imperatives come to the forefront as public health authorities grapple with methods of epidemic control" (p. 443).

The determination of an ethical course in the care and treatment of persons with AIDS and in the control and prevention of the disease requires that the health care professional make decisions on several para-

"The Ethics of Caring for Patients with HIV or AIDS," *American Journal of Occupational Therapy* 44, March 1990, pp. 239-242. Ruth Ann Hansen, Ph.D., is chair of the American Occupational Therapy Association's Standards and Ethics Commission and associate professor at Eastern Michigan University, Ypsilanti. Copyright © 1990 by the American Occupational Therapy Association, Inc. Reprinted with permission.

meters. Some of the questions that must be answered are as follows:

1. How should resources be allocated to care for AIDS patients? What amount of funding should be designated for HIV and AIDS research?

2. What are the best methods of disease control?

3. Does the patient have the right to decide who should be informed?

4. Does the health care professional have an obligation to inform persons who test positive for HIV and to report these persons as carriers of the disease?

5. Do health care professionals have the duty to treat persons with AIDS? Do health care professionals have the right to refuse to treat such patients?

Some of the more pressing ethical dilemmas for health care professionals arise in the treatment of persons with AIDS or HIV. The tough decisions that must be made regarding the treatment of persons who have contagious, life-threatening diseases, however, are not new. The care of persons with plague, typhus, malaria, polio, leprosy, and tuberculosis has caused concern and fear. During a plague in Florence in 1348, Boccaccio wrote of his frustrations in finding no cure for the disease (Winwar, 1955). He particularly bemoaned the fate of physicians who in caring for their patients contracted the disease and perished. The modern-day epidemic of AIDS, however, carries more of a stigma because of its association with homosexuality and drug abuse.

Allocation of Resources

How should we use available personnel and materials? What kind and quantity of medical resources should we expend? The treatment of persons in the final stages of the disease raises questions about when, how, and if to resuscitate, the use of certain surgical procedures, and the "initiation or withdrawal of assisted ventilation or artificial nutrition" (Milliken & Greenblatt, 1987, p. 447). Such decisions are common in the treatment of terminally ill patients, but they are made more difficult in cases of AIDS due to the relatively young age of the patients. Moreover, the expense involved in the use of universal precautions has contributed to the skyrocketing cost of health care provision and health care insurance.

Another critical financial concern is the amount of money needed to support research efforts to find a cure and effective methods of prevention for the disease. James D. Watkins, chair of the Presidential Commission on the Human HIV Epidemic, during a media briefing about the commission's report, estimated that more than $3 billion would be needed annually to support an adequate national research effort ("Pessimistic Outlook," 1988). Some people vigorously oppose the allocation of such large sums of taxpayers' money to find a cure for a disease that affects a relatively small percentage of the population (Kilpatrick, 1988).

Disease Control

Some of the more apparent methods to control the spread of AIDS are (a) universal mandatory testing for HIV, (b) forced isolation of all persons with AIDS and perhaps of all HIV carriers, (c) the practice of tracing and contacting sexual partners and those with whom the infected person has shared needles, and (d) education. Each of these methods, however, has inherent problems.

Universal mandatory testing. Methods by which to screen large numbers of people already exist. Besides the problem of false-positive and false-negative results, however, is the question of how test results would be used. Mass screening programs have serious personal and societal implications. Although mass screening would allow HIV carriers to receive early counseling and drug therapy, such counseling does not ensure the cessation of promiscuous behavior. Additionally, if positive test results are reported to a public agency (e.g., public health department), the infected person may be ostracized by his or her family and friends.

Forced isolation. Persons with HIV or AIDS may face forced isolation from society, just as persons with tuberculosis did approximately two decades ago. In Cuba, persons with AIDS are forcibly detained (Betancourt, 1988). Although these persons, under the jurisdiction of the Ministry of the Interior, are asked to voluntarily report to an isolation facility, if they do not comply they are taken there by force. This response to the AIDS epidemic raises concerns about the individual's rights.

One might believe that forced confinement is possible only in countries considered less democratic than the United States. But even in this country, some legal and health professionals have been debating the legitimacy of confining to psychiatric institutions those HIV-positive persons who engage in promiscuous sexual activity (Appelbaum, 1988). Appelbaum noted the distinction between quarantine and civil commitment laws. Some states permit the quarantine of persons with transmittable infectious diseases. Quarantine facilities are unavailable in certain areas, however, and because the laws have fallen into disuse, they are not easily invoked. Conversely, civil commitment laws are used regularly to detain persons considered dangerous to the general public. Although Appelbaum discussed the inappropriateness of the use of civil commitment to confine persons with HIV or AIDS, he believed that there would be continuing pressure from public officials to use the mental health system for this purpose unless other means of detention are created (Appelbaum, 1988).

Informing others. In June 1988, the American Medical Association (AMA) issued a policy report outlining the steps that a physician should follow in informing third parties that a patient is infected with HIV. The report stated that the physician should first encourage the patient to inform third parties who may be at risk. If this fails, the physician should notify public health authorities. Finally, if the authorities do not act, the physician should directly inform and counsel those persons who are endangered ("AMA Takes Stand," 1988).

The AMA has also urged states to establish systems by which they can trace and contact sexual partners of HIV-positive persons, much like the methods used to contact the sexual partners of persons with venereal disease. This policy has drawn sharp criticism from gay activists, who believe it to be an oversimplified solution to a complex problem. Jeff Levi, executive director of the National Gay and Lesbian Task Force, maintains that the problem requires a flexible approach rather than one standard procedure for the notification of partners ("AMA Takes Stand," 1988).

Education. The least invasive disease control strategy is education. Examples of such efforts are former Surgeon General Koop's mailing of an educational pamphlet to all U.S. citizens and the showing of short informational clips on national television. Although these materials are developed in the interest of increasing public understanding and awareness, I have found that some persons consider these materials to be a serious invasion of their privacy and an affront to their values. Nonetheless, the perceived threat of AIDS is so great that the otherwise conservative Reagan administration provided funding for the preparation and wide distribution of these materials.

Professionals' Duty To Treat AIDS Patients

Fear and ignorance. Because a cure or a preventive vaccine does not exist, some health care professionals question their duty to treat persons with AIDS. They express their fear both actively and passively by refusing to provide certain types of care or by providing only that care that does not necessitate close physical contact with the patient. Some of this fear evolves from a lack of knowledge or mistrust of the information provided. Although research has shown that HIV infection can only be transmitted perinatally, through infected blood or blood products, or through unprotected sexual activity, doubt still exists among health care professionals. For example, in a 1987 study of nurses and physicians conducted at New York's Beth Israel Medical Center, 64 percent of the respondents were unsure or did not believe that they had been given accurate information about the risk of contracting HIV ("Ignorance About AIDS," 1988).

The American Medical Association in 1987 publicly stated that physicians have a duty to treat the sick and that this duty prevails even when the patient has a transmissible and lethal disease such as AIDS ("Medical Association," 1987). I believe that the same duty holds for all health care workers. In their chapter entitled "Ethical Issues in AIDS," Murray and Aumann (1987) stated, "The moral force of professional commitment means nothing if it applies only when safe and convenient. . . . Exaggerated fears of a minimal danger of contracting AIDS are no excuse for failing to live up to professional vows" (p. 142).

Prejudice. Some health care professionals have reacted negatively to the sexual preferences or drug abuse of some AIDS patients. These reactions are then used to rationalize their avoidance of persons with AIDS. In a study conducted at Beth Israel Hospital in New York, approximately 11 percent of the nurses and 4.5 percent of the physicians considered AIDS to be "God's punishment" to homosexuals ("Ignorance about AIDS," 1988).

Implications for Occupational Therapists

We as occupational therapists may proclaim that we know better and that we have no ethical conflicts when working with and for persons who have HIV or AIDS. A recent survey of 119 occupational therapists (Atchison, Beard, & Lester, 1990), however, indicated that 41 percent of the respondents feared AIDS more than any other disease, 36 percent feared contracting AIDS during routine care of patients with AIDS, and 36 percent feared transmitting the virus to their family and friends.

Although occupational therapists are guided by a professional code of ethics (American Occupational Therapy Association [AOTA], 1988), the code does not provide specific methods for the resolution of ethical dilemmas. Rather, it provides guidelines and a general description of behaviors that are considered desirable for all occupational therapists. Principle I, for example, states that the therapist must "protect the confidential nature of information gained from educational, practice, and investigational activities unless sharing such information could be deemed necessary to protect the well-being of a third party" (AOTA, 1988, p. 795). The determination of when and with whom to share information to protect the patient or others is difficult and is one that is particularly complex when the patient has HIV or AIDS.

Hansen, Kamp, & Reitz (1988) provided one strategy of analysis for the resolution of ethical dilemmas. Additionally, Hansen and Kyler-Hutchison (1989) provided the following five-step process by which the therapist can select a defensible solution:

1. Who are the "players" in the dilemma?
2. What other facts/information do you need?
3. What are the actions which might be taken?
4. What are the consequences (ethical, medical, and/or legal) of each action?
5. Choose an action or combination of actions that you would recommend and can defend.

Either method may prove useful to the therapist who is grappling with the dilemmas that arise when caring for the patient with HIV or AIDS.

I believe that occupational therapists face the same ethical dilemmas regarding HIV and AIDS as do other health care professionals. We must consider many factors when determining which solution is the best for the patient, for the occupational therapist, and for society. The resolution of these ethical concerns, like many other concerns that health care workers face, is influenced by the personal and professional values of all of the persons involved. We must remember, however, that the cultural, social, and political climates strongly influence the final determination of an appropriate course of action. We are bound by the ethical code of our profession to care for all who require our services. Although the decision to treat a person infected with HIV or AIDS is a personal one, we must also consider our moral responsibility and professional accountability and must understand that very little personal risk is involved. The refusal to care for a person with HIV or AIDS because of prejudice or fear is clearly an ethical violation. Equally unethical is subtle discrimination, such as a premature discharge or referral or the choice of a less effective treatment method so as to diminish the need for close physical contact. The ethical care of our patients requires the careful and thoughtful consideration of our own values and attitudes and of the values and needs of all concerned.

Currently, our most effective weapon against AIDS is the diminishment of the fears of health professionals and of society at large. We can best accomplish this by providing everyone with accurate information about HIV and AIDS. This requires frequent updates, because research is continually providing us with a new understanding of the disease's mechanisms and with the most effective precautionary measures (Heyward & Curran, 1988). Our duty as occupational therapists is to be knowledgeable about HIV and AIDS and to share this knowledge with our colleagues and patients.

Acknowledgments

I thank Virginia Dickie for her guidance and suggestions. Portions of this article were taken from my paper entitled "Ethical Dilemmas Related to AIDS," presented at the First World Congress on Allied Health in Elsinore, Denmark, June 16, 1988.

This article is dedicated to the memory of my friend John who died in December 1988.

References

AMA takes stand on AIDS-related issues. (1988, August 5). *Psychiatry News*, 1, 20, 21.

American Occupational Therapy Association. (1988). Occupational therapy code of ethics. *American Journal of Occupational Therapy, 42,* 795-796.

Appelbaum, P. S. (1988). AIDS, psychiatry, and the law. *Hospital and Community Psychiatry, 39,* 13-14.

Atchison, B. J., Beard, B. J., & Lester, L. (1990). Occupational therapists and AIDS: Attitudes, knowledge, and fears. *American Journal of Occupational Therapy, 44*, 212-217.

Betancourt, E. F. (1988, February 11). Cuba's callous war on AIDS. *New York Times*, p. 10.

Hansen, R. A., Kamp, L., & Reitz, S. (1988). Two practitioners' analyses of occupational therapy practice dilemmas. *American Journal of Occupational Therapy, 42*, 312-319.

Hansen, R. A., & Kyler-Hutchison, P. L. (1989, April). *Light at the End of the Tunnel: Resolving Dilemmas*. Workshop presented at the American Occupational Therapy Association's 69th Annual Conference, Baltimore.

Heyward, W. L., & Curran, J. W. (1988). The epidemiology of AIDS in the U.S. *Scientific American, 259*, 72-81.

Ignorance about AIDS, homophobia still strong among health professionals. (1988, June 17). *Psychiatry News, 11*, 25.

Kilpatrick, J. J. (1988, June 9). AIDS is neither an epidemic nor tragedy, so why are we making such a fuss? *Detroit Free Press*, C-10.

Medical association says doctors must treat AIDS patients. (1987, November 13). *Ann Arbor News*, B2.

Milliken, N., & Greenblatt, R. (1987). Ethical issues in the AIDS epidemic. In J. F. Monagle & D. C. Thomasma (Eds.), *Medical Ethics: A Guide for Health Professionals* (443-459). Rockville, MD: Aspen.

Murray, T., & Aumann, G. (1987). Ethical issues in AIDS. In V. Gong & N. Rudnick (Eds.), *AIDS: Facts and Issues* (141-153). New Brunswick, NJ: Rutgers University Press.

Pessimistic outlook on AIDS reports. (1988, June 11). *Science News*, 372.

Winwar, F. (Trans.). (1955). *The Decameron of Giovanni Boccaccio*. New York: Random House.

Chapter 8

Ethics and Treatment of HIV Infection

Edmund D. Pellegrino

Treatment of human immunodeficiency virus infection poses some of the most difficult dilemmas in clinical medicine. As new data on natural history, treatment, and prevention appear, some new ethical questions are raised and older ones reexamined. This review focuses on the ethical impact of recent research, particularly the availability of early treatment.

The most significant recent findings include the potential effectiveness of the early use of zidovudine (formerly known as azidothymidine [AZT]) in delaying the emergence of the acquired immunodeficiency syndrome (AIDS) and the use of sulfamethoxazole and aerosolized pentamidine isethionate in preventing opportunistic infections.[1-3] In addition, zidovudine has shown some reversing effect on AIDS dementia in children.[4] Dideoxyinosine seems effective in zidovudine-resistant and intolerant patients. Other more promising and more sophisticated therapies are in the offing.[5]

None of these measures is curative, but they change the physician's approach to management dramatically. Early diagnosis, early treatment, and monitoring must replace fatalistic resignation. Patients are eager for access to medication. Activists and legislators call for rapid distribution of new drugs to all who need them. Earlier ethical debates about testing, confidentiality, and autonomy have been reopened, since early treatment is impossible without frequent testing. Patients now must be told about treatment possibilities. They are free to reject medication, but how absolute are their claims to confidentiality and autonomy when early testing and treatment might avert the disease in their contacts? The American Medical Association has already recommended that all contacts of human immu-

"Ethics," *JAMA*, May 16, 1990, pp. 2641-2642. Edmund D. Pellegrino, M.D., is at the Kennedy Institute of Ethics, Georgetown University, Washington, DC.

nodeficiency virus-positive patients be notified and urged to be tested and treated.

Do patients have an obligation to seek treatment to protect sexual contacts and reduce the social and economic costs of treating overt AIDS?[6] How vigorously should physicians urge treatment? When are physicians obliged to disclose test results to significant others? What are their ethical and legal responsibilities if they do not? Is the potential good from treatment such that routine testing without consent is now defensible in high-risk populations, or in all hospital admissions? Do the potential benefits of testing outweigh the right of autonomy, the expense, and the possibility that some will be dissuaded from seeking medical help? How will physicians know who is in the early stage of the infection and who is a candidate for treatment without routine testing? Were the Congress under a moral obligation to pass antidiscrimination legislation, as recommended by the President's Commission, some of these dilemmas would be easier to resolve.[7]

Equally vexing are the questions of social ethics that widespread availability and accessibility of expensive treatment entail. Currently, the 1200-mg daily dose of zidovudine costs $6,400 annually, with the recently recommended dose of 600 mg daily costing about half that amount.[8] Who should pay, since many AIDS victims are poor or ineligible for Medicaid? Should society take a strictly utilitarian approach of "the most care for the most people" and allocate its resources to other purposes, or should drugs be made available at public expense to all without discrimination?[9] Do drug manufacturers have obligations to reduce profits in the face of the needs of AIDS patients?

If treatment is to become readily available to all who need it, it will have to be better integrated into the health care system than at present. The burden of care will have to be better distributed among physicians and hospitals, since at present only a minority treat the bulk of AIDS patients. Physicians will also be obliged to be better prepared for the care of patients with AIDS and its complications. Other patients will have to accept the fact that AIDS patients will be treated in community hospitals. Communities must be prepared to support the care for those who are unable to pay. Questions of just allocation of resources between AIDS and non-AIDS patients have already arisen.[10]

The possibility of treatment underscores the obligation of health professionals to treat all patients. It also highlights the neglected question of ethical obligations of society and patients to the health professions.[11] The fact of psychological "burnout" must be recognized and provided for.[12] When accidental needle sticks occur, physicians and other health professionals have a moral claim for mandatory testing of patients so that early treatment can be instituted and the trauma of uncertainty removed.[13] How firm is the reciprocal obligation of AIDS patients to be tested in such cases? How should their strong moral claim to confidentiality and autonomy be balanced against the welfare of the health professional?

The fatal nature of AIDS and the suffering of its victims constitute powerful arguments for making experimental agents available as soon as possible. This pressure has effected a "speedup" in clinical trials. The National Institutes of Health has proposed a "parallel track" system that would retain the randomized trial as standard but permit bypassing this method if, in the opinion of an expert panel, a drug appears promising and has an acceptable toxicity.[14] Similarly, the Food and Drug Administration has very recently approved acceleration of the process of approval for children, which has been understandably more rigorous than with adults.

Less rigorous testing criteria for experimental drugs seem ethically justifiable in patients with full-blown AIDS. If death is delayed or prevented, effectiveness will be clear. But with asymptomatic patients the uncertainties of the natural history of this infection make evaluation very difficult, even in the best-designed experiment.[15] However, the dangers of uncontrolled trials must not be ignored — false expectations, delay in identifying effective drugs, unanticipated toxicity, clandestine trials, and failure to study basic mechanisms of drug action.[16] The recent data on viremia and its relationship to activity should permit a better staging of the disease and more precise evaluation of treatment.[17, 18]

These questions are further complicated when trials are conducted on pregnant women or neonates. Should all women be offered testing, or just those in high-risk groups? Should such testing be mandatory as some have urged? What is the physician's liability if testing and treatment are not offered? Is routine testing in pregnancy preferable to voluntary testing, since it avoids questions of life-style? Should treatment be offered before evaluation? How will evaluation be carried out?

All these questions force a reexamination of the statistical, epistemological, and design assumptions that underlie clinical trials. The demand of activists that persons with AIDS be involved in experimental design may be helpful. The presence of persons with AIDS may enhance resolution of some of the serious dilemmas and motivations experienced by scientists and may also serve to promote the understanding that well-designed experiments are in the interests of patients themselves.

If, as seems possible in the future, a vaccine becomes available for testing, the difficulties will be compounded by the need for rigorous design and controls. Perhaps by that time some consensus will have emerged on how to balance compassion and science in the short- and long-term interests of patients with AIDS.

Until a vaccine does become available, education and counseling remain the mainstays of primary prevention. Because of the increase in human immunodeficiency virus infection in drug users, many countries have introduced needle exchange.[19] The hope is to decrease transmission among intravenous drug users by allowing safe disposal of infected equipment and encouraging entry into treatment programs.[20] The ethical issue is whether such programs encourage substance abuse or are even feasible, given the many uncontrollable variables in the behavior of intravenous drug users.[21] Results so far are inconclusive. Four studies in Tacoma, Washington; Sydney, Australia; and Sweden report no increase in drug use; three from the United Kingdom and Sweden report a reduction in needle sharing, while other studies show no effects or even an increase in risk behavior.[22] Given these uncertainties, the objections of minority and religious communities, and the difficulties of design, evaluation, and expense, initiation of such programs on a national scale is ethically debatable.

The ethical issues surrounding treatment of human immunodeficiency virus infection are far from resolved. As new information appears, continuous reassessment of the ethical issues — old and new — is a necessity. Clinicians will need to make ethical decisions on a daily basis in a climate of ethical uncertainty and change for some time to come.

Notes

1. Centers for Disease Control. Guidelines for prophylaxis of *Pneumocystis carinii* pneumonia for persons infected with human immunodeficiency virus. *MMWR*. 1989; 38 (suppl S-5): 1-9.

2. For some of the promising new therapeutic possibilities, some unevaluated, some in the process of evaluation (e.g., interferon alfa, AZDU (3'-azido-2', 3'-dideoxyuridine), gp 160-based AIDS vaccine, zidovudine in human immunodeficiency virus-infected pregnant women, zidovudine in asymptomatic patients and patients with AIDS-related complex, and probenecid), see the September 1989 and July 1989 issues of *NIAID AIDS Agenda*.

3. AZT delays HIV progression in asymptomatic and ARC patients. *NIAID AIDS Agenda*. September 1989:1.

4. Culliton BJ. AZT reverses AIDS dementia. *Child Sci*. October 6, 1989; 246:23-24.

5. Palca J. New AIDS drugs take careful aim. *Science*. 1989; 246:1559-1560.

6. Winkenwerder W, Kessler AR, Stolec RM. Federal spending for illness caused by the human immunodeficiency virus. *N Engl J Med*. 1989; 320:1598-1603.

7. *Report of the Presidential Commission on the Human Immunodeficiency Virus Epidemic*. Washington, DC: Presidential Commission on the Human Immunodeficiency Virus Epidemic; 1988. Publication 1988 0-214-701:QL 3.

8. Staver S. MDs hesitate to change AZT dosage. *Am Med News*. February 9, 1990:14-16.

9. Penslar RL, Lamm RD. Who pays for AZT? *Hastings Cent Rep*. September-October 1989; 19:30-32.

10. Rogers DE. Federal spending on AIDS — how much is enough? *N Engl J Med*. 1989; 320:1623-1624.

11. Pellegrino ED. HIV infection and the ethics of clinical care. *J Leg Med*. 1989; 10:29-45.

12. Le Bourdais E. Hopelessness and helplessness: treating the doctors who treat AIDS patients. *Can Med Assoc J*. 1989; 140:440-443.

13. AIDS and HIV update: acquired immunodeficiency syndrome and human immunodeficiency virus infection among health-care workers. *JAMA*. 1988; 259:2817-2818. Leads from the *MMWR*.

14. Dr. Fauci proposes parallel track system to expand access to drugs. *NIAID AIDS Agenda*. July 1989:1.

15. Fauci AS. AIDS—challenges to basic and clinical biomedical research. *J Assoc Am Med Coll*. 1989; 64:115-119.

16. Benjamin Freedman and the McGill/Boston Research Group. Non-validated therapies and HIV disease. *Hastings Cent Rep*. May/June 1989; 19:14-20.

17. Ho DD, Moudgil T, Alam M. Quantitation of human immunodeficiency virus type I in the blood of infected persons. *N Engl J Med*. 1989; 321:1621-1625.

18. Coombs RW, Collier AC, Allain JP, et al. Plasma viremia in human immunodeficiency virus infection. *N Engl J Med*. 1989; 321:1626-1631.

19. *MMWR Update: Acquired Immunodeficiency Syndrome Associated With Intravenous Drug Use—United States 1988*. Atlanta, Ga.: Centers for Disease Control; 1989.

20. Van Den Hoek JAR, Van Haastrecht HJA, Coutinho RA. Risk reduction among intravenous drug users in Amsterdam under the influence of AIDS. *Am J Public Health*. 1989; 79:1355-1357.

21. Schoenbaum EE, Hartel D, Drowyn P, et al. Risk factors for human immunodeficiency virus infection in intravenous drug users. *N Engl J Med*. 1989; 321:874-879.

22. See also 34 abstracts, 32 with numerical data dealing with needle swapping, in *Program for the Fifth International Conference on AIDS, Montreal, June 1989*.

Chapter 9

Women and AIDS

Carole A. Campbell

Introduction

The first cases of acquired immunodeficiency syndrome (AIDS) in the United States were recognized and described in 1981. The appearance of AIDS in disparate groups, linked only by probable routes of transmission, was among the first pieces of evidence suggesting an infectious cause. AIDS was first described among homosexual men in 1981.[1] In the following year it was recognized in intravenous (IV)-drug users[2] and Haitians.[3] Also in 1982 AIDS was reported in recipients of blood or blood products,[4,5] infants born to mothers at risk[6], and heterosexual partners of persons with AIDS.[7] Initially it was thought that the newly appearing female AIDS cases were the result of transmission through IV-drug usage. Soon it was realized that these women had become infected through heterosexual contact with an infected male. More female AIDS cases resulting from heterosexual transmission began to appear in 1983 and the percentage of female cases in that category has continued to increase yearly from that time. This trend in heterosexual transmission may serve as a good marker for future trends. AIDS in women also is of special interest because women with AIDS or with human immunodeficiency virus (HIV) infection are the major source of infection of infants with AIDS.[8] Trends in AIDS in women may help to determine future trends in pediatric cases.

This article describes the epidemiology of AIDS in women in the United States. Emphasis is given to the significant growth in the proportion of

"Women and AIDS," *Social Science and Medicine*, 30 (4), 1990, pp. 407-415. Carole A. Campbell, Ph.D., is professor of sociology, California State University, Long Beach. Reprinted with permission from Pergamon Press Ltd., Oxford, England.

women with AIDS in the heterosexual transmission category from 1982 to 1988. Routes of perinatal transmission are described. AIDS tends to present critical fertility and reproductive issues for women. Some of these issues are examined in this article. The special problems that women with AIDS face are addressed. AIDS education efforts aimed at women are examined. Attention is directed to the way in which women's involvement in the AIDS epidemic is associated with the traditional female role.

AIDS Cases in Adults in the United States

As of January 2, 1989, women comprised 9 percent or 6983 of the total 81,418 adult AIDS cases in the United States. A large majority of these women are in their child-bearing years with 79 percent between ages 13 and 39.[9]

AIDS tends to affect minority women more than minority men since a greater percentage of men with AIDS are white. About half (52 percent) of the women with AIDS are black and 19 percent are Hispanic. AIDS cases have occurred 14 times more frequently among Hispanic women than among white women.[10]

The major transmission category for women with AIDS is IV-drug usage. Fifty-two percent of female cases fall in this category. This category has been the major route of transmission for women since the onset of the disease. This transmission category is the principal link to other adult populations through heterosexual transmission and to children through perinatal transmission.

Heterosexual contact with an infected male is the second largest transmission category for women. Thirty percent of female cases fall in this category. This category can include sexual contact with male IV-drug users, males infected by blood products and males who are bisexual. Female IV-drug users and sexual partners of male IV-drug users make up the largest number of HIV-infected women of child-bearing age. It is particularly noteworthy that in 1982, 14 percent of female cases were from heterosexual contact with an infected male.[9] The proportion of women with AIDS in the heterosexual transmission category has increased annually in the last 6 years. In comparison to female cases, a much smaller proportion (2 percent) of male AIDS cases are in the heterosexual transmission category. Male cases have not shown such a significant increase in the heterosexual category over this time period. Men with AIDS outnumber women with AIDS in all transmission categories except heterosexual transmission.

Transmission from blood transfusions comprises 11 percent of female cases. In comparison, 2 percent of male cases fall in the transfusion category. Although the male percentage is lower, the number of male cases exceeds the number of female cases in the transfusion category, in contrast to the heterosexual transmission category.

The final transmission category for women is that of undetermined risk. Seven percent of female cases fall in this category. The undetermined risk category includes those persons for whom no specific risk is identified. It also includes persons for whom risk information is incomplete due to death or refusal to be interviewed. Persons who are lost in follow-up efforts are also in this category. The Centers for Disease Control does not separately tabulate persons who report only heterosexual contact with a prostitute or sex with multiple partners. Such persons are included in the undetermined risk category.[8] In comparison to female cases, a smaller proportion (3 percent) of male AIDS cases are in the undetermined risk category.

The percentage of total cases that the undetermined risk category comprises for both males and females has not fluctuated dramatically over the last 6 years. It should be emphasized though that the percentage of female cases in this category started at 14 in 1982 which is considerably larger than the male percentage at 2. The percentage of female cases of undetermined risk has remained consistently larger than the percentage of male cases over the last 6 years. In 1981 women comprised 3 percent of all AIDS cases. Female AIDS cases now comprise 9 percent of the total number of cases and the male to female ratio of AIDS cases is 11:1.8

At the present time a heterosexual woman in the United States faces a greater risk of becoming infected with HIV through sexual intercourse than does a heterosexual man. There is a larger pool of men infected by other means such as IV-drug use and homosexual contact. Since a greater proportion of men are infected, a women is more likely than a man to encounter an infected partner. The relative efficiencies of male-to-female versus female-to-male transmission also may be relevant here.

HIV infection has occurred in a high percentage of women exposed only occasionally to semen from a single man. To date no cases of transmission through artificial insemination have occurred in the United States, but four of eight Australian women who received semen from a single infected donor became infected.[11] Infected semen had been injected directly into the uterus through a catheter. In similar cases of only occasional exposure, 10 out of 17 women became infected through vaginal intercourse with one infected man.[11]

Pediatric AIDS Cases and Routes of Perinatal Transmission

Pediatric AIDS cases follow a racial distribution similar to that of women since most are the result of perinatal transmission from infected mothers. These cases also follow a similar geographic distribution with the majority of both pediatric and female cases being in New York, New Jersey and

Florida.[8] There is a strong overlap between geographic areas of IV-drug use among women and HIV prevalence among infants.

Between 1982 and 1986 the increase in the number of women with AIDS in the IV-drug, heterosexual and unidentified risk categories was closely paralleled by the increase in pediatric patients whose mothers were in those risk groups. A majority (78 percent) of pediatric AIDS cases are a result of perinatal transmission.[8]

The frequency of transmission from an infected mother to her fetus or newborn infant ranges from 25 to 50 percent.[11] Uninfected as well as infected infants have been born to mothers who previously have given birth to an infected child. The actual rate of perinatal transmission is difficult to determine because there are no laboratory tests that reliably establish HIV infection in newborns. As is the case with other infections, newborns naturally carry antibodies passively acquired transplacentally from their mothers. They may test positive for HIV antibody but actually may not be infected themselves. There is no way to distinguish maternal antibodies from antibodies in an infant infected with HIV. It takes up to 15 months for maternal antibodies to disappear. Newborns produce a limited antibody response to HIV because of their physiologically depressed immune systems. Laboratory diagnosis of HIV in children aged under 15 months currently is based on virus isolation from lymphocyte cultures and on antigen capture in serum. Virus culture from blood or other tissues is an expensive and cumbersome technique and is not always reliable.[12] Antigen capture is not sufficiently sensitive and is not always reliable either.[12] In order for an infant's true HIV status to be determined, it is necessary to follow the infant during the first 15 months in order to detect the loss of maternal antibody and the development of serologic or virologic markers of infection.

Evidence for intrauterine transmission, as opposed to intrapartum transmission, comes from a case where an infected mother gave birth to an infected child in a cesarean delivery. Further evidence is found in the isolation of HIV from cord blood[13] and fetal tissues.[10] Facial malformation has been found in some infants, suggesting that infection occurred between the twelfth and sixteenth week of gestation.[13]

Immunosuppression naturally accompanies pregnancy as a means to prevent the body from rejecting the fetus. Pregnancy, especially during the last 3 months, is a relatively immunosuppressed condition. It appears that increasing maternal immunosuppression facilitates perinatal transmission. Preliminary results from a large study in Zaire found an association between a low T-helper to T-suppressor ratio in the mother and early laboratory and clinical infection in the infant.[14] The development of AIDS or AIDS-related complex (ARC) in perinatally infected children is significantly associated with the presence of symptomatic HIV infection in their mothers,[15] but perinatal transmission may occur in the absence of severe maternal disease.

The effect of pregnancy on existing HIV infection has not been clearly established though two studies have found a high frequency of AIDS and ARC among women during the months after delivery.[16, 17] The critical variable here is duration of infection and it is not known in most cases. Information on the effect of pregnancy on HIV infection would be highly valuable in terms of counseling women.

Data about the timing during pregnancy or the perinatal period of transmission of HIV to the fetus or newborn are not generally available. Moreover, it is not known whether intrapartum transmission occurs as it can with the herpes virus. Only intrauterine and postnatal transmission have been documented. It is not known whether cesarean delivery decreases or increases the risk of transmission. Such information would be helpful to infected women.

Three cases of transmission of HIV from mother to infant through breast milk have occurred.[10] The mothers contracted HIV through postpartum blood transfusions. In these cases the infants would not receive transplacental anti-HIV antibody before birth and breast feeding appears to be the most likely route of transmission. However, it should be stressed that transmission has not always occurred when infected mothers have breast fed their infants. The risk of transmission through breast milk appears to be small compared to the risk through intrauterine transmission. It could be the case that breast feeding after acquisition of HIV, as in the case of a postpartum transfusion, carries a higher risk of viral transmission.

Information on HIV antibody prevalence available from 27 studies of women in settings related to women's health and child-bearing gives some sense of the current rate of infection among women of reproductive age.[18] These studies were conducted in 19 inner-city areas in 12 states. Rates from 11 to 30 percent were found among pregnant IV-drug users. For women who didn't use IV-drugs, prevalence rates ranged from a fraction of 1 percent in most areas to 2.6 percent in New York City. A study of newborns in Massachusetts using the newborn's blood as an indicator of the mother's serologic status found that one of every 476 or 2.1/1000 women giving birth in Massachusetts was positive for HIV antibody.[19] A study testing infants' cord blood in an inner-city hospital in Brooklyn found an even higher prevalence of HIV infection, a rate of 20/1000.[20] A study of newborns' blood specimens conducted in New York State in late 1987 found the prevalence of infection outside the metropolitan area of New York City to be 1.3/1000 and the rate for New York City, 16.4/1000, or 1/61 infants.[21]

The rate of HIV infection in women of reproductive age can serve as a good indicator of the course of the epidemic. Since these women became infected directly through IV-drug usage or indirectly through heterosexual contact with male IV-drug users or bisexual men, they serve as an important bridge group. In addition, perinatal acquisition of HIV by infants of infected mothers is associated with a high probability of infant morbidity and mortality. There is a high rate of disease progression in perinatally infected children during the first year of life.[10]

AIDS and Reproductive Issues

AIDS presents some extremely complex fertility and reproductive decisions for women. Since the majority of children are infected perinatally, prenatal testing for HIV has been recommended as a means of preventing AIDS in children. Prenatal testing is complicated by the fact that not all pregnancies are planned. Women don't always have or take control over conception and many pregnancies happen more by default than intent. Prenatal testing will be effective only for those pregnancies that are planned. Even so, it's not clear that knowledge of antibody status will prevent women from having children. Childbearing for some women is such a strong cultural expectation that a 25-50 percent chance of having an infected child may be acceptable odds. Risk-taking and pregnancy can be compared to risk-taking and AIDS since neither fertilization nor infection are certain.

Many infected women, however, do not know that they are infected when they are pregnant. They may learn of their own infection only after they give birth to an infected child since pediatric AIDS cases become manifest early in life with about half appearing during the first year. Infected mothers often have to deal not only with the consequences of their own illness but also those of their child's at the same time.

Women undergoing artificial insemination need to be aware of the possible risk of infection they face. Most licensed sperm banks now test semen and the American Fertility Society has guidelines that exclude high-risk men from donating. Some banks require that the donor be HIV negative both at the time of donation and 60 days later before his sperm will be used. Some sperm banks even test 90 days later. Some physicians prefer fresh semen because they claim that it results in impregnation more effectively. At present there really are not enough data to show whether fresh or frozen semen gives different pregnancy rates. Most artificial insemination is handled by private physicians with their own sources of sperm. These sources may not always test for HIV. The Congressional Office of Technology Assessment's 1988 study surveyed 1500 physicians and found that physicians who conduct the entire artificial insemination process themselves do not always check thoroughly for the AIDS virus or for genetic disorders.[22] Only about half the doctors performing the procedure test in advance for the AIDS virus or for genetic disorders. In 1987, 172,000 women sought pregnancy through artificial insemination and 65,000 babies were born through this process.[22] The Food and Drug Administration set voluntary testing guidelines for physicians in February of 1988 and now is considering implementing regulations. Some professionals in the insemination field feel that the study has blown the problem out of proportion and stress that there haven't been any cases of AIDS transmitted through artificial insemination in the United States.

Because AIDS has been so strongly linked with sex, it is hard for some women even to recognize a past insemination as a possible risk factor. Pregnancy is usually foremost on the minds of women undergoing artificial insemination, not risk of HIV infection. Even though pregnancy might not result from artificial insemination, HIV could be transmitted from infected sperm in this process nonetheless.

There are limits to the usefulness of amniocentesis since it cannot determine if a fetus is infected with HIV. It is not possible to tell if antibodies are the fetus's own or the mother's. But even if it were possible to detect HIV infection with certainty, transmission could occur at a later stage in pregnancy after amniocentesis had been conducted. Abortion at this stage may not be an option. Moreover, transmission possibly may take place at birth. Amniocentesis thus doesn't offer the same safeguards for HIV infection as it does for other diseases. The HIV maternal antibody test, as compared to other fetal tests such as amniocentesis, is not a good predictor of future infant health.

Reproductive rights of women surface again with the AIDS issue. A central issue is the right of an infected woman to be pregnant. The right to become pregnant and to maintain a pregnancy could be seen as part of a woman's right to control her body. However, as more child-bearing women become infected and give birth to infected children, child-bearing could come under the surveillance of the state. Women of child-bearing age could be among the first groups to undergo mandatory testing as part of an attempt to control women's reproductive choices. The widespread practice of safe sex could serve to drastically reduce the birth rate.

Reproductive rights take on a new meaning when applied to AIDS and AIDS tends to turn the abortion issue on its head. The state traditionally has expressed an interest in preserving and protecting the rights of the fetus. This interest was most clearly demonstrated in the 1973 Roe v. Wade decision when the Supreme Court recognized a woman's right to choose an abortion. The court ruled that a woman's right to privacy must be weighed against the state's interest in protecting the future life of the fetus. The state's interest in fetal survival tends to diminish, however, when the mother is infected with HIV.[23] The state's duty to protect potential life tends to shift to the interest of protecting society from another person with AIDS. In this view, seropositive women do not have the right to become pregnant and should be sterilized automatically. Seropositive pregnant women do not have the right to maintain a pregnancy and should undergo abortions. Sterilization and abortion would be advocated for health reasons alone. Conservatives though might be opposed to this view on grounds that pregnant women should remain pregnant because every fetus, even a defective fetus, has the right to life and ultimately to an AIDS death. Abortion for HIV infections may be opposed on ground that it is a step towards abortions for a wide range of defective fetuses.[24]

Counseling given for abortions in AIDS pregnancies is quite different from counseling for abortions for other diseases such as Down's syndrome, since in an AIDS pregnancy the mother herself already is infected with the virus. She will need to take precautions in order to protect herself from further development of the virus. Moreover, should she decide to go forth with the pregnancy, she herself may not live to be able to raise the child. However, the situation of an infected women is similar to that of woman carrying a Down's syndrome child in one sense. Usually these women are seeking termination not of an unwanted pregnancy but of a wanted pregnancy that was actively sought until learning the possible outcomes.

Special Problems Faced by Women with AIDS and at Risk for AIDS

The rapid loss of health associated with AIDS has implications for both males and females afflicted with the disease. Correspondingly, loss of health often can bring on loss of employment and loss of employment in turn has implications for finances and health insurance.

Although little social class information on persons with AIDS exists, it probably could be safely inferred from data on race and AIDS that women with AIDS are more poor than men with AIDS since women are more likely to be black and Hispanic. These women often suffer from poverty and discrimination without the added weight of AIDS. They are not always able to control the nature and the quality of their health care.

Some inferences from data on IV-drug users as an AIDS patient group also could be made. IV-drug users usually develop the more lethal opportunistic infections than other patient groups and thus have a shorter life expectancy.[25] Often these individuals have other complicating underlying conditions – tuberculosis, hepatitis and cirrhosis among them. Their immune systems are extremely suppressed because of these diseases and also because of the effect of the drugs themselves. Their conditions usually require hospitalization and cannot easily be treated on an outpatient basis. As a patient group, these individuals are usually unemployed and thus do not have group health insurance. As a result, they do not have a family physician and their first contact with the health care system is often in the emergency room. Their disease is usually in a fairly advanced state by the time it is even diagnosed. This patient group usually does not have access to experimental drug therapy. Moreover, these individuals lack equal access to home health care since many home care attendants are not willing to go into poor neighborhoods.

Demographic information on female IV-drug users indicates that these women are more likely to have young children and to be the sole support of these children.[26] The career of addicted women is different from that of addicted men. As compared to men, these women face a narrowing of life options, including fewer friendships and limited education and employment opportunities.[27] Fewer drug treatment programs exist for female IV-drug users than for male IV-drug users, both in absolute numbers and in proportion to need.[26] Most treatment centers will not house women who are pregnant or women with children.

HIV antibody prevalence is three to four times higher among prostitutes who acknowledge IV-drug use than among those who do not.[18] The lives of women who use drugs and who engage in prostitution may be complicated further by their illegal survival activity and incarceration. Prostitutes who use IV-drugs are often street prostitutes and are most often subject to arrest.[28] A large number of street prostitutes are black and Hispanic women. This is partly related to poverty but it is also due to racism which prevents these women from working in brothels, casinos, escort services, and massage parlors.[29] These agencies usually almost exclusively employ Anglo and Asian women.[30] Addicted street prostitutes may buy drugs rather than condoms with what little money they earn. They might not always remember to use condoms because of the drugs' effects. Moreover, they are not in a strong position to enforce condom use with customers. Prostitutes are at risk of becoming infected with HIV from their boyfriends or husbands who are sometimes IV-drug users and who generally do not use condoms.[31]

Few resources exist for prostitutes who want to leave prostitution. Legislation for mandatory HIV antibody testing of women arrested for prostitution has been passed in several states. The actual intent of mandatory testing is to get women out of prostitution. Ironically though, the effect may be to limit their occupational mobility even more.[32] A prostitute who has been arrested already has a difficult time getting out of prostitution because of the criminal record she acquires. Her criminal record is made worse because of the more serious criminal penalties associated with her HIV status.

With most illnesses, it is the mother who assumes the caregiver role in the family. But with AIDS, the mother herself may be ill since most pediatric cases are the result of perinatal transmission. She may have to plan for the welfare of her children after her own death. There is no inclusive coordinated care system in place for women who become ill. As compared to infected males, infected women who seek AIDS-related services usually seek services not only for themselves but for their children as well.[33] Currently adult residential or long-term care facilities are not able to handle pediatric cases and pediatric facilities cannot accommodate mothers of sick children. There is a pressing need for "family" homes that would allow mothers and children to remain together.

Women with AIDS may find themselves dealing with institutions that respond in ways that reinforce the traditional role of women. The institution of welfare has been seen as instilling feelings of dependency, passivity, resignation, and powerlessness in women.[34] Similarly, physicians' diagnoses and treatments may reinforce the traditional sex role of women.[35, 36, 37] Sexism in the response from obstetrician-gynecologists also has been addressed.[38, 39] Since AIDS has affected men predominantly, women with AIDS may not find physicians especially responsive to their illness. Physicians may be slow to recognize the symptoms of AIDS in women and the disease may be in a fairly advanced stage before it is even diagnosed. The potential for misdiagnosis exists as well.

An AIDS diagnosis itself can further inculcate the female stereotype since it carries with it a great deal of powerlessness and uncertainty for women. Infected women may not have the same support system and sense of community as infected men. As a result, women with AIDS may feel isolated and alone and may keep their infection secret for fear of discrimination against them or their families. They may not have the support of an extended family like they may have in other health crises because of the stigma associated with AIDS. Mothers with infected babies may feel a tremendous sense of guilt and grief about infecting their children. Infected women who don't have children often just deal with the loss of their child-bearing potential.

Women's responses to AIDS often places them in the traditional role of nurturer and caregiver. Even when the mother herself is not infected such as in the case of a son's homosexually transmitted AIDS, she is often the one to assume the family caregiver role. Women in the role of mothers, wives, sisters and daughters are usually the ones to provide care.[33, 40] Male family members are the most resistant to homosexually transmitted AIDS — fathers tend to be least supportive of all and brothers also may have negative reactions.[41] The stress of the disease is very often shifted onto women.

The demands of caregiving can be extremely isolating for women. Mothers are used to sharing their knowledge about childhood diseases but are not always able to do this with AIDS because of the stigma it carries. For some mothers, though, the caregiving role has been cathartic. Two mothers, for example, wrote books about their sons' struggles with AIDS.[42, 43] Mothers also have organized support groups for other mothers caring for children with AIDS. Women affected by AIDS tend to seek out therapy and support groups more than do men. The national Hemophiliac Foundation has found that few hemophiliac men with AIDS will go to therapy or attend support groups.[44] It's much more common for the wives of these men to be involved in such activities.

Many AIDS support services currently available arose out of gay men's health concerns and thus have a predominantly male focus. Some women may feel uncomfortable with discussing their concerns about AIDS in support groups with men. Mothers of grown children with AIDS are not always comfortable in mixed groups and sometimes have expressed a need to be only with other mothers.[40]

The epidemiology of female AIDS cases brings together disparate groups of women—IV-drug users, transfusion recipients and sex partners of IV-drug users, transfusion recipients and hemophiliacs. Although what they all have in common is AIDS, their differences may be greater than this similarity. Not all women will find comfort in support groups. Women of different socio-economic backgrounds may vary in the amount of comfort they feel in group therapy settings. Poor women, in comparison to middle class women, are not always able to "talk it out" endlessly and may not find much relief in this type of therapy.[45]

Some of the special situations that AIDS presents for women have been discussed in this section. As the number of female cases continues to rise, an even greater strain may be placed on family social services. There may be more of a need for welfare services for mothers and children if these mothers are no longer able to work. There may be even more of a need for foster care for children whose mothers have died from AIDS. As the number of HIV-infected children continues to rise, there may be an additional need for special day-care services.

AIDS Education Efforts Aimed at Women

The emphasis that has been placed on risk of transmission through IV-drug usage may be misleading. More recent attention has been given to female nonintravenous drug users, in particular, the heavy users of the refined form of cocaine known as "crack."[46] These women may exchange sexual favors for crack but since there is no monetary transaction, they may not consider themselves prostitutes. Yet, they face a risk of infection from the high number of unprotected sexual exposures they have. Since efforts toward prevention have aimed at IV-drug users and prostitutes, female cocaine users who do not see themselves as belonging to these groups may not protect themselves or modify their behavior. Because of the highly addictive nature of crack, these women who exchange sex for crack are seen as a new generation of prostitutes.[47] Moreover, as compared to heroin, crack heightens sexuality and makes users vulnerable to HIV infection.[47]

Success of AIDS education efforts will depend first of all on whether outreach efforts reach women at risk. Women who use IV drugs are among the most difficult to reach since their lifestyles are often transient, unstable and impoverished. These women often take risks in their day-to-day survival. They constantly face risks of overdose, poor health, and physical violence. AIDS then is just one risk among many for them. They may have other priorities and constraints in their lives. In order to be effective, educators must put AIDS in perspective in relation to these priorities and constraints.

A majority of female sex partners of male IV-drug users do not use drugs.[48] These women may not realize the risk they face through sexual relations with their partners. IV-drug users are usually identified when they seek treatment or when they're arrested but since these women do not use drugs, they don't come in contact with treatment centers or with the criminal justice system. Even if these women are reached with AIDS information, they may not be able to be assertive and insist on using condoms since they are already in a subordinate relationship and are especially vulnerable to physical abuse. Their insistence on using condoms could bring on a risk of physical violence. These women may be reluctant to introduce condoms because they are dependent on their male partners for economic support.

Condom use is a particularly sensitive issue among minorities. Using condoms sometimes threatens minority males' sense of masculinity.[45] The position of the Catholic church on condoms also has influenced some minority group members' views. In addition, condom use has been interpreted by some minorities as having genocidal implications.[33, 45] AIDS preventive education could be seen as feeding into racist agendas by promoting the message that blacks and Hispanics should stop having children altogether. It is, therefore, important that educational efforts be culturally sensitive.

AIDS prevention education must also recognize the impact of cultural attitudes toward gender roles. Male Hispanic adolescents, influenced by the role of "Machismo," may feel that impregnating a woman is proof of virility and manhood. The female counterpart of Machismo, "Marianismo," requires that young Hispanic females defer to these males.[49] This deference makes it difficult for these young women to introduce safe sex practices.

There are also gender-related misperceptions surrounding condom use. A survey of attitudes and sexual practices of adolescents in San Francisco[50] reflects these misperceptions. Females in the study were uncertain about males' views on using condoms, although males reported quite positive views about using them. Educational interventions will need to target these types of misperceptions in order to increase the use of condoms among young women. Unprotected anal sex is sometimes practiced by young women who want to remain virgins until marriage.[51]

AIDS educational efforts will need to reach this group of women whose behavior is at risk.

Because AIDS has largely affected males, women with AIDS have been made to fit into a male profile. AIDS education efforts haven't targeted women as much as other persons at risk. Women are frequently absent in AIDS brochures. When the media have included women, they usually focus on white women, despite the fact that a vast majority of female cases are black and Hispanic.[52] Recent articles on heterosexual risk that have appeared in popular magazines target a white middle-class readership. Pictures that accompany these articles show mainly white women.

The distinction between women as "infectors" and women as "infectees" can be made and it becomes evident that far more attention has been given to women as infectors than to the very real risks that they face as infectees.[52] Initially there was a lack of attention to the problem of AIDS among women until there was concern that prostitutes were spreading the disease.[53, 54] Prostitutes seem to have gotten far more attention for their role in infecting customers than for the serious risk of infection they face.[29, 30, 33] Moreover, little attention has been given to the role the customer plays in the act of prostitution, although he is usually the initiator of the transaction. Mandatory testing of prostitutes could serve to protect the customer more than the prostitute since the prostitute may be antibody negative, but there is no assurance that the customer is.[32]

Despite women's vulnerability to AIDS, there has been a general lack of attention to the seriousness of the problem of AIDS in women. Data on women and AIDS are not routinely collected or reported. For example, figures on the total number of women who are pregnant and who have AIDS or who have died from AIDS are not available. Nor is there much data on parity and AIDS. Health departments in some states collect data on pregnancy and parity of female AIDS cases, but no composite profile reflecting the total number of cases exists. These data would be valuable in assessing the future course of the epidemic. It also would be helpful to know more about the personal lives of female AIDS cases, including their family situations, resources, and the special problems they face.

Thus far clinical trials of the experimental drug, azidothymidine (AZT), largely have involved gay men. Hemophiliacs, IV-drug users and persons infected through heterosexual contact haven't been included in these trials. Little data exist about the effects of drug therapy on HIV infection in women.

Although women haven't been targeted with AIDS education as much as men, many health professionals see the hope of controlling the AIDS epidemic as relying a great deal on the effort of women. Women have been found to seek health care more readily than men[55,56] and to take preventive health steps more than men.[57] There is some debate on this issue and some feminists have questioned the idea of directing AIDS preventive education at women since men are largely the ones doing the infecting.[45] AIDS prevention, just like birth control, is made a female responsibility and in this way, women are kept in the caregiver role. Targeting women with AIDS education is defended by some public health professionals who feel that women have a more sharply defined sense of the future and are more responsible about health issues than men.[45] These professionals tend to think that what success can be achieved against AIDS very much depends on women's response. Women also play an important role in the socialization of their children and in this role may be involved in educating their children about AIDS.

Conclusion

The debate over whether AIDS will explode into the heterosexual community as it did in the homosexual community seems more to be over whether AIDS will affect heterosexual men and women equally. The high rate of heterosexual transmission of HIV for women underscores the need for sexually active women to be aware of the risk they face from partners who they do not know well. The high rate of transmission from undetermined risk tends to suggest that women may not know about the past IV-drug or bisexual practices of their partners. Sexually active women with more than one lifetime partner are advised to reduce their risk of HIV infection by using condoms during intercourse. Celibacy, of course, will prevent infection but it is not a viable option for many women.

Prevention of HIV in women will require that women be assertive about condom use. It is projected that AIDS will move down in age and adolescents have been identified as a probable "next" risk group for the disease. The high rate of teenage pregnancy in the United States tends to suggest that condoms are not being used consistently. It is therefore essential that young women especially be informed about condoms and be encouraged to use them if they are sexually active.

Since early 1987 the AIDS epidemic has leveled off among white gay men in Los Angeles County, San Francisco and New York City, the three cities hit earliest and hardest by the disease.[58] This leveling off in the number of new cases is believed to reflect the adoption of safer sex practices by white gay men in these cities. There has been an increase in AIDS cases among IV-drug users. This increase will have consequences for females who are themselves IV-drug users or the sexual partners of IV-drug users. Moreover, this increase among IV-drug users has relevance for future trends in pediatric AIDS cases resulting from perinatal transmission. The increase in AIDS cases among IV-drug users already is reflected in the number of pediatric AIDS cases. In fact, children comprise the fastest growing group of AIDS cases.[59]

This article has described the ways in which AIDS is associated with the traditional feminine stereotype. As AIDS cases continue to increase, the burden of AIDS care will fall more and more on women if sex roles in AIDS care persist in patterns established so far.

Prevention of HIV infection in women will require that they not only take a more assertive role over their own health, but also a more assertive role in making public policy on AIDS. Although women are experienced in lobbying for other public health programs, they have been notably absent from the public health dialogue on AIDS. The data on heterosexual risk for women highlight the need for women to organize and to take preventive steps.

Notes

1. Centers for Disease Control. Pneumocystis pneumonia. *Morbid. Mortal. Weekly Report*, 30, 250-252, 5 June, 1991.

2. Centers for Disease Control. Update on Kaposi's sarcoma and opportunistic infections in previously healthy persons—United States. *Morbid. Mortal. Weekly Report*. 31, 294-301, 11 June, 1982.

3. Centers for Disease Control. Opportunistic infections and Kaposi's sarcoma among Haitians in the United States. *Morbid. Mortal. Weekly Report*, 31, 353-361, 9 July, 1982.

4. Centers for Disease Control. Update on acquired immune deficiency syndrome (AIDS) among patients with hemophilia A. *Morbid. Mortal. Weekly Report*, 31, 644-652, 16 July 1982.

5. Centers for Disease Control. Possible transfusion-associated acquired immune deficiency syndrome (AIDS)—California. *Morbid. Mortal. Weekly Report*, 31, 652-654, 10 Dec., 1982.

6. Centers for Disease Control. Unexplained immunodeficiency and opportunistic infections in infants—New York, New Jersey, California. *Morbid. Mortal. Weekly Report*, 31, 665-668, 17 Dec., 1982.

7. Centers for Disease Control. Immunodeficiency among female sexual partners of males with acquired immune deficiency syndrome (AIDS)—New York. *Morbid. Mortal. Weekly Report*, 31, 697-698, 7 Jan., 1983.

8. Centers for Disease Control. *AIDS Weekly Surveillance Report—United States*, 2 Jan., 1989.

9. Guinan M. E. and Hardy A. Epidemiology of AIDS in women in the United States, 1981 through 1986. *J. Am. Med. Ass.* 257, 2039-2042, 17 April, 1987.

10. Curran J. W., Jaffe H. W., Hardy A. M., Morgan W. M., Selik R. M. and Dondero T. J. Epidemiology of HIV infection and AIDS in the United States. *Science* 239, 610-616, 5 Feb., 1988.

11. Allen J. R. and Curran J. W. Prevention of AIDS and HIV infection: needs and priorities for epidemiologic research. *Am. J. Publ. Hlth* 78, 381-386, April 1988.

12. Amadori A., Giaquinto C., Zacchello F., DeRossi A., Faulkner-Valle G. and Chieco-Bianchi L. *In vitro*-production of HIV-specific antibody in children at risk of AIDS. *Lancet* 1, 852-854, 16 April, 1988.

13. Friedland G. H. and Klein R. S. Transmission of human immunodeficiency virus. *New Engl. J. Med.* 317, 1125-1135, 29 Oct., 1987.

14. Nzilambi N., Ryder R. W. and Behets F. Perinatal transmission in two African hospitals. *Third International Conference on AIDS*, Washington, D.C., June 1987.

15. Mok J. Q., Giaquinto C., DeRossi A., Grosch-Worner I., Ades A. E. and Peckham C. S. Infants born to mothers seropositive for human immunodeficiency virus, preliminary findings from a multicentre European study. *Lancet* 1, 1164-1168, 1987.

16. Minkoff H., Nanda D., Mendez R. and Fikrig S. Pregnancies resulting in infants with acquired immunodeficiency syndrome or AIDS-related complex: followup of mothers, children and subsequently born siblings. *Obstet. Gynec.* 69, 288-291, 1987.

17. Scott G. B., Fischl M A., and Klimas N. mothers of infants with the acquired immunodeficiency syndrome, evidence for both symptomatic and asymptomatic carriers. *J. Am. Med. Ass.* 253, 363-366, 1985.

18. Centers for Disease Control. Human immunodeficiency virus infection in the United States: a review of current knowledge. *Morbid. Mortal. Wkly Rep.* 36, 1-48, 18 Dec., 1987.

19. Hoff R., Berardi V. P., Weiblen B. J., Mahoney-Trout B. S., Mitchell M. L. and Grady G. F. Seroprevalence of human immunodeficiency virus among childbearing women. *New Engl. J. Med.* 318, 525-530, 3 March, 1988.

20. Landesman S., Minkoff H., Holman S., McCalla S., and Sijin O. Serosurvey of human immunodeficiency virus infection in parturients. *J. Am. Med. Ass.* 258, 2701-2703, 1987.

21. Lambert B. One in 61 babies in New York City has AIDS antibodies, study says. *The New York Times* 1, 13 Jan., 1988.

22. Lichtblau E. Artificial insemination data raises fears. *Los Angeles Times*, 1, 14, 10 Aug., 1988.

23. Franke K. Turning issues upside down. In *AIDS: The Women* (Edited by Rieder I. and Ruppelt P.), pp. 226-232. Cleis Press, San Francisco, Calif., 1988.

24. Murphy J. Women with AIDS. In *AIDS: Principles, Practices, and Politics* (Edited by Corless I. B. and Pittman-Lindeman M.), p. 74. Hemisphere, New York, 1988.

25. Porter P. Minorities and HIV infection. In *The AIDS Epidemic* (Edited by O'Malley P.), pp. 371-379. Beacon Press, Boston, Mass., 1989.

26. Shaw N. and Paleo L. Women and AIDS. In *What To Do About AIDS* (Edited by McKusic L.), pp. 150-151. University of California Press, Berkeley, Calif., 1986.

27. Rosenbaum M. *Women on Heroin*, p. 132. Rutgers University Press, New Brunswick, NJ, 1981.

28. James J. Prostitution: arguments for change. In *Sexuality Today and Tomorrow* (Edited by Gordon S. and Libby R.), pp. 110-113. Duxbury Press, North Scituate, Mass., 1976.

29. Richardson D. *Women and AIDS*, pp. 43-44. Methuen, New York, 1988.

30. Leigh C. Further violations of our rights. In *AIDS: Cultural Analysis, Cultural Activism* (Edited by Crimp D.), pp. 177-181. MIT Press, Cambridge, Mass., 1988.

31. Centers for Disease Control. Antibody to human immunodeficiency virus in female prostitutes. *Morbid, Mortal. Wkly Rep.* 36, 157-161, 27 March, 1987.

32. Campbell C. Prostitution and AIDS. In *Behavioral Aspects of AIDS* (Edited by Ostrow D. G.). Plenum Press, New York. In press.

33. Stevens P. C. U.S. Women and HIV infection. In *The AIDS Epidemic* (Edited by O'Malley P.), pp. 381-401. Beacon Press, Boston, Mass., 1989.

34. Campbell C. Women, work and welfare. Unpublished MA thesis. University of Colorado, 1979.

35. Smith-Rosenberg C. and Rosenberg C. The female animal: medical and biological views of women and her role in the nineteenth century. *J. Am. Hist.* 60, 332-341, 1973.

36. Barker-Benfield B. The spermatic economy: a nineteenth century view of sexuality. *Feminist Stud.* 1, 45-74, 1972.

37. Wood G. D. The fashionable disease: women's complaints and their treatment in nineteenth century America. *J. Interdis. Hist.* 4, 25-32, 1973.

38. Lambert H. Biology and Equality: a perspective on sex differences. *Signs* 4, 97-117, 1980.

39. Scully D. and Bart P. A funny thing happened on the way to the orifice. In *The Sociology of Health and Illness* (Edited by Conrad P. and Kern R.), pp. 350-355. St. Martin's Press, New York, 1981.

40. Richardson D. *Women and AIDS*, p. 34. Methuen, New York, 1988.

41. Brown B. Creative acceptance: an ethics for AIDS. In *AIDS: Principles, Practices and Politics* (Edited by Corless I. and Pittman-Lindeman M.), p. 230. Hemisphere, New York, 1988.

42. Peabody B. *The Screaming Room*. Oak Tree, San Diego, Calif., 1986.

43. Moffatt B. C. *When Someone You Love Has AIDS*. NAL Penguin, New York, 1986.

44. Norwood C. *Advice for Life. A Woman's Guide to AIDS Risks and Prevention*, pp. 139-140. Pantheon, New York, 1987.

45. Gross J. The bleak and lonely lives of women who carry AIDS. *The New York Times* 27, Aug., 1987.

46. Sterk C. Cocaine and HIV seropositivity. *Lancet* 1, 1052-1053, 7 May, 1988.

47. Bowser B. Crack and AIDS: an ethnographic impression. *Multicult. Inquiry Res. AIDS* 2, 1-2, Spring 1988.

48. DesJarlais D. C. Heterosexual partners: a risk group for AIDS. *Lancet* 2, 1346-1347, 1984.

49. Worth D. and Rodriques R. Latina women and AIDS. *Rad. Am.* 20, 63-67, 1987.

50. Kegeles S. M., Adler N. and Irwin C. E. Sexually active adolescents and condoms: changes over one year in knowledge, attitudes and use. *Am. J. Publ. Hlth.* 78, 460-467, April 1988.

51. Kelly J. AIDS conference reports. *The National News* 4, Sep./Oct. 1988.

52. Wofsy C. Human immunodeficiency virus infection in women. *J. Am. Med. Ass.* 257, 2074-2076, 17 April, 1987.

53. Patton C. *Sex and Germs*, p. 41. South End Press, Boston, Mass., 1985.

54. Treichler P. A. AIDS, gender and biomedical discourse: current contests for meaning. In *AIDS, The Burdens of History* (Edited by Fee E. and Fox D.), pp. 190-266. University of California Press, Berkeley, Calif., 1988.

55. Graham S. Socio-economic status, illness and the use of medical services. *Milbank Meml Fund Q.* 35, 58-66, Jan. 1957.

56. Blackwell B. L. Upper middle class adult expectations about entering a sick role for physical and psychiatric dysfunctions. *J. Hlth Hum. Behav.* 8, 83-95, June 1967.

57. Freeborn D. K., Pope C. R., Davis M. A and Mullooley J. P. Health status, socioeconomic status and utilization of outpatient services for members of a prepaid group practice. *Med. Care* 15, 115-128, Feb. 1977.

58. Steinbrook R. AIDS slowdown in three key cities seen. *Los Angeles Times* 1, 26, 6 Dec., 1988.

59. Heyward W. L. and Curran J. W. The epidemiology of AIDS in the U.S. *Scient. Am.* 259, 78, Oct. 1988.

Chapter 10

HIV and Intravenous Drug Users

Marsha F. Goldsmith

Investigators for almost a decade have been gathering data on infection with the human immunodeficiency virus (HIV) among intravenous drug users (IVDUs) as avidly as a user seeking a fix. Yet for all the statistics amassed and all the adjustments in risk behavior documented, no turnoff from this particular dead-end avenue is in sight.

At the seventh international conference on AIDS, Jonathan Mann, M.D., director of the International AIDS Center, Harvard AIDS Institute, Boston, said infection among drug users is one of several reasons to avoid complacency about the pandemic.

"Only 5 percent to 10 percent of the world's injecting drug users have thus far become HIV infected," Mann said, "and yet needle sharing remains a common practice. The potential, therefore, remains for new explosive epidemics in communities of injecting drug users."

Among hundreds of presentations on the subject at the conference, Mann chose a few to illustrate his point.

From London, Adam N. Crosier, M.D., Center for Research on Drugs and Health Behavior, Charing Cross and Westminster Medical School, reported that the HIV prevalence rate in a representative sample of 534 people who injected heroin, cocaine, or amphetamines was 13 percent. Before 1990, the prevalence rate in a similar population was no more than 6 percent. Crosier says the study indicates that while the risk behaviors remain unchanged, the prevalence of HIV among IVDUs in London appears to be increasing.

In Paris, Natalie Rude, M.D., at the Institut National de la Santé et de la Recherche Médicale (INSERM), undertook a study to determine

"A Sticky Issue: HIV and the IVDU," *JAMA*, August 18, 1991, pp. 1053-1054. Marsha F. Goldsmith writes for *JAMA*.

whether a deficit in the incidence of AIDS—the difference between reported cases and projections based on earlier trends—was occurring among homosexuals, heterosexuals, or intravenous drug users. Rude found that while an incidence deficit was occurring among homosexuals, there was no falloff in the actual incidence compared with projections for heterosexuals and IVDUs.

The Municipal Health Service in Amsterdam backed a study reported by Jan Fennema, M.D., and colleagues that compared HIV infection rates in IVDUs in three methadone programs with rates in IVDUs interviewed on the street in that city. The researchers found that projections of infection for a whole community of injecting drug users cannot be based on a convenient sample. In this case, the predicted seroprevalence was 21 percent and the observed seroprevalence in the drug-using community was 37 percent.

Why Do They Start?

In an interview in Florence, Don C. Des Jarlais, Ph.D., director of research, Chemical Dependency Institute, Beth Israel Medical Center, New York, said that the number of injecting drug users in the United States is about the same as it was a decade ago. "We've had some people quit, some people die, but we've also had some people start," he said. "AIDS isn't going to get people to stop using drugs any more than AIDS is going to get people to stop having sex."

Approximately 40,000 cases of AIDS in the category "IVDU" have been reported to the Centers for Disease Control. About 12,000 additional cases have been reported in the "homosexual or bisexual IVDU" category.

As to why anyone would start injecting anything in the face of antidrug propaganda that covers a broad front, Des Jarlais—whose global research efforts attest to his expertise on this subject—has an answer that may startle some well-intentioned people. "Much of what is being done in the name of drug education goes directly against the experience of young adults," he says.

"People who start injecting drugs are typically very experienced in drug use by noninjection. They've been sniffing heroin or cocaine and have had more positive than negative experiences. Their drug use can be fairly heavy but it has not been all bad. When they are shown some supposedly scary pictures and hear people say 'This is your brain on drugs,' they just laugh it off, because that's not the way they feel when they take drugs," says Des Jarlais.

Another factor the antidrug forces find difficult to combat is that most people who start to inject drugs have a relative or close friend who is already injecting, says Des Jarlais, "so they have a role model, and that's probably a person whose drug use is more pleasurable than it is painful."

Americans are accustomed to seeing intravenous drug users portrayed as societal outcasts, but Des Jarlais says 23 percent of those he studied in New York recently were employed. "A good percentage of them are regular working people," he says. "Some of them are upper middle-class professionals."

How Can They Stop—or Be Safer?

Des Jarlais says that he and his colleagues in other countries who have been studying drug use for the past ten years have learned a lot. "We've learned that drug users are really pretty good at changing their drug use behavior. They're quite good at adopting safe injection procedures. They're less good at changing their sexual behavior—using condoms—but they're still ahead of most heterosexuals in the United States and the world.

"We've also learned," he continues, "that providing safe injection programs, bleach distribution, syringe or needle exchange, or over-the-counter sales of equipment, is a good way of getting drug users into treatment to reduce or stop their use. There's no contradiction," he states emphatically. "Safe injection programs serve as a good recruiting system for getting people into drug abuse treatment."

There has been at best a small expansion of drug treatment programs for Americans who want to quit, Des Jarlais says sadly. "It's tough to quit without a program—think about the people who can't quit smoking. It has not come close to where you could provide treatment to everybody that wanted it and needed it. That's still a faraway goal."

Politics and Prevention

Early this month, the National Commission on AIDS, of which Des Jarlais is a member, issued a report that said one of the most important factors in curbing the spread of AIDS is to get drug users into treatment programs. The commission criticized the Bush administration for not recognizing the link between AIDS and drug use. It called this failure "bewildering and tragic."

Addressing the issue of needle exchange programs for the first time, the commission endorsed them as one means of stemming HIV infections among IVDUs and their sexual partners—and their children. The administration remained unconvinced, but the issue is unlikely to go away.

With the exception of part of Sweden, all the Western European countries allow the legal sale and possession of sterile injection paraphernalia. Most large European cities also have some form of syringe exchange programs where used equipment can be exchanged for sterile equipment, while at the same place counselors are available to talk about risky drug and sexual behavior, give out condoms, refer people to medical service, or steer those who are interested into drug treatment programs. These programs are government run in most of the countries and in Australia, although some are run by private nonprofit groups.

In the United States, Seattle and Tacoma have moderate-sized programs that appear to be attaining their goals, Honolulu has started one, and New Haven recently reported the success of its new needle exchange program. Such programs are carried out on a semilegal basis in other cities, such as New York (*JAMA* 1988; 260:2620-2621) and San Francisco.

There was a report at the conference in Florence on an unsanctioned street-based needle exchange program in San Francisco that goes by the name of Prevention Point. John Watters, Ph.D., assistant professor in the Institute for Health Policy Studies at the University of California, San Francisco, and colleagues say it is effective.

The researchers studied 1400 injecting drug users, who were tested for HIV, in three San Francisco neighborhoods. They found that when drug users visit the needle exchange program at least twice a month, they are three times less likely to share needles than users who do not frequent the program.

Results of a study released last month by the Addiction Research Foundation in Canada also demonstrate that free distribution of clean needles is limiting the spread of HIV in that country's largest cities. James Rankin, M.D., the foundation's director of medicine, said the percentage of injecting drug users who test positive for HIV in Toronto "is among the world's lowest in areas where drugs are a problem."

That figure is 4.6 percent, in contrast with 60 percent in New York and 15 percent to 20 percent in other large US cities. The Canadian federal government helps fund the needle exchange programs, which exist also in Montreal and Vancouver.

Canada began its needle distribution program in 1989, despite the concern of many officials that it would increase intravenous drug use. Now, Randall Coates, M.D., University of Toronto, says, "there is no indication that it has increased illegal drug use."

At the AIDS conference two months ago, Des Jarlais concluded on a note that seems to presage the recent U.S. National Commission report. He said: "We've come an awful long way in 10 years in terms of learning how to promote risk reduction in drug users. We've come a modest way in terms of generating political support for AIDS prevention. If we don't get better at generating political support, we can look for the situation to continue to get worse in this country. We will have more drug injectors infected and more heterosexual and more perinatal transmissions of HIV."

Chapter 11

HIV-Infected Professionals and Patient Rights

Norman Daniels

In July 1991, the Centers for Disease Control (CDC) issued new guidelines for professionals, who may be infected with the human immunodeficiency virus (HIV) or hepatitis B, performing invasive procedures. The guidelines call for infected professionals to refrain from "exposure-prone" procedures, a category to be defined by the "medical/surgical/dental organizations and institutions at which the procedures are performed."[1] Concerned about liability, one New York hospital board decided that removing sutures was an exposure-prone procedure (exceeding the CDC's intent). They discharged an emergency department physician and notified patients that they might have been treated by an HIV-infected health care worker. One patient, angry because of risk he had faced, called the hospital, shouting, "You took away my right to choose!"[2] The patient is not alone: a *Newsweek* poll says 90 percent of people want to know their physician's HIV status.[3]

The infected emergency department physician, insisting on his right to work, defended his practice of informing only those patients he thought could "handle" news of his status by stating, "They don't have the right to know if I'm not affecting their health."[4] The American Medical Association (AMA) disagrees: because physicians must "Do no harm," they should find out their HIV status, and, if infected, they must either cease performing invasive procedures or disclose their condition to their patients.[5]

Do these CDC and AMA policies capitulate to public fears and prejudice? Do they violate the rights of HIV-infected professionals, who qualify as "handicapped" under the Americans With Disabilities Act of 1990?[6, 7]

"HIV-Infected Professionals, Patient Rights, and the 'Switching Dilemma,' "*JAMA*, March 11, 1992, pp. 1368-1371. Norman Daniels, Ph.D., is professor of philosophy at Tufts University, Medford, Massachusetts.

Or do they properly respect patient rights to be informed of or to be protected against the risks of HIV transmission? These issues will be debated in medical centers and legislatures nationwide, since Congress has thrown enforcement of the CDC guidelines to the states. Because professional organizations refused to supply lists of exposure-prone procedures, in November 1991, the CDC issued draft revisions of its guidelines, recommending that local committees review the risk imposed by infected workers on a case-by-case basis.[8] The AMA similarly modified its guidelines.[9] Since local discretion could lead to variable, inequitable decisions, it is imperative that the basic issues be understood.

Unfortunately, the usual way of framing the problem is seriously flawed. The standard approach assumes that, for any given level of risk, we have a clear ranking of patient rights against the rights of infected surgeons or dentists. The problem then seems largely empirical, not moral: determine the level of risk and then consult that ranking to see which right takes precedence at that level of risk. If the probability of HIV transmission is very high—clearly "significant" in the technical sense as specified by anti-discrimination law (the Americans With Disabilities Act of 1990)—then there is no controversy; significant risks limit the rights of handicapped professionals. But at the level of risk estimated by the CDC,[10] there is no clear ranking of the conflicting rights. Patient rights advocates claim the right to know even about risks that advocates for the rights of handicapped workers consider insignificant. Knowing the risk thus does not tell us whose rights take precedence.

The policy dilemma must be resolved on other grounds, which I shall provide. Before turning to my central argument, I want to note and reject two strategies for sidestepping the problem about conflicting rights. The first strategy suggests that we can ignore patient rights since it is irrational to worry about such small risks. The second strategy asserts that professionals have obligations to avoid imposing risks that supersede their rights as handicapped workers and are independent of patient rights.

Is It Irrational for Patients To Worry about HIV Risks?

The CDC estimates that the probability of transmission from a known HIV-infected surgeon to a patient is between one in 40,000 and one in 400,000 (the estimated risk from dentists, which I do not discuss here, is nearly ten times lower).[10] In order to address the issues raised if the CDC estimate is correct, I shall ignore the controversial assumptions and important uncertainties surrounding the underlying statistical model. For simplicity of reference I shall (arbitrarily) round off the estimate of surgical risk to one in 100,000 (similar to a recent estimate of one chance in 83,000 per hour of surgery).[11] If we multiply the estimate of surgical risk by a conservative estimate of the incidence of HIV among health care workers (0.5 percent), we discover that a patient undergoing an invasive procedure performed by a surgeon of unknown HIV status faces a risk of one in 20 million of becoming infected with HIV.

Is it irrational for patients to worry about these risks of HIV transmission when they routinely accept much greater risks elsewhere? For example, the one in 20 million risk of becoming infected during an invasive procedure performed by a surgeon of unknown HIV status equals the probability of death from bicycling 0.8 km (risk of accident), travelling 31 km by air or 24 km by car (risk of accident). The risk of HIV infection is only one-tenth the chance of being killed by lightning, one-fourth the chance of being killed by a bee, and half the chance of being hit by a falling aircraft.[12] The one in 100,000 risk of transmission from an infected surgeon equals the probability of death we face bicycling 3.2 km each way to school for one month, commuting 24 km round-trip by car for a year.

Similarly, our chance of dying from anesthesia during an operation is roughly 10 times our chance of being infected by a surgeon known to be infected with HIV. A mother who approves a penicillin injection for her toddler with pharyngitis accepts a one in 100,000 risk of death from anaphylactic shock.[13] In one study, the most successful coronary artery bypass graft surgeon surveyed had a 1.9 percent mortality rate, while the least successful had a 9.2 percent mortality rate.[14] Patients selecting the least successful surgeon thus face 7,300 times the extra risk of death posed by an HIV-infected surgeon.

This strategy for debunking patient fears about HIV transmission should be rejected. Insisting that people should respond only to the underlying probabilities of death when they assess risks is strongly paternalistic. It implies that we have a clear conception of what is good for us only if we pay attention solely to our chances of death. There is nothing irrational, however, about bicycling great distances to stay fit while refusing the risks of diet sodas, or about wanting to control risks by driving, even though it is riskier than flying.

Similarly, the mother who knows that her toddler faces a one in 100,000 risk of death from penicillin might conclude that the benefits outweigh the risks. But if her child needed surgery and she knew that the surgeon was infected with HIV, she could avoid that risk solely at the cost of switching surgeons. Although her switching may reflect the phobic fear she has of HIV—a fear exaggerated by stigma or prejudice—it may also reflect a rational risk-benefit calculation. It costs her more to live with her fear of HIV than it does to switch to another surgeon. Switching can thus be rational even when we all tend to ignore comparable risks in other contexts. Also, even if prejudice increases our fear, we cannot simply dismiss the fear as pure prejudice since there is a real mechanism for transmission.

Must Professionals Avoid Imposing "Identifiable Risk"?

The AMA claims that "physicians who are HIV positive have an ethical obligation not to engage in any professional activity which has an *identifiable risk* of transmission of the infection to the patient [emphasis added]."[5] This claim is much too strong. Physicians and other health professionals may be carriers of infectious agents that might have a serious impact on patient health. Even if the chance of infection is remote, it represents an identifiable risk. If we take the AMA claim literally, no surgeon should ever operate. Broadening the "no identifiable risk" requirement to include other mechanisms for harming patients, including all the factors that might affect physician performance such as stress, fatigue, side effects of medication, substance abuse, and family problems, clearly makes the unacceptably strong requirement even stronger.[15] It would oblige every surgeon who generally performed worse than the best surgeons to refrain from operating all but the most successful coronary artery bypass graft surgeons impose a greater identifiable extra risk on their patients than HIV-infected surgeons do.

Perhaps the AMA should only have claimed that physicians have a duty not to impose *avoidable* identifiable risks. If surgeons are unaware of the risks they impose as a result of stress or family problems, then they cannot avoid them. Similarly, it might be too costly to remove all surgeons from practice who have less than optimal success rates. But this modification of the AMA position is still inadequate. If we devote sufficient resources and effort, we can avoid many seemingly unavoidable risks. If, however, we interpret "avoidable" to mean "avoidable given an appropriate weighing of the benefits and costs," then the AMA position may no longer imply that infected professionals should refrain from practice: the costs of removing them may well outweigh the benefits. In any case, other avoidable risks, such as those imposed by the least successful coronary artery bypass graft surgeons, arguably are more cost-effective to eliminate than the risks from HIV-infected surgeons.

Strictly speaking, I have not shown that surgeons have no professional duty to refrain from exposure-prone procedures, but I have shown that the AMA has not demonstrated there is such a duty. We should also reject the AMA argument that professionals must err on the side of protecting patients because risks are uncertain. To be sure, the CDC estimate may be wrong. Nevertheless, setting aside the best risk estimate we have while emphasizing uncertainty may unwittingly augment public fears.

Why the CDC Estimate Does Not Tell Us Which Rights Take Precedence

If the CDC estimate was significant from the perspective of advocates of the rights of handicapped workers, there would be no controversy. But these advocates argue persuasively that the risk is not significant in the sense required by employment discrimination law. To be significant in the relevant sense, a risk must not be "speculative," and must be more than "remote" or "minute" or a "mere elevation" of the risks usually tolerated in the setting. We must not have singled out this risk in contrast to other larger ones we routinely tolerate. These criteria count heavily against considering HIV transmission risks significant.

Risk is thus judged in a highly objective way, focusing on the underlying probabilities of harm, when we are thinking about the rights of handicapped workers. We are motivated to focus on objective risks because of the situation in which we appeal to those rights to protect them. We must protect them against the subjective beliefs about risks appealed to by employers, fellow workers, or customers, who must rationalize their reluctance to accommodate handicapped workers. The pragmatics of affirming these rights thus leads us to discount subjective views of risk and to insist on high, objective standards, shifting the burden of proof to those who claim there are risks. If the CDC estimate of risk was much higher, all would agree significant risk was present. But the low CDC estimate suggests that we had better ignore the exaggerated fears of patients. Giving in to them, like giving weight to the subjective fears of fellow workers or employers, would mean abridging the rights of handicapped workers to equal opportunity.

Strikingly, patient rights take exactly the opposite perspective, affirming subjective and rejecting objective assessment of risks. The point of appealing to patient rights is to protect patients against "expert" judgments by physicians who may be so sure the risks they impose are worth taking that they fail to inform patients about them. To preserve the right of patients to decide what risks are worth taking means refusing to let expert or objective assessments of risks and benefits carry the day and requiring instead that the subjective assessment by the patient be decisive. This emphasis on consent is in accordance with our general attitude toward distributing the benefits and burdens of risk taking. It is only because employers or other workers try to hide behind their subjective views of risks in order to deny equality of opportunity to handicapped workers that we must insist on objective assessments of risk.

In general, we require informed consent from patients only for risks a reasonable person would want to know, not to all risks. Since the overwhelming majority of patients want to know the HIV status of their physicians, and since switching behavior is not irrational for them, as I have shown, it seems patients should have such information. Similarly, although courts have sometimes ruled that physicians need not disclose remote or minute risks, this exception may not be relevant in this case. We ordinarily need not disclose such risks because there are too many of them to discuss and there is no reason to believe a reasonable person would care about them. But patients want to know about the risks of HIV, and they will act on that knowledge.

The problem reduces to this: a risk that is not (objectively) significant, judging from within the pragmatics of the rights of handicapped workers, is viewed (subjectively) as serious and material by patients. The issue cannot be settled simply by saying, "The probability is only one in 100,000." An independent argument that establishes which rights, and thus which view of risks, should be given priority, would resolve the problem. I am not aware of any such general argument showing how we should rank these rights.

How We Can All Be Worse Off if We Each Try To Do Better: The Switching Dilemma

We are often in situations like this: if we each try to do better, we all do worse. For example, suppose we are fishermen. If all other fishermen respect a limit on catches, I can do better by exceeding the limit. If others violate the limit, I can still do better by catching more. Of course, if we all try to catch the most fish we can, we each catch less because the fish population collapses. A situation with this structure is known to economists as a public goods or "commons" problem; to game theorists, it is a type of "many person prisoners' dilemma."[16] (The term is taken from a famous example involving two separated prisoners, each given the choice of confessing for a lighter sentence. Each can serve less time by confessing, whatever the other does, but if both confess, they each serve more time than if neither confesses.)

This situation results in what I call the switching dilemma. Suppose all of us refrain from switching behavior, that is, from demanding information about the HIV status of surgeons and then switching to uninfected surgeons. Then we will all be better off for several reasons. If we want to reduce the risk of HIV transmission, resources are spent more effectively on education and infection control, including the development of improved methods and compliance, than on locating and avoiding or removing infected surgeons. Moreover, services provided by such surgeons will still be available to us, but at lower risk, and patients with HIV will have better access to care since surgeons will have less reason to fear treating them. Our fear of contagion will diminish in the long run because we cost-effectively share the burden of reducing the risks of transmission. Of course, if others refrain from switching behavior, thereby providing all the benefits I just described, but I can get information about my surgeon's status and switch, then I can do even better, further reducing my fear of catching HIV at low cost to me. (I am here "free riding," since I am getting the benefit of others' refraining from switching behavior without paying the price [in fear] of refraining myself.) Similarly, if everyone else is demanding the information needed to locate and avoid or remove infected surgeons, then the benefits that would result from cooperating around better strategies are lost, and I would do even worse by not switching. I can thus do better by switching whatever everyone else does. Since everyone else reasons this way, we will all switch and thus everyone will do worse.

My claim that we face a switching dilemma rests on important empirical assumptions, e.g., that (1) there are more cost-effective ways to reduce the risks of HIV transmission from professionals to patients than locating infected surgeons and avoiding them or removing them; (2) costs of enforcing the CDC guidelines will be high; (3) the guidelines open the door to demands for mandatory testing of physicians and patients, e.g., by liability insurers; (4) physicians who face CDC or AMA restrictions will have more fear of treating HIV patients; and (5) fears of contagion are likely to be reduced more over time by emphasizing infection controls rather than by seeking out infected surgeons, since fewer cases of transmission will result. If we also assume that the CDC and AMA guidelines involve some enforced switching, substituting practice restrictions for patient switching behavior, then they produce many of the bad effects described in the switching dilemma, at least on a reduced scale.

The switching dilemma tells us that we will each be worse off if we give unrestricted play to patient rights to engage in switching behavior, or if we adopt policies that are equivalent to people so exercising those rights. The switching dilemma gives us adequate reason to restrict those rights and to avoid such policies. Instead we should (1) improve compliance with existing infection control measures, including those in nonhospital settings; (2) invest in research and development to improve infection control compliance and methods; (3) encourage voluntary testing and treatment of practitioners who suspect they are at risk; (4) resist efforts to impose restrictive measures aimed at managing liability, such as insurers' efforts to require testing; (5) continue monitoring HIV and hepatitis B transmission, so that better estimates of risk are obtained; and (6) use education and strong leadership by the scientific and medical establishment to reduce the public perception that transmission risks are serious.

Ignoring practice restrictions in favor of these policies also has risks. Some cases of transmission will be discovered, making it look like the public was not protected. But if the assumptions behind the switching dilemma are correct, including the CDC risk estimate, then these policies will lead to fewer cases of transmission than focusing on practice restrictions.

Though these six policies are generally endorsed by the AMA and CDC, they undercut them through their emphasis on finding and restricting infected professionals. Even the most recent guideline revisions retain that emphasis, although in a contradictory fashion. They require that infected professionals come forward to be assessed for their competency to abide by infection controls. Why focus on infected professionals? Anyone so incompetent should be subject to restrictions. Focusing on infected professionals, however, sets us up for the switching dilemma.

The policies endorsed here are compatible with protecting the rights of infected workers, but in pushing us toward them, the switching dilemma depends on no claim that these rights have priority. Nor do we invoke the kind of strong paternalism that seemed objectionable earlier. There is no claim that it is irrational for patients to prefer switching behavior. Rather, even though it would be rational for individuals to exercise their patient rights, each of us will be worse off if we all do so. This is true even if such rights have priority over the rights of handicapped workers. Therefore, it is better for each of us to accept a restriction on those rights under these special conditions. Realizing that we must avoid the switching dilemma thus allows us to solve the policy problem while sidestepping the apparently intractable problem of ranking conflicting rights.[17]

Notes

1. Centers for Disease Control. Recommendations for preventing transmission of human immunodeficiency virus and hepatitis B virus to patients during exposure-prone invasive procedures. *MMWR*. 1991; 40 (No. RR-8):1-9.

2. Wolff C. Doctor with AIDS virus evokes anger and pathos. *New York Times*. July 29, 1991; 140:B1-B2.

3. Gross J. Many doctors infected with AIDS don't follow new U.S. guidelines. *New York Times*. August 18, 1991; 140:1,20.

4. Wolff C. New rules on AIDS produce first resignation of a doctor. *New York Times*. July 27, 1991; 140:A1.

5. American Medical Association. *AMA Statement on HIV-Infected Physicians*. January 17, 1991.

6. The Americans With Disabilities Act of 1990. Pub L No. 101-336, 104 Stat 327.

7. Parmet W. Discrimination and disability: the challenge of the ADA. *Law Med Health Care*. 1990; 18:331-345.

8. Centers for Disease Control. Revised recommendations for preventing transmission of human immunodeficiency virus and hepatitis B virus to patients during invasive procedures. Draft. November 27, 1991.

9. Leary W. AMA backs off on an AIDS risk list. *New York Times*. December 15, 1991; 140:38.

10. Centers for Disease Control. Estimates of the risk of endemic transmission of hepatitis B virus and human immunodeficiency virus to patients by the percutaneous route during invasive surgical and dental procedures. Draft. January 30, 1991.

11. Lowenfels AB, Wormser G. Risk of transmission of HIV from surgeon to patient. *N Engl J Med*. 1991; 325:888-889.

12. Wilson R. Analyzing the daily risks of life. *Technol Rev*. 1979; 81:41-46.

13. Landesman S. The HIV-positive health professional: policy options for individuals, institutions, and states: public policy and the public — observations from the front line. *Arch Intern Med*. 1991; 151:655-657.

14. O'Connor GT, Plume SK, Olmstead EM, et al. A regional prospective study of in-hospital mortality associated with coronary artery bypass grafting. *JAMA*. 1991; 266:803-809.

15. Barnes M, Rango NA, Burke GR, Chiarello L. The HIV-infected health care professional: employment policies and public health. *Law Med Health Care*. 1990; 18:311-330.

16. Taylor M. *The Possibility of Cooperation*. New York, NY: Cambridge University Press, 1987.

17. My research on "Justice and AIDS Policy" is supported by grant RH-20917 from the National Endowment for the Humanities, Washington, D.C., and grant 1 R01LM05005 from the National Library of Medicine, Bethesda, Md. I would also like to give special thanks to Stephen White, Ph.D., and Ronald Bayer, Ph.D., for discussion of key ideas presented in this article.

Chapter 12

Attitudes toward the Care of Persons with AIDS

Martin F. Shapiro
Rodney A. Hayward
Didier Guillemot
Didier Jayle

The pandemic of infection with human immunodeficiency virus (HIV) has confronted health care professionals with potential exposure to a new and deadly disease, while they provide care for persons whose life-styles may differ dramatically from their own.[1,2] The disease has produced an array of societal responses. Some of these, such as controversies over job and housing discrimination, can add considerable social complexity to the provision of care. Others, such as calls for obligatory testing of patients and providers, may profoundly affect relationships between those who render care and those who receive it.[3,4]

At the same time, it is likely that the cultural values and public discourse in a society encountering the pandemic may profoundly affect physicians' responses to it. Homosexuality and HIV disease itself have elicited very different public responses in different societies. Publicly expressed concerns about the disease, those afflicted, and the risk of contagion are likely to affect the views of many people, including those who provide medical care.

"Residents' Experiences in, and Attitudes toward, the Care of Persons with AIDS in Canada, France, and the United States," *JAMA,* July 22/29, 1992, pp. 510-515. Martin F. Shapiro, M.D., is a member of the Department of Medicine, UCLA, Los Angeles; Rodney A. Hayward, M.D., is in the Department of Medicine and Health Services Management and Policy, University of Michigan, Ann Arbor; Didier Guillemot, D.E.S., is at the Association Prévention SIDA, Paris; Didier Jayle, M.D., is with the Centre Régional d'Information et Prévention de SIDA, Paris.

Similarly, legal, religious, literary, and other cultural perspectives on such matters vary dramatically across societies and are likely to color the attitudes of many who come in contact with those known to be HIV infected.

Physicians-in-training often are in the front lines of those providing such care and are the practitioners most likely to acquire the knowledge and competency needed to attend to the medical needs of HIV-infected patients in the future.[5,6] Some studies of the attitudes of American physicians, including residents, toward HIV care have identified some physicians who are reluctant to treat patients with the disease.[7,8] These studies have not given us much insight into whether the relatively high rates of such negative attitudes in the United States are an inevitable consequence of confronting an epidemic of this sort. Any finding that health professionals in other societies are responding less negatively to those with the acquired immunodeficiency syndrome (AIDS) should add an additional stimulus to efforts to determine whether any of the factors responsible for such attitudes are amenable to educational intervention.

We undertook this study to explore these phenomena among medical and family practice residents in three countries with large numbers of reported cases of AIDS: Canada, France, and the United States. Specifically, we were interested in the residents' experiences with, and attitudes toward, the care of persons with HIV infection.

Samples

We surveyed residents in all three countries who were either in their last year of training or in their last year prior to undertaking further subspecialization. The methods for the US survey and some results from it have been reported.[7] It included all residents who had matched in three-year internal medicine or family medicine programs in the 1986 National Residency Match in ten states: Illinois, Kansas, and Missouri in the Midwest; New Jersey and New York in the Northeast; Alabama, Georgia, and North Carolina in the South; and California and Washington in the West. The two eastern states and California have the highest rates of AIDS in the country. New York and New Jersey also have the highest proportions of intravenous drug users in their AIDS populations.[9] The Canadian survey included all residents in the third year of internal medicine residencies (as identified by each university's program director) or in the second year of two-year family medicine residencies (as identified by the Canadian College of Family Practice). For the French survey, we obtained lists of all residents in internal medicine and family medicine from the Direction Régionale des Affaires Sanitaires et Sociales for three regions with distinct profiles of HIV infection: Île de France (Paris and environs: high incidence of AIDS, mostly among homosexuals), Nord-Pas-de-Calais (Lille, Calais, and environs in the north: low incidence) and Provence-Côte d'Azur (Marseilles,

Nice, Montpellier, and environs in the south: intermediate incidence with a high proportion of cases among intravenous drug users).[10] We randomly sampled residents in their second year of residency, stratifying for specialty and region (family medicine residency lasts two years; after two and a half years, internal medicine residents choose areas of further specialization).

Survey Methods

The American survey was conducted from January to June 1989, the Canadian survey from February to June 1989, and the French survey from October 1989 to August 1990. (The longer period of data collection in France was necessitated by a national strike by the residents.) Questionnaires were sent to the hospitals in which Canadian and American residents were based and to the hospitals to which French residents currently were assigned. (French residents rotate to a different hospital in their region every six months.) The first mailing was accompanied in the United States and Canada by a $2 cash payment (which has been shown to improve response rates).[11]

The survey items were developed using the assistance of past research,[2,12] and unstructured interviews with health professionals. It was pilot tested for clarity and internal consistency on a small number of recent graduates of residency programs. Most attitudes and opinions were measured on five-point scales (strongly agree, somewhat agree, unsure, somewhat disagree, and strongly disagree).

Response Rates

Of the 685 Canadian residents surveyed, 542 (79.1 percent) responded. Of the 2,917 US residents surveyed, 1,745 eligible residents responded, 976 did not, and 196 residents were initially identified as being ineligible (identified as not being senior family or internal medicine residents in the specified programs). Of the 149 US residents in a nonresponders' survey, 48 (32.2 percent; 95 percent confidence interval [CI], 24.7 percent to 39.7 percent) were found to have changed programs or specialties. We therefore estimated that another 314 nonresponders (95 percent CI, 241 to 387) were not eligible, leaving a final sample of 2,407 eligible residents, among whom 72.5 percent responded to the survey.[7] Among the 694 French residents sampled, questionnaires were returned from their hospitals as undeliverable on two occasions for each of 49 residents who were no longer working at those hospitals. Of the remaining 645 individuals, 361 (56.0 percent) returned a completed questionnaire.

Nonresponder Surveys

Random samples of eligible nonresponders were surveyed in the United States (n = 101) and France (n = 96) to assess whether a response bias had occurred and to obtain an estimate of the number of nonresponders who were eligible for the study. In the United States, these subjects were asked to complete a one-page questionnaire that requested information about their personal characteristics and attitudes. We then made follow-up telephone calls to those who failed to respond. Of 101 eligible residents in the US nonresponder survey, 77 (76 percent) responded. As noted previously,[7] there were trends for nonresponders to be less likely to plan to specialize further, but no substantial difference was found for other demographic characteristics or key attitudes about AIDS.

The French nonresponder survey, which included one-third of all those who had not completed the questionnaire, was conducted entirely by telephone. We were able to complete interviews with 79 (83 percent) of 96 subjects. The results indicate that French nonresponders were slightly older, less conservative, and more likely to be in family medicine. There were only minor differences in variables for which the main survey identified differences between the French sample and those from Canada and the United States. Projecting these rates onto all nonresponders would not have changed the significance of any of the differences among French, Canadian, and American residents.

Analytic Methods

Bivariate comparisons of subgroups were done using x^2 testing for categorical variables and *t* tests for ordinal variables (a Bonferroni correction for multiple comparisons was used for all comparisons among the three countries). The distribution of residents in the three countries differed by age, sex and specialty. Americans were older and were more likely to be male and specializing in internal medicine than those in Canada and France. To determine whether results were confounded by demographic differences between residents in the different countries, we constructed a series of logistic regression models using each attitude as a dependent variable and using the residents' country as a dichotomous independent variable. Adding variables for other resident characteristics (age, sex, program specialty, anticipated percentage of future professional time spent providing general primary care, and amount of contact with HIV-infected patients) to these models did not substantially affect the magnitude of the associations (as indicated by the ß coefficient for the variable indicating country) or the level of statistical significance.

Results

American residents were more likely to have cared for inpatients with AIDS than were those in the other two countries. In addition, in all three countries, residents in internal medicine were more likely than family medicine residents to have cared for large numbers of inpatients with AIDS ($P < .05$). The majority of family medicine residents in each country reported that fewer than 5 percent of their general medicine admissions had the disease. Most of the residents in each country had provided at least some care for ambulatory patients with AIDS, with the exception of the Canadian family practice residents, among whom 39 percent had done so.

While the American residents had somewhat more extensive experiences caring for patients with AIDS, they were also much more likely to have had the experience of a surgeon or subspecialist refusing care to their patients. Overall, 13 percent of Canadian, 8 percent of French, and 39 percent of American residents reported that a surgeon had refused care to at least one of their HIV-infected patients. A similar pattern was seen for refusals by subspecialists. As was the case for other findings, controlling for amount of the residents' contact with patients with AIDS did not affect these international differences.

Needle-stick injuries were common in all three countries, with about three-fourths of the Canadian and American residents reporting at least one needle-stick contaminated by a patient's blood. Needle-sticks from patients known to have HIV infection were reported by internal medicine residents about twice as often as by those in family practice in each country, in contrast to the frequency of needle-sticks from patients with hepatitis, which did not differ by specialty. The rates of HIV needle-stick injuries also differed by country: for internal medicine residents, the rates were 4 percent in Canada, 10 percent in France, and 14 percent in the United States. These differences between countries persisted after controlling for the amount of contact with AIDS patients. When needle-sticks from patients possibly infected with HIV were taken into account, these figures more than doubled.

A majority of future primary care providers (those expecting to spend more than half their time in primary care) in each country believed that their training had been deficient in AIDS ambulatory care. Consistent with this finding, a substantial proportion in each country indicated that they did not feel competent in the ambulatory area of patients with AIDS. Self-perceived competence was much lower in France and Canada than in the United States. Most residents did not consider AIDS to be a disease that should be relegated to the care of subspecialists: Less than 20 percent in each country believed that it was too complex for physicians in their specialty. However, future primary care providers in France were more likely to plan to refer AIDS patients to specialists.

Although the great majority of residents indicated some sense of obligation to fulfill professional responsibilities to all patients, some did not have strong convictions in this regard. American physicians were the least likely to feel a strong sense of obligation to treat regardless of patients' sexual orientation or possible HIV infection. Whereas Canadian physicians were more likely than French physicians to believe that it is unethical to refuse care for a patient with AIDS, French physicians were more likely to believe that discrimination based on sexual orientation was unethical.

French and American physicians were more likely to believe strongly that it is unethical to discriminate against patients on the basis of race, religion, or sexual orientation than because the patients might have AIDS. A little over one-third of residents in each country strongly supported the notion that surgeons had a right to know a patient's HIV status before operating.

Most residents viewed their experiences in HIV care positively: 61 percent in France, 69 percent in Canada and 75 percent in the United States considered taking care of AIDS patients to be an excellent educational experience. At the same time, many expressed the view that they would prefer not to take care of persons with AIDS or in groups at increased risk for AIDS. When the residents were asked a series of questions about whether they would not take care of certain categories of patients if given a choice, there were striking differences among the countries: 2 percent of French, 6 percent of Canadian, and 11 percent of American residents would choose not to provide care to homosexual men. Four percent of French, 14 percent of Canadian, and 23 percent of American residents would choose not to care for persons with AIDS, about the same rates in each country as would not take care of homosexual men with AIDS. The highest rates of refusal were for intravenous drug users. The proportions of residents in each country who indicated that they would choose not to live in an area with a high prevalence of AIDS were similar to those who would choose not to care for AIDS patients, with the highest rate in the United States (22 percent) and the lowest rate in France (4 percent). American residents also were more likely to express the view that caring for AIDS patients is dangerous (37 percent vs. 21 percent in Canada and 24 percent in France, $P < .05$).

Comment

Human immunodeficiency virus-related disease has affected the medical profession profoundly. The epidemiology of the disease has been very different in the developed and developing worlds and has presented unique problems in each. In developing countries, the disease has occurred widely among the heterosexual population and is sometimes spread by the use of medical supplies and unscreened blood products.[13] The principal problem in these countries is the lack of meaningful resources to mount effective prevention programs and the near complete inability to secure resources for treatment.[14]

On the other hand, in Europe and North America, where resources are plentiful, the disease is occurring most often in populations frequently disenfranchised by society: Homosexual men and intravenous drug users.[9,10] Physicians, being human, bring to their medical work the foibles, anxieties, and deficiencies that characterize the human species. There is no requirement in the medical school admissions policies of any nation, to our knowledge, that the physician be sensitive to the problems of these groups. When members of these groups acquire an illness that often is related to behaviors in which they have engaged, and of which many physicians do not approve, it becomes easier for such physicians to discount the responsibility to provide them with medical care.

The emergence of AIDS is a milestone of sorts for medicine. Throughout the millennia, physicians have placed themselves at a certain amount of risk when providing care to persons with contagious diseases. Indeed, some of the stature of the profession undoubtedly is related to that activity. With the emergence of antisepsis and then of antibiotics, it became possible for physicians to imagine that the risks associated with medical practice would wither away.[15]

The entrance of AIDS into the picture appears to have changed that. While there have been very few reports of persons being infected with HIV in the course of medical work, they have been widely discussed, and more surely will occur. Anyone entering the practice of medicine 50 years ago knew that he or she ran the risk of contracting certain diseases. In contrast, few of the graduates in the quarter century prior to the first report of AIDS had cause to give much thought to any substantial risk of becoming ill in the line of professional duty. When AIDS appeared, it did so in a situation in which at least the perception existed that the disease is risky to those providing care, and it emerged in patients engaging in behaviors of which many physicians did not approve. This made it easier for some to assume a posture that countenances the possibility of not providing care. Such views may be exacerbated by recent sentiments that physicians should undergo mandatory testing, should be obliged to inform patients of the results, and should refrain from many professional activities at the pain of imprisonment, all of which implies relative ease of transmission of the disease in the clinical setting in the absence of any data to support that concept.[6,16]

The current study illuminates the terrain on which the practitioners of tomorrow are learning about caring for persons with AIDS. It is evident that most of the residents are encountering AIDS patients, but most often in the inpatient setting. Many have had experiences that might make them less inclined to care for patients with AIDS. A majority in the United States and Canada have experienced needle-stick injuries. The rates are somewhat lower in France, although responsibilities for drawing blood and performing procedures are comparable to those in Canada and the United States, and training in needle-stick avoidance does not appear to differ. In each country, an alarming proportion reported having had a needle-stick from a patient who may have been infected with HIV. The rates of needle-stick injuries identified by surveying residents are higher than those from standard surveillance data, since many episodes go unreported.[17,18,19] Only in the United States did the majority of residents feel clinically competent in AIDS care, and the majority in each country believed that their training in the ambulatory management of AIDS has been deficient. This latter point is of concern, since so much of AIDS care now occurs in the ambulatory setting, given the development of antiretroviral therapy and effective prophylaxis for *Pneumocystis carinii* pneumonia.

The residents were far from unequivocal in their beliefs concerning a professional obligation to provide these patients with care. Still, the majority of residents in all countries did recognize such an obligation, and strongly so. While the majority, if given a choice, would choose to care for persons with AIDS, many residents would not. Antipathy to caring for AIDS patients has been noted in previous reports on American physicians,[7,8,12] but no previous study has compared such attitudes in different countries. We found striking differences among the three countries in the proportions expressing negative sentiments in these respects. The French were least likely to want to avoid care of homosexual men, persons with AIDS, and intravenous drug users; the Americans were most likely, and the Canadians were intermediate. The fourfold to sixfold differences in these variables suggest major differences in social norms regarding tolerance of those with alternative life-styles. There were some regional differences in the United States. The two western states were the least unwilling to treat: attitudes toward HIV care there were similar to those in Canada. The attitudes of the French, on the other hand, did not overlap with any subgroup in the United States.

These large differences cannot be attributed to the higher prevalence of AIDS in the United States. Residents in all three countries have similar levels of responsibility for AIDS patients in their hospitals. Controlling for the amount of contact physicians had with AIDS inpatients did not substantially affect our results. The international differences in willingness to care for persons with AIDS may be related to such factors as level of tolerance and sense of professional responsibility, which may differ among the three countries' medical cultures, but this clearly is a subject meriting further investigation. Further research should address whether the dramatic differences in attitudes among residents of the three countries are related most strongly to fear of contagion of AIDS, to homophobia or dislike of intravenous drug users, to feelings of futility in caring for persons with the disease, of difficulty in providing such care, or to different levels of feelings of professional responsibility to care for all kinds of patients. Similarly, such research should explore the relationship of these views to degrees of religiosity and to political orientation. Such studies might help to identify any factors that are amenable to educational interventions.

The striking international differences identified in this study imply that the relatively high rate of negative attitudes toward HIV care in the United States is not an inevitable consequence of physicians confronting a disease that presents them with some personal risk. The much lower rates of unwillingness to care for persons with AIDS in these other countries present American medicine and medical education with a stark challenge that needs to be addressed.

The study similarly provokes questions about general societal attitudes. Some research has examined public perceptions of persons with AIDS and of members of groups at risk,[20] but work comparing attitudes in Europe and North America is scant.[21] Certainly, the prevailing cultural norms differ and, in many respects, they appear to contribute to an environment in which there is less tolerance in the United States toward persons who are infected with HIV. For example, homosexuals are not excluded from the military in France or Canada but are in the United States. Conservative religious groups appear to be far less politically influential in Canada or France than in the United States, where, in some cases, they have been observed to be unsympathetic to many of those with AIDS. Public concern about contagion has resulted in exclusions from schools in some cases in the United States, events that have not had similar prominence in France or Canada. In France, the political right wing, led by Le Pen, has promoted anti-AIDS feelings in the country at times, as have some conservative politicians in the United States. Our study suggests that more systematic examination of the attitudes toward the disease and groups at risk and the response to the epidemic in different countries would be a very fruitful area for sociological investigation.

These results should be interpreted with caution. The results are self-reported and are therefore limited to the recall and validity of residents' responses. They are the views of residents, not practitioners. The fact that residents encounter these patients at their worst, when they are sick in bed, may make them less inclined to see them as people, thereby making it easier to reject a responsibility to care for them. We included respondents from only three French regions and ten American states, but they were selected to be representative of their countries both demographically and in terms of AIDS occurrence. The survey methods and timing varied slightly, but it is unlikely that this substantially affected the results. Although the response rate was not universal, it was acceptable in all three countries, and the nonresponder surveys in the two countries with the lowest response rates revealed only small differences between responders and nonresponders in responses for key attitudes studied.

We conclude that, while most residents acknowledge a responsibility to care for patients with HIV, intended and actual refusals of care were commonly reported but varied considerably from one country to another. The lower level of antipathy toward AIDS patients in France and Canada presents a clear challenge to medical educators in the United States and underlines the importance of addressing the higher level of unwillingness to care for AIDS patients there. It appears that an important component of future educational efforts in this area should be discussions of professional ethics and responsibilities[3] and discussions of strategies for decreasing the risk of needle-stick injuries.[17-19]

Notes

1. Gerberding JL, Littell C, Tarkington A, Brown A, Schecter WP. Risk of exposure of surgical personnel to patients' blood during surgery at San Francisco General Hospital. *N Engl J Med*. 1990; 322: 1788-1793.

2. Douglas CJ, Kalman CM, Kalman TP. Homophobia among physicians and nurses: an empirical study. *Hosp Community Psychiatry*. 1985; 36: 1309-1311.

3. Northfelt DL, Hayward RA, Shapiro MF. The acquired immunodeficiency syndrome is a primary care disease: the need for ambulatory care education. *Ann Intern Med*. 1988; 109: 773-775.

4. Hayward RA, Kravita RL, Shapiro MF. Program directors' attitudes towards residents' care of patients with AIDS. *J Gen Intern Med*. 1991; 6: 18-26.

5. Bayer R. *Private Acts, Social Consequences: AIDS and the Politics of Public Health*. New York, NY: The Free Press; 1989.

6. Gostin L. HIV-infected physicians and the practice of seriously invasive procedures. *Hastings Cent Rep*. 1989; 19: 32-39.

7. Hayward RA, Shapiro MF. A national study of AIDS and residency training: experiences, concerns and consequences. *Ann Intern Med*. 1991; 114: 23-32.

8. Gerbert B, Maguire BT, Bleecker T, Coates TJ, McPhee SJ. Primary care physicians and AIDS: attitudinal and structural barriers to care. *JAMA* 1991; 266: 2837-2842.

9. *HIV/AIDS Surveillance Report*. Atlanta, Ga.: Centers for Disease Control; 1989: 1-16.

10. Surveillance du SIDA en France (situation au 30 Septembre 1991). *Bull Epidemiol Hebdomadaire*. 1991; 44: 187-194.

11. Mizes J, Scott E, Fleece L. Roos C. Incentives for increasing return rates: magnitude levels, response bias, and format. *Public Opinion Q*. 1984; 48: 794-800.

12. Link RN, Reingold AR, Charap MH, Freeman K, Shelov SP. Concerns of medical and pediatric house officers about acquiring AIDS from their patients. *Am J Public Health*. 1988; 78:455-459

13. Piot P, Plummer FA, Mhalu FS, Lamboray JL, Chin J, Mann JM. AIDS: an international perspective. *Science*. 1988; 239:573-579.

14. Prual A, Chacko S, Koch-Weser D. Sexual behavior, AIDS and poverty in Sub-Saharan Africa. *Int J STD AIDS*. 1991; 2:1-8.

15. Zuger A, Miles SH. Physicians, AIDS, and occupational risk: historic traditions and ethical obligations. *JAMA*. 1987; 258:1924-1928.

16. Centers for Disease Control. Recommendations for preventing transmission of human immunodeficiency virus and hepatitis B to patients during exposure-prone invasive procedures. *MMWR*. 1991; 40 (suppl RR-8):1-9.

17. Edmond M, Khakoo R, McTaggart B, Solomon R. Effect of bedside needle

disposal units on needle recapping frequency and needlestick injury. *Infect Control Hosp Epidemiol.* 1988; 9:114-116.

18. Morgan DR. Needlestick injuries: how can we teach people better about risk assessment? *J Hosp Infect.* 1988; 12:301-309.

19. Gerberding JL, Henderson DK. Design of rational infection control policies for human immunodeficiency virus infection. *J Infect Dis.* 1987; 156:861-864.

20. Pollak M, Dab W, Moatti J-P. Systèmes de réaction au SIDA et action préventive. *Sci Sociales Santé.* 1989; 7:111-135.

21. Conner G, Richman CL, Wallace S, Tilquin C. AIDS knowledge and homophobia among French and American university students. *Psychol Rep.* 1990; 67:1147-1152.

Chapter 13

Costs of HIV/AIDS

Marsha F. Goldsmith

Nearly 1 percent of the annual health care budget of the United States —
$5.8 billion — is the estimated cost of treating all Americans with HIV infec-
tion in 1991. By 1994, this country will be spending almost twice that
much — at least $10.4 billion annually — for such care.

These figures have been developed by Fred J. Hellinger, Ph.D., Agency
for Health Care Policy and Research, Department of Health and Human
Services, Washington, D.C. He presented them at a plenary session of the
Seventh International Conference on AIDS, held in Florence, Italy.

Hellinger's study is the first to assess the costs of treating everyone who
is infected with HIV, not only people with full-blown acquired immunodeficiency syndrome (AIDS). He says that estimates based on treating just
the latter group understate the medical care costs of the pandemic, because
expensive new therapies designed for asymptomatic seropositive people, to
forestall the worst effects of the disease, are increasingly being approved
for use.

The economist estimates that the average cost of treating an HIV-
infected person who doesn't have AIDS is $5,160 per year, whereas the
average cost of treating a person with AIDS is $32,000 per year ($24,000
for inpatient hospital care and $8,000 for other services). He calculates the
lifetime cost of medical care for a person with AIDS at $86,333.

This precise figure exceeds the diagnosis-to-death estimates of $40,000
to $70,000 that were made by previous researchers, Hellinger says, because
persons with HIV disease are living longer and more of them are taking
prophylactic treatment against opportunistic infections.

"Costs in Dollars and Lives Continue To Rise," *JAMA,* August 18, 1991, p. 1055
and "Costs of HIV/AIDS Rise, Care Disparities Increase," *JAMA,* September 9,
1992, p. 1246. Marsha F. Goldsmith writes for *JAMA.*

Although some physicians with large practices of HIV-infected people suggest that only the most highly motivated, best-informed patients are likely to press for the newest possible prescriptions, Hellinger has based his study on total numbers of HIV-seropositive persons.

He has derived his projections of the number of AIDS cases that will occur in the next several years using Centers for Disease Control (CDC) data from January 1984 to September 1990. The projections are as follows: 63,000 cases of AIDS will be diagnosed in the United States this calendar year, 74,000 in 1992, 87,000 in 1993, and 101,000 in 1994. (As of June 30, [1991] the total number of cases reported to the CDC since June 1981 was 182,834.) Hellinger predicts that the number of HIV-infected people without AIDS who receive care during each of these years will equal twice the number of AIDS cases diagnosed during the year—thus, 126,000 in 1991 and so forth.

Care for the Impoverished

Given these dire predictions, it came as no surprise to conference delegates to learn from Dennis Andrulis, M.D., of the National Public Health and Hospital Institute in Washington, D.C., that public hospitals in the United States find their AIDS programs full to bursting.

Andrulis presented data amassed from survey questionnaires returned in 1989 by 700 community and teaching hospitals, part of an ongoing national survey. Because many patients with a diagnosis of AIDS do not have private health insurance, he said, they now account for 28 percent of the costs and 36 percent of the financial losses of public hospitals.

The plight of these institutions is already well known (*JAMA.* 1987;257: 1437-1444, 1571-1575, 1698-1701, and 1850-1857). To enable them to bear their increasing burden, Andrulis says, "extra money must be found."

Buttressing Andrulis' argument was another report on the role of public hospitals, from Stephen Crystal, Ph.D., Institute for Health, Rutgers University, New Brunswick, New Jersey. Crystal and his AIDS Research Group found that as persons with AIDS become sicker they rely more on hospital clinics rather than on private physicians.

The study, based on 107 persons with AIDS interviewed throughout New Jersey, revealed that 37 percent of the sample used hospital clinics for outpatient medical care before they were diagnosed with AIDS, but by the time of the interview, this was true of 79 percent. The percentage who used only private physicians declined from 42 percent to 17 percent. Crystal says these changes appear to reflect the impoverishment that often accompanies worsening illness in the United States.

Moreover, the public hospital patients often were not receiving the care private patients can demand. Fewer were receiving zidovudine, for example, and even when they began therapy with the antiviral drug, many dropped

CL { MACRO VIEW
   { MICRO VIEW

out of treatment because there was no way they could have their cell counts monitored or adverse effects treated.

Crystal said, "The care of persons with HIV illness dramatizes several of the ironies in the US health care system. Despite spending more of its GNP than any other country on health care, we do not have access to care by many individuals in need."

Calling for reassessment of the role played by Medicare and Medicaid in the lives of these patients and for strengthened antidiscrimination and insurance policy continuation rules, Crystal pointed out that "ironically, access is easier to the most expensive care, inpatient hospitalization, while the outpatient care that could keep a patient out of the hospital, or extend life and improve function with preventive antiviral therapy, is more difficult to access."

No Panacea in AIDS Picture

These predictions from experts who look at the numbers — both of costs and consumers of medical care — are serious enough as concerns only the United States. A global view presents even more grounds for dismay. However, whether they are motivated by feelings of denial or genuine belief that the worst is over, reports have been surfacing in the popular press that tend to downplay what more unflinching observers say may be the worst plague in history.

The World Health Organization's James Chin, M.D., said in Florence, "The HIV/AIDS pandemic clearly poses formidable problems for the future. All of the methods used to project HIV infections and AIDS cases indicate, for both the short and long term, substantial increases in total men, women, and children who will become infected, progress to AIDS, and subsequently die."

Chin said that "during the 1980s, it was estimated that the global cumulative total of adult AIDS cases was about one million. In contrast, during the 1990s, an additional nine million adult AIDS cases are projected."

He called for better surveillance and estimation of the disease worldwide, to monitor HIV/AIDS prevalence and trends and to increase support of health care and social welfare systems.

In his closing presentation at the conference, Jonathan Mann, M.D., whose positions include that of professor of epidemiology and international health at the Harvard University School of Public Health, Boston, Massachusetts, warned that "public complacency is rising and societal commitment to HIV/AIDS is declining." He said, "The pandemic not only remains volatile, dynamic, and unstable, but it is gaining momentum and its major impacts in all countries are yet to come."

As in any war, the costs of the global battle against AIDS can be measured in personnel and material. Although more physicians and nurses directly engaged in caring for persons with HIV infection and acquired immunodeficiency syndrome are needed in many areas, it is the lack of money for prevention and treatment options that frustrates the best intentions of many engaged in the struggle.

At the Eighth International Conference on AIDS, held in Amsterdam, the Netherlands, Daniel Tarantola, M.D., of the Global AIDS Policy Coalition at the Harvard School of Public Health addressed this issue. He presented figures that he and colleague Charles Cameron, M.B.A., M.P.H., gathered for 1990 and 1991 that he says will apply to 1992 as well, since no major increases are expected to occur in the near future.

Tarantola and Cameron estimate that it now costs the world between $2.6 billion and $3.5 billion annually to care for people with AIDS. Although disparity between rich and poor parts of the world is a given, the contrast is glaring, plunging downward from $32,000 spent on each person with AIDS in the United States each year to $22,390 in Western Europe to $2,000 in Central America and South America to $393 in sub-Saharan Africa.

More than half of all the people infected with AIDS are in Africa, but less than 2 percent of the money spent on the disease globally is expended there. "Of the world total spent on adult AIDS care in 1992," says Tarantola, "$2.37 billion are expected to occur in North America alone and $100 million in Africa."

Fred Hellinger, Ph.D., of the U.S. Agency for Health Care Policy and Research, said at a different session that costs in the United States are going up rapidly. The cumulative cost of treating everyone in the country with HIV infection is expected to rise 48 percent, from $10.3 billion annually to $15.2 billion annually, between 1992 and 1995. He attributes the projected increase to greater use of services by more people with both HIV infection and AIDS.

Hellinger's current U.S. figures, which he says are the latest available, are even higher than those cited by Tarantola. He says the $32,000 spent on each person with AIDS last year rose to $38,000 this year primarily because of a steep increase in the use of outpatient services and the addition to the AIDS armamentarium of such new and costly drugs as glanulocyte macrophage colony stimulating factor (GM-CSF) for treating neutropenia ($1,000 per week), erythropoietin for anemia ($200 per week), and didanosine (DDI) ($40 per week). The average cost of treating HIV infection in each person who doesn't have AIDS nearly doubled, from $5,100 to $10,000.

Chapter 14

Risk of Suicide among Persons with AIDS

Timothy R. Coté
Robert J. Biggar
Andrew L. Dannenberg

Throughout history, suicide has been a uniquely human response to the misery of illness and perceptions of inescapable death. Increased rates of suicide among persons with serious illness have been well documented;[1,2,3] these risks are especially high when the illness includes a psychiatric disorder.[4,5,6]

The acquired immunodeficiency syndrome (AIDS) is a uniformly fatal condition.[7] Persons with AIDS (PWAs) are frequently depressed and, in some cases, have suicidal ideation.[8] Marzuk et al.[9] found 12 PWAs who committed suicide in New York City in 1985, yielding a rate 66 times higher than in the city's general population. Kizer et al.[10] found 12 PWAs who committed suicide in California in 1986, yielding a rate 21 times higher than in the general population. Since these early reports, advances in therapy have led to new strategies for preventing common opportunistic infections and antiretroviral therapies that delay progression of the disease itself. Also, during this time social stigma against PWAs may have decreased.

The National Center for Health Statistics routinely compiles multiple causes of death recorded on US death certificates.[11] Since 1987, these certificates have included standardized codes for AIDS.[12] These codes identify 70 percent to 90 percent of all AIDS-related deaths.[13] The existence of this

"Risk of Suicide among Persons with AIDS," *JAMA* October 21, 1992, pp. 2066-2068. Timothy R. Coté, M.D., and Robert J. Biggar, M.D., are members of the National Cancer Institute, Viral Epidemiology Section, Rockville, Maryland; and Andrew L. Dannenberg, M.D., is at the Injury Prevention Center, Johns Hopkins University School of Hygiene and Public Health, Baltimore.

data set permitted an examination of suicide risks, methods, and trends among PWAs nationwide.

Methods

The National Center for Health Statistics multiple-cause mortality tapes from 1987 through 1989 were examined for reports of AIDS and suicide on the same death certificate. A record of a suicide by a PWA was defined as one with coincident codes for both causes of death without regard to hierarchy (underlying, immediate, contributory, or intermediate).

We calculated person-years of observation and expected numbers of suicides among PWAs by methods similar to those used by Marzuk et al.[9] Age-, sex-, and race-specific person-years of observation of PWAs who lived at least one day in the period 1987 through 1989 were computed using the Centers for Disease Control public-use AIDS data set. Published evaluations of national AIDS surveillance estimate that the data set holds more than 80 percent of cases of AIDS that occur nationally.[14] Person-years at risk of suicide in 1987 through 1989 were computed for each case report as the time from date of AIDS diagnosis or January 1, 1987 (whichever was later), to date of death or December 31, 1989 (whichever was earlier). For example, a PWA diagnosed on July 1, 1987, who died on June 30, 1988, would contribute one-half person-year for the 1987 calculation of relative risk and one-half year for the 1988 calculation. Rates of suicide among PWAs were expressed as suicides per 100,000 person-years of observation of PWAs.

Age-, sex-, and race-specific observations of suicide among the general population were tabulated from death certificates whenever an International Classification of Diseases (ICD) code for suicide appeared in any position and an ICD code for AIDS did not appear in any position. Rates were computed using midyear 1987 to 1989 intercensal estimates. Each person in each midyear population was assumed to contribute one person-year of observation. No adjustment to the population base was made for time at risk lost by PWAs or those who committed suicide from 1987 through 1989 because these correction factors would be smaller than any error associated with intercensal population estimates. After computing age- and race-standardized rates of suicide among male PWAs, we divided by the rate of the general male population to determine the standardized mortality ratio (SMR).

Results

In 1987 through 1989 there were 165 death certificates with both AIDS and suicide listed as causes of death. Persons with AIDS who committed suicide were 99 percent male, 87 percent white, 12 percent black, and 1 percent other races. Their median age was 35 years with a range from 20 to 69 years. There were no statistically significant differences in the age, sex, or race distribution of PWAs who committed suicide compared with all PWAs alive during 1987 through 1989. Suicides among PWAs were widely distributed in the United States: California (30 percent), Florida (11 percent), Texas (5 percent), and New York (4 percent) had the most cases, but suicide among PWAs occurred in 41 other states and the District of Columbia. We found only one woman with AIDS who committed suicide; therefore, we limited further analyses to men.

Drug poisoning (35 percent), firearms (25 percent), and suffocation (13 percent) were the most common methods of suicide. We found excess proportions of suicides by self-poisoning with drugs for PWAs and by firearms among all men; adjusting for age and race did not change these results. The risk of suicide was most elevated for self-poisoning with drugs (SMR, 34.7) and jumping from high places (SMR, 26.7).

A total of 98,473 person-years of observation of male PWAs occurred from 1987 through 1989. Therefore the crude suicide rate among PWAs was 167 per 100,000 person-years. In 1987 through 1989, a total of 72,940 suicides among male non-PWAs occurred during 357,396,494 male person-years of observation, yielding a crude suicide rate of 20.4. When adjusted for age and race, male PWAs had a rate of suicide 7.4 times higher than men in the general population ($P < .001$). This risk decreased over time: it was 10.5 in 1987, 7.4 in 1988, and 6.0 in 1989 (x^2 test for trend, $P < .05$).

Comment

We have confirmed that PWAs have an elevated rate of suicide. In our nationwide study, suicide was found to occur among PWAs of all ages, throughout most regions of the United States, and the rate for male PWAs was 7.4-fold higher than for men in the general population. Among male PWAs, poisoning with drugs was both the most common method of suicide and the method with the greatest increased risk relative to men in the general population. Death certificates do not indicate the type of drugs used, but we speculate that many of these suicides resulted from overdoses of prescribed medications. Suicides by heroin are often coded as accidental intoxications;[15] this is less likely for suicides by prescription medications.

Also of importance is our finding that the rate of suicides declined significantly between 1987 and 1989. This improvement may have resulted from renewed hope brought by advances in medical care introduced over this time period, such as antiretroviral therapy and prophylaxis against common opportunistic infections. Lessening social stigma toward PWAs and more available psychiatric support for PWAs also may have resulted in decreased suicide rates.

The use of multiple-cause death certificate data to determine the number of PWAs who commit suicide engenders biases that may have caused us to underestimate the association of these two causes of death. First, death certificates are designed to report the cause of death, not to list all co-morbidities. Therefore, a person who committed suicide should not have AIDS listed unless the certifying official both knew the decedent had AIDS and decided that AIDS may have had a role in the suicide. Both AIDS[16] and suicide[17,18] are conditions for which death certificate underreporting has been well documented; these joint effects may be multiplicative when seeking certificates with both diagnoses. Another bias that may have caused underestimation of increased suicide risk among PWAs is an acknowledged incompleteness of ascertainment of death in AIDS surveillance data. Incomplete death reporting would inflate totals of person-years of observation for PWAs and consequently understate suicide rates and relative risks of suicide of PWAs. However, some biases may have led to overestimating suicide risk among PWAs. Most of the PWAs studied were homosexual men or intravenous drug users. Ideally, determination of the relative risk for suicide among PWAs would rest on comparisons to individuals from the same risk group, not to the general population. Such data were not available.

In this study, we have confirmed that PWAs are at increased risk for suicide. However, the declining trend in suicide rates between 1987 and 1989 is particularly encouraging, perhaps reflecting greater optimism among PWAs about both their quality of life and their chances for long-term survival or a lessening of social stigma against PWAs. Nevertheless, ongoing psychological assessments of suicidal risk should become a standard practice in the care of PWAs. These assessments should be carefully considered when potentially lethal medications are prescribed. If suicidal ideation is recognized, PWAs will require the same psychological and social support as other persons at risk for suicide.

Notes

1. Abrams HS, Moore GL, Westervelt FB. Suicidal behavior in chronic dialysis patients. *Am J Psychiatry*. 1971; 127:119-124.

2. Schoenfeld M, Myers RH, Cupples LH, et al. Increased rate of suicide among patients with Huntington's disease: implications for preclinical testing of persons at risk. *Am J Med Genet*. 1986; 24:305-311.

3. Marshall JR, Burnett W, Brasure J. On precipitating factors: cancer as a cause of suicide. *Suicide Life Threat Behav*. 1983; 13:15-27.

4. Black DW, Warrack G, Winokur G. The Iowa Record Linkage Study III: excess mortality among patients with functional disorders. *Arch Gen Psychiatry*. 1985; 42:82-88.

5. Black DW, Warrack G, Winokur G. The Iowa Record Linkage Study II: excess mortality among patients with organic mental disorders. *Arch Gen Psychiatry*. 1985; 42:78-81.

6. Black DW, Warrack G, Winokur G. The Iowa Record Linkage Study I: suicides and accidental deaths among psychiatric patients. *Arch Gen Psychiatry*. 1985; 42:71-75.

7. Berkelman RL, Heyward WL, Stehr-Green JK, Curran JW. Epidemiology of human immunodeficiency virus infection and acquired immunodeficiency syndrome. *Am J Med*. 1989; 86:761-770.

8. Holland JC, Tross S. The psychosocial and neutropsychiatric sequelae of the acquired immunodeficiency syndrome and related disorders. *Ann Intern Med*. 1985; 103:760-764.

9. Marzuk PM, Tierney H, Tardiff K, et al. Increased risk of suicide in persons with AIDS. *JAMA*. 1988; 259:1333-1337.

10. Kizer KW, Green M, Perkins CI, Doebbert G, Hughes MJ. AIDS and suicide in California. *JAMA*. 1988; 260-1881.

11. Israel RA, Rosenberg HM, Curtin LR. Analytical potential for multiple cause-of-death data. *Am J Epidemiol*. 1986; 124:161-179.

12. *International Classification of Diseases, Ninth Revision, Clinical Modification*. 4th ed. Washington, DC: US Dept of Health and Human Services; 1991. DHHS publication (PHS) 91-1260.

13. Buehler JW, Devine OJ, Berkelman RL, Chevarley FM. Impact of the human immunodeficiency virus epidemic on mortality trends in young men, United States. *Am J Public Health*. 1990; 80:1080-1086.

14. Buehler JW, Berkelman, RL, Stehr-Green JK. The completeness of AIDS surveillance. *J Acquir Immune Defic Syndr*. 1992; 5:257-264.

15. Grow M, Haffner HT, Besserer K. [Fatalities in drug-dependent patients: suicide or accident?] *Versicherungsmedizin*. 1989; 41:188-191.

16. Gertig DM, Marion DS, Schechter MT. Estimating the extent of underreporting in AIDS surveillance. *AIDS*. 1987; 5:1157-1164.

17. Moyer LA, Boyle CA, Pollock DA. Validity of death certificates for injury-related causes of death. *Am J Epidemiol*. 1987; 130:1024-1032.

18. Goodman RA, Herndon JL, Istre GR, Jordan FB, Kologham J. Fatal injuries in Oklahoma: descriptive epidemiology using medical examiner data. *South Med J*. 1987; 82:1128-1134.

Chapter 15

AIDS Vaccines: What Chance of a Fair Trial?

Phyllida Brown

Imagine you are the health minister of a poor country where AIDS has affected every family you know. One in three adults in your city is infected with HIV and growing numbers of children are left without parents. Everyone knows that a vaccine is urgently needed. Next, suppose that a promising candidate vaccine emerges—almost certainly from the West. It is possible that your country could agree to participate in trials of that vaccine to see whether it works. However hopeful that might seem, it would also entail enormous ethical and scientific problems.

How, for example, would your government ensure that any vaccine proven to work would continue to be available to your country, regardless of its cost, after a trial ended? How would the organizers of the trial take steps to explain the risks, as well as the potential benefits, to participants? How confident could you be that the strain or strains of HIV on which the vaccine was based would protect you against the strains in your region?

These questions may be hypothetical now, but they will not remain so for long. Trials of potential vaccines against HIV could begin in parts of Africa, Southeast Asia and Latin America in as little as five years. No one has firm plans yet, but a number of developing countries want trials, and teams in American and European institutions are already working with some of them.

As yet, there is no vaccine ready to be tested for its ability to protect against HIV infection. Nevertheless, several candidate vaccines are now

"AIDS Vaccines: What Chance of a Fair Trial?" *New Scientist*, April 27, 1991, pp. 33-37. Phyllida Brown is a news writer for *New Scientist.* Reprinted with permission of *New Scientist*.

being put through their paces in healthy volunteers, mainly in the U.S., to evaluate their safety—phase 1—and the kind of immune response they produce—phase 2. While researchers know they still face important obstacles in the design of a vaccine, they will face even greater ones in future if they do not start preparing the ground now for phase 3, the test of whether a vaccine works. So they are preparing.

In Uganda, for example, Britain's Medical Research Council (MRC) is working at the request of the Ugandan government with scientists in Entebbe at the Uganda Virus Research Institute and others, to build up data on infection in the population and the strains of HIV that are present. Geoffrey Schild, head of the MRC's AIDS Directed Program, has recently said that Uganda "could be one of the appropriate sites for some of the eventual trials of a vaccine's effectiveness." And a dozen universities in the U.S. supported by the National Institutes of Health (NIH) are training researchers from developing countries with possible vaccine trials in mind. The participating countries in the NIH's scheme include Haiti, Brazil, Peru, Thailand, Uganda and Zimbabwe. The U.S. Department of Defense also has collaborative projects with researchers in many countries, through the Walter Reed Army Institute of Research in Rockville.

But is it right that the world's poorest populations should be the testing grounds for vaccines against a disease that affects people everywhere? At its worst, might this approach not look like "safari research"—the exploitation of the vulnerable by the unscrupulous? "That's exactly what we are trying to avoid," says David Heymann, head of research at the World Health Organization's Global Program on AIDS. In fact the WHO, the NIH and others are so sensitive to this issue that they are holding meeting after meeting, some of them closed, to discuss it. Next month in Geneva, the WHO's Vaccines Development Steering Committee, which represents member states, will finalize new guidelines for any country doing research on people, particularly in vaccine trials.

Many epidemiologists think that trials will have to happen in the developing world, for example in Africa, because it is there that the virus is spreading most rapidly through the adult populations of many cities. In order to test whether a vaccine protects against HIV, scientists need to compare the rate of new infections in vaccinated individuals with the rate in others who have received a placebo, over a given period, in an area where the risk of being infected is high. The higher the incidence of new infections each year, the fewer the participants and the shorter a trial need be before the vaccine is either proven or found wanting.

The effect of the incidence level on the size of a trial is not trivial. For example, in a population where "only" two people per thousand become infected in a year, a trial would need to involve between 8,000 and 40,000 people, depending on how well a vaccine was thought to work and how stringent the statisticians wanted to be with their analyses. By contrast, in a population where one in three people become infected each year, a trial could involve only hundreds of individuals.

But despite the relatively low incidence of infection in the rich countries overall, some individuals are at high risk of infection, for example intravenous drug users and the uninfected partners of HIV-positive people. Last year, a working party on HIV vaccines for the European Community (EC) said that such groups might be possible participants in a trial in Europe. And privately at least, some scientists think it should be equally possible to find such a group in the cities of North America.

Jaap Goudsmit, director of the Human Retroviruses Laboratory at the University of Amsterdam, and a member of the EC working party, says there are advantages in doing a trial in the West. First, the researchers will already have done long-term studies on the group and will have baseline information on the rate of new infections. Secondly, they will probably know more already about the prevalent strains of HIV in that population. In Africa, by contrast, much of this information has yet to be collected.

"I think it could be done in Amsterdam among drug users," says Goudsmit. Although the incidence of HIV in this group appears to have dropped sharply with the advent of needle-exchange schemes and intensive counselling, people still take risks and the rate has reached a plateau at around 5 percent. Yet even with several cities combined, there might be "room" for only one such trial. The MRC believes that no more than one phase 3 trial, if any, would be feasible in Britain.

Some scientists think it would be difficult to keep track of intravenous drug users. Ironically, the very behavior that puts such people at risk of infection, and therefore makes them eligible for a trial, is illegal. Would drug users be deterred from returning for checkups and tests through fear that their participation might bring them into contact with the law? In medical jargon, this translates into "problems of compliance and follow-up." As the EC working party put it: "Structured cohorts of individuals who are both at risk for infection and reliable for continuous follow-up might be difficult to establish."

Mary Lou Clements, director of the Center for Immunization Research at Johns Hopkins University, agrees that there might be difficulties in monitoring drug users. (Johns Hopkins is one of the NIH's units for phase 1 and 2 trials, and also trains researchers from developing countries.) But, she says, studies by researchers in Baltimore have shown that proper cooperation and follow-up with this group is possible. "And they have got around some of the confidentiality issues," she says. "But we really haven't planned trials in this population in the U.S. as yet."

Some scientists question the implicit assumption that participants in trials in developing countries would somehow be more cooperative and easier to follow up. Bruce Forrest, clinical trials coordinator for AIDS vaccines at the MRC, says that the problems of follow-up could be equally serious wherever a trial was done. For example, people not used to the West's medical ideas might see little point in visiting the clinic for regular checkups if they felt well.

Mike Bailey, HIV/AIDS adviser to Save the Children, says: "How can anyone suggest that an African study population would be more compliant? That must mean you are going to place all sorts of impositions on what they are allowed to do. People in Africa expect to move about, between cities and rural areas, to markets, to work, to visit relatives." Clements agrees that "it won't be any easier" to do trials in Africa than in the U.S.

Meanwhile, developing countries want to get on with trials as soon as they can. The WHO is supportive, says Heymann: first, because the problem is at least as serious, if not more so, for them as anyone else, and secondly, because researchers need to make sure they can protect against the less-known strains of HIV that are prevalent in Africa. Staff from the WHO are already inspecting a number of possible test sites in countries that have requested trials, says Heymann. Until specific sites are chosen, no one is naming names, but a good guess might include Bangkok as well as several central African cities. "Finally six or seven sites will be selected by the steering committee," says Heymann. Once that is done, and it will probably be within months, the WHO will hold another planning meeting involving the other main research bodies, such as the NIH and the MRC, to agree on training programs for local researchers and other ways in which the Western collaborators could strengthen the infrastructure of the country involved. For example, laboratory facilities will almost certainly need improving.

Money and Ethics

The WHO is short of money, however, and it is unlikely to be the only sponsor of trials. This year, the Global Program on AIDS is running on funds only three-quarters of its projected budget, despite the rapidly worsening pandemic. Schild at the MRC is convinced that the WHO should be the sole umbrella organization to coordinate trials, and the sole body to set criteria for vaccines. But other, more wealthy agencies, particularly the NIH, are also keen to take an active role that they see as complementary to the WHO's efforts. Dale Lawrence, senior scientific adviser for the vaccines branch at NIH says: "We are encouraging a thorough review of the international possibilities and how we might best use our resources in collaboration with others to find safe, ethical and meaningful ways to test vaccines." Heymann says the organization sees the participation of other bodies positively. "We're certainly not trying to exclude other people," he says.

The WHO's main ethical concerns, says Heymann, are that vaccines should meet internationally agreed on safety standards: That any country conducting a trial must have a national policy for AIDS and a system of healthcare that will provide advice, counselling and medical treatment as well as the test vaccine; that phases 1 and 2 should already have been done in the vaccine's country of origin, and then, probably, repeated in the country involved; and that the country should have been able to collect and isolate the prevalent strains of HIV in its population.

All countries will be encouraged to use an ethical "check list" and contracts between the Western collaborators and the host country's scientists. "We are working right now to develop the check list," says Heymann. This will ask, for example, whether the country has a proper procedure for obtaining informed consent from individuals before they join a trial. What is understood by informed consent is, of course, the nub of the whole problem. For example, someone who cannot read will have to have the potential risks and benefits of participating explained to them only verbally.

In vaccine trials anywhere in the world, people will have to be told, for example, that there is a fifty-fifty chance they will get a placebo, and that the vaccine is unproven and therefore affords no license to let down their guard against risky behavior such as unprotected intercourse.

"One would have to use the appropriate means of informing people," says Clements. "It would probably be verbal consent, and then you need some way of verifying that they do understand." Staff would also need to be educated to a higher standard. "The counselling's far greater than with any other type of vaccine," says Clements.

There is a risk that private foundations or eminent scientists could finance trials and bypass the international guidelines. "It's always a real possibility," admits Heymann. But, he says, "We are not a police organization." Nzilambi Nziia, joint director of Project SIDA in Kinshasa, Zaire, is no stranger to this risk. "Everywhere when we go to AIDS conferences people are pushing for trials; and we say that we are not ready," he says. No one can enforce guidelines, agrees Clements. Would pharmaceutical companies be tempted to rush trials of their candidate vaccines? Clements thinks that any company that did would be "very unwise"; the FDA has warned all American companies in no uncertain terms against rushing into poorly designed trials, she says. But she admits that it could happen elsewhere.

Just as the rich countries are sensitive to suggestions that they are about to embark on safari research, the poor countries are equally sensitive to suggestions that they might allow it. In Zaire, for example, the chairman of the national ethical committee, Rila Kapita at Mama Yemo Hospital, Kinshasa, has made it clear that his committee will scrutinize any proposal for a trial. Zaire is sensitive about vaccine trials after the controversy created by Daniel Zagury, a French researcher who injected himself and some Zairean children with an experimental preparation. AIDS researchers in Kinshasa are loath to discuss Zagury, but privately they distance themselves from his work. Instead, Project SIDA is discussing possibilities for future trials with U.S. researchers.

In fact it is a Zairean who has just written a hypothetical protocol for a phase 1 and 2 trial in Zaire. Kayembe Kalambayi from the University Clinic in Kinshasa has just returned home after a spell studying at Johns Hopkins in Clements's team, funded by NIH money. He worked with the Americans on the safety trials in the U.S. of one candidate vaccine, a recombinant form of gp160. "We're encouraging him to get on as quickly as possible," says Clements.

Under a separate scheme, the NIH's international arm, the Fogarty International Center, is paying for the training of epidemiologists and others, from participating countries in the developing world, in AIDS research in the U.S.. For example, Case Western Reserve University in Cleveland, Ohio, is training researchers from Uganda; the University of Washington in Seattle trains Kenyans, Thais, Senegalese and Zimbabweans.

One of the most urgent priorities is to ensure that the world's widely variable strains of HIV are collected. No one knows how much the variation between strains within and between different geographical areas will matter for an effective vaccine, because no one knows exactly what part of the immune response to HIV is correlated with protection from disease. But in the meantime, some information on what strains are where is long over-due.

With this in mind, the WHO has recently begun to set up a network of primary laboratories in developing countries to collect samples of HIV. Where facilities are limited, the isolating of the strains may have to be done by a laboratory in the West. Then the strains will be stored as an international repository with existing "strain banks," partly in the U.S. at the NIH and partly in Britain. The strains can then be sequenced and scientists can find out whether antibodies to one strain can neutralize another.

In Amsterdam, Goudsmit is coordinating a project with Rafael Najera from the Charles III Institute, Madrid, sponsored by the EC to collect and test strains from across Europe and the Soviet Union. "We want to see if you can actually cross neutralize virus from Portugal with serum from Denmark, for example," says Goudsmit. So far, he and his colleagues have collected 50 strains, but they hope to get about 200. This June [1991] in Madrid, the Europeans will meet with colleagues from the Walter Reed Army Institute for Research and other researchers from the U.S. to discuss their work so far, then the American Institute will exchange strains with the Europeans. Walter Reed's laboratories all over the world have been collecting strains for several years. Finally, the WHO will receive the strains.

This is a crucial step for vaccine developers. Until very recently, most companies making vaccines had been restricted to working with American or European isolates, such as LAV/IIIB, MN and SF2. With access to a wider range, they may be able to find out more about the necessary components of broadly protective vaccines. At Chiron in California, researchers have tested recombinant gp120 vaccine, based on strain SF2 in the laboratory against a range of strains, including all the usual North American ones but also two from the Caribbean and two from Zaire. One of the Zairean strains, NDK, is highly virulent and kills cells 10,000 times more efficiently that IIIB.

A Vaccine for All

Larry Kurtz of Chiron says antibodies to the gp120 were capable of neutralizing all these strains. "We are not making a vaccine just for San Franciscans, we are making a vaccine hopefully for the whole world," he says. Just suppose the Chiron vaccine turned out to be effective. How would the company deal with the issue of its cost for the world's poor? "We would acknowledge that there should be a mechanism in place whereby people can afford to buy it," says Kurtz. So far, only one realistic mechanism has been proposed.

This issue will not go away in the coming years. But in the meantime, trial planners will face many other practical problems. There is the question of exactly what we mean when we talk of protecting people with a vaccine. Do we mean protection from infection, or do we just mean protection from disease? The difference is a big one, in the case of HIV. Most vaccines seem to work by limiting the invading organisms' attack to the immediate site of entry, then overwhelming infection. In the case of HIV, this could be a disaster. If any virus survives anywhere in the body, the person may remain healthy but will technically be infectious to others. So vaccinated individuals who continued to practice risky behavior might be safe themselves, but would be infecting others.

How should researchers measure the success or failure of a vaccine? If they wait to use progression to AIDS as a measure of failure, they will have to keep a trial running for many years, because of the slow course of the disease. If they use other markers of success or failure, such as declining levels of T4 cells, they will be able to end a trial at an earlier stage but they will still need to follow up the participants for several years, says Forrest, to be certain of the outcome. It would also be necessary to have an independent body to watch the trial's progress. This body, unlike the researchers or the vaccinees, would have access to the data during the trial and could advise its coordinators to discontinue the trial immediately if, for example, the vaccine was shown to be successful or had adverse effects.

In the end, everyone is hoping for a vaccine, or several vaccines, that are affordable to everyone and effective all the time. Whether it takes five years or 20, most scientists are now much more confident that they can design the product. Whether the world can devise a fair way to distribute it is another matter.

III

SOCIETY AND AIDS

Responses and Strategies

Q: what can rel/ch
do to shape
attitudes?
How effective a
force?

Depends on
people's view of rel/ch

Chapter 16

Public Opinion and AIDS

Robert J. Blendon
Karen Donelan
Richard A. Knox

In the 1980s, the United States found itself confronting the acquired immunodeficiency syndrome (AIDS), a new epidemic disease with the potential to affect millions of lives and irrevocably alter the practice of medicine and public health. As the potential magnitude of this deadly epidemic became more widely understood, there was an outpouring of public fear and concern expressed in a range of response from compassion to outright hostility. The American experience with AIDS to date suggests that public attitudes about AIDS can play a crucial role in shaping the nation's response on a number of critical issues, including the need for increased national spending for AIDS research and treatment, US discrimination laws, immigration and tourism policy for persons infected with human immunodeficiency virus (HIV), compulsory HIV screening of all health care professionals and hospital patients, the content and form of preventive educational efforts, and the distribution of condoms in public schools or of clean needles to drug addicts.

In 1988, we published an overview of then current public opinion data about AIDS.[1] In this discussion, we review the results of more recent national opinion surveys to reveal some common themes in the public's attitudes about AIDS as the nation faces its second decade of caring for afflicted persons and tries to slow the escalation of the epidemic. First, we

"Public Opinion and AIDS: Lessons for the Second Decade," *JAMA*, February 19, 1992, pp. 981-986. Robert J. Blendon, Sc.D., and Karen Donelan, Ed.M., are with the Harvard Program on Public Opinion and Health Care, Department of Health Policy and Management, Harvard School of Public Health, Boston; and Richard A. Knox, M.S., is with the *Boston Globe*.

present data on general attitudes about the severity of the epidemic and the public's perceptions of personal risk, and we update trends on discriminatory attitudes toward people with AIDS. Second, given this climate of opinion, we look at the realities of shaping AIDS policy in the 1990s.

Data and Methods

Data reviewed in this article were compiled by the authors from several sources including the POLL database and archives at the Roper Center for Public Opinion Research in Storrs, Connecticut, the National Center for Health Statistics (NCHS), Louis Harris and Gallup Poll subscription services, and print and broadcast media and through agreements with several private survey and media organizations. All sources were monitored from 1988 to 1991 to identify national public opinion surveys about the AIDS epidemic and related issues such as drug abuse and sexual orientation.

The data reported herein come from twenty national public opinion surveys conducted between 1989 and 1991 and from twelve other national surveys reviewed by the authors in 1988.[1] These earlier data are presented herein for historical or comparison purposes. These survey efforts were undertaken by the federal government and several private survey organizations using different research instruments and designs. Each involved telephone interviews of randomly selected adults. The AIDS supplement to the National Health Interview Survey[2] has been conducted annually since 1987 using personal interviews with approximately 10,000 respondents each year; all other surveys were conducted by telephone with between 1,000 and 3,000 individuals.

All such surveys are subject to sampling error. Results may differ from what would be obtained if the whole population had been interviewed. The size of this type of error varies with the number of people in the survey and with the magnitude of the differences in the responses to each question. The sampling error for a survey of 1,200 respondents is approximately ±3 percent for each question.[3] Results based on telephone surveys tend to underrepresent the views of members of the population less likely to have telephones, particularly individuals with low income. During this period 5 percent to 7 percent of households in the United States were without telephones and were excluded from these surveys.

A limited number of findings from these surveys can be reported in this article. Findings were chosen for review based on: (1) their relevance to a number of trends in public attitudes previously reported, (2) their relevance to key policy choices about AIDS facing our nation, (3) their consistency with other survey findings on the same topic, (4) our assessment that survey instruments did not use obviously biased or confusing wording of questions, and (5) their timeliness (if only one finding is reported on a given issue, it is the most recently available measure).

Results

Perception of risk. Americans remain concerned about the AIDS epidemic and about contracting the virus. This attitude may be abetted by personal experience: the proportion of Americans who know someone with AIDS has nearly doubled since 1987. However, the vast majority of the public perceive their personal risk of becoming infected as low or nonexistent, which probably blunts the nation's sense of urgency about addressing the epidemic.

More than eight in ten Americans (82 percent) report in surveys that AIDS is a "very serious" problem for all people living in the United States, and 71 percent see the epidemic becoming worse in the next three years.[4] However, in annual surveys since 1980 that ask Americans to name the nation's most important problems, AIDS has never been listed by more than 5 percent of the population and has never ranked among the top five problems.[5] In response to another type of question, though, a plurality (45 percent) believe it is the worst health problem our society faces; cancer ranks a distant second with 18 percent.[6] However, the proportion that ranks AIDS first on this list has declined since 1987, when 68 percent rated the disease as the nation's most important health problem.[7]

Americans recognize that AIDS is a major societal problem, but this concern is probably muted by the fact that the majority have not been touched personally by the epidemic. Today, somewhere between one in five and one in six Americans report knowing someone with HIV disease, a proportion that has increased substantially over the last decade. In 1983 only 2 percent of Americans said they knew someone with AIDS or the AIDS virus[8]; by 1987 that proportion had grown to 9 percent,[7] and by 1991 it had risen again to 17 percent.[9,10]

Perhaps because of their limited contact with persons affected by this epidemic, the majority of Americans do not see themselves as being at significant personal risk of contracting the disease. In national surveys conducted from 1987 through 1991, the number of Americans who express concern that they will get AIDS has not changed dramatically, with about two in ten saying they are "very concerned" and six in ten saying they are "not very concerned" or "not at all concerned."[3,6,10,11,12] Perhaps more informative than these measures of personal concern about getting the virus are data from National Center for Health Statistics NCHS) surveys showing that in 1990, nearly three in four Americans (72 percent) said they felt at no personal risk of getting AIDS or the AIDS virus, and an additional 21 percent say their risk was low. Only 4 percent said they were at high or medium risk, which corresponds rather closely to the 2 percent who meet one of the six risk groups outlined in the NCHS survey for self-risk assessment.[2] In fact, the percentage of people who perceive themselves to be in a high-risk group for AIDS has declined since these surveys were initiated in 1987.[13]

In another survey where comparative data are available, perception of risk does appear higher in groups in which disease incidence is higher. In 1990, 25 percent of the total population said they felt at risk of contracting AIDS, but larger proportions of persons aged 18 to 39 years (34 percent) and of blacks and Hispanics in the same age groups (43 percent and 39 percent, respectively) indicated that they felt at risk.[4]

Behavioral change. Despite major public health education efforts, today more than half of Americans report that they are not taking any personal precautions against becoming infected with AIDS. However, those who perceive themselves to be at risk of contracting the disease are substantially more likely than others to take preventive actions.

Since the majority of Americans are not concerned about their personal risk of contracting AIDS, it is not surprising to find that 53 percent of the public report they are not taking any precautions against getting the disease.[4] Importantly, however, this proportion has declined since 1987, when 83 percent said they had not changed their behavior in response to the threat of the epidemic.[7] When the 42 percent of the general population who say they are taking precautions are asked what precautions they have actually taken, 31 percent say they are using condoms, 40 percent are limiting the number of sexual partners, 5 percent are not sharing needles, and 24 percent are avoiding high-risk individuals (only one answer was recorded for each respondent).[4]

There is encouraging evidence that AIDS prevention educational efforts are having measurable impact. Persons who perceive themselves to be at high risk, and those in demographic groups with higher prevalence of HIV disease, are more likely than the average American to be protecting themselves against AIDS. Compared with the 42 percent of all Americans who say they are practicing prevention, 57 percent say they are taking action among those who say they feel very much or somewhat at personal risk of getting AIDS, as are 53 percent of people aged 18 to 39 years, 52 percent of unmarried persons, and 62 percent of black Americans. Males are more likely than females to say they are using condoms but are not more likely to say they are doing something to prevent transmission of AIDS.[4]

On the other hand, a substantial proportion of Americans acknowledge they are at risk of contagion but admit not taking any personal action to reduce that risk. Although condom use is promoted by public health professionals as the most effective form of prevention of HIV transmission (other than abstinence from sexual activity), condoms are used by only 31 percent of those who say they are practicing prevention methods. Among both the general population and those who perceive they are at risk of getting AIDS, limiting the number of sexual partners is more frequently reported than condom use as the primary method of prevention.[4]

One problem may be with the public's perception of the efficacy of condom use in preventing HIV transmission. Data from the NCHS indicate that only 26 percent of Americans believe condoms are "very effective" in preventing the spread of the AIDS virus during sexual activity, 53 percent think they are "somewhat effective," 4 percent say that condoms are "not at all effective," and 17 percent believe they do not have enough information to say whether condoms are effective.[2]

Attitudes toward people with AIDS or HIV infection. As the epidemic progresses, Americans display increasing tolerance toward people with AIDS in their workplaces, schools, and communities, and the majority support the federal antidiscrimination legislation enacted in 1990. Substantial proportions, however, express little compassion for persons who have contracted the disease through sexual or drug use practices.

In 1988, we reported that one in four or five Americans was unwilling to have contact with people with AIDS in workplaces, schools, and communities.[1] Several studies conducted between 1989 and 1991 indicate that the proportion of Americans who express these hostile attitudes is gradually decreasing. Survey trends reported in 1991 show a substantial decline, from 51 percent in 1987 to 33 percent in 1991, in the proportion of Americans who agreed that "it's people's own fault if they get AIDS."[6,7]

The public does have the perception that the AIDS epidemic has led to discrimination against people in different risk groups, particularly homosexuals, and the majority (65 percent) support the antidiscrimination legislation enacted in 1990.[4] Sixty-one percent (compared with 49 percent in 1987) believe that AIDS has caused unfair discrimination against homosexuals,[1,4] although less than a majority (44 percent, down slightly from 52 percent in 1985) believe the government would be doing more about the epidemic if it did not primarily affect homosexuals.[1,14] About four in ten Americans think the epidemic is causing unfair discrimination against blacks, Hispanics, and Haitians, only slightly less than the proportion of minorities themselves who echo these sentiments.[1,5]

Disturbing predictions of growing intolerance toward those with AIDS are not being borne out in the course of the epidemic. Rather, hostility toward those with AIDS has either declined or remained the same during this period. For example, while 25 percent of Americans said in 1987 that employers should have the right to fire a worker with AIDS, this figure was 21 percent in 1991. Surveys show that in 1990 the proportion agreeing with that statement had fallen as low as 13 percent. Surveys find there has been a substantial decrease between 1987 and 1991 in the number of people who say they would refuse to work alongside a person with AIDS, from 25 percent to 16 percent.[6,7] Similarly, only 9 percent now believe children with AIDS should not be allowed to attend school, compared with 39 percent in 1985.[3,15] The proportion of Americans who believe in enacting quarantine or isolation measures declined from 20 percent to 10 percent between 1987 and 1991.[6,7] The proportion who would support a landlord's decision to evict a tenant with AIDS declined from 17 percent to 10 percent in same period.[6,7]

Increased tolerance of people with AIDS in public places does not necessarily mean that people with AIDS are viewed with sympathy, however. A great deal of national attention has increased empathy for people who have contracted the disease from transfusions of blood or blood products or other routes not related to life-style choices. It appears that this awareness has led to increased compassion for all people with AIDS.

National surveys conducted in 1990 and 1991 show that only 6 percent of Americans say they disagree with the statement that people with AIDS should be treated with compassion.[4,10] However, in the 1990 survey that number increased to 27 percent if the individual contracted the disease through homosexual activity, 30 percent if the disease was transmitted through use of illegal drugs, and 24 percent if transmission occurred because a person had sexual relations with a drug user. As previously noted, people who contracted AIDS through blood transfusions, though they represent only 2 percent of AIDS cases, appear to play a major factor in the generally sympathetic view of all people with AIDS — only 3 percent do not view people in this group with compassion.[4] Even in these measures, however, time and the more widespread nature of the epidemic have led to considerable change in attitudes. In 1988, 72 percent expressed "not much" or no sympathy for people who got AIDS through use of illegal drugs, 60 percent for those who got AIDS through homosexual activity, and 20 percent for all people with AIDS.[16]

A 1990 survey underscores that the level of intolerance and concern that still exists about AIDS among Americans can have an important impact in the daily lives of persons who suffer from this disease. Survey respondents were asked to rank several types of facilities on a six-point scale of acceptability in their own neighborhoods (6 = would welcome, 1 = would not welcome). Fourteen types of facilities were included. Group homes for AIDS patients ranked eleventh among fourteen items on the list, with only three in ten saying they would welcome such a facility in their neighborhood. Only factories, garbage landfills, and prisons ranked lower in desirability.[17]

These data should be viewed in the broader context of Americans' general attitudes toward individuals who are at high risk for contracting AIDS. For example, since 1973 annual surveys reveal very little change in the proportion of Americans who think that homosexual relations are wrong.[18,19] In fact, another pair of surveys shows that between 1977 and 1991 the public perception that homosexual relations should not be legal has actually increased from 43 percent to 54 percent.[20,21] Despite indicators that Americans are becoming less likely to express hostility toward people with AIDS, it is clear that persons with this disease will continue to confront the problem of prejudice, especially if they are in a risk group that is identifiable and unacceptable to substantial numbers of Americans.

Attitudes toward official policies. A majority of Americans agree that the government is not doing enough about the problem of AIDS and either disapprove of the way President Bush is handling AIDS policy or do not know what he is doing about it. Three in four Americans do not believe that our current level of national spending on AIDS is hampering efforts to respond to other diseases and do not support diverting funds from the AIDS epidemic to other disease treatment or research.

Surveys conducted in 1990 and 1991 show that approximately six in ten Americans believe the government is not doing enough about AIDS.[6,14] Only 29 percent rate the president [Bush] as excellent or good at handling the problem, and 67 percent say his efforts are only fair or poor.[22] There are indications, however, that Americans recognize that recent years have brought increased federal expenditures to address the AIDS epidemic. While in 1987 nine in ten Americans favored increased government spending on AIDS,[23] those numbers declined to about seven in ten in 1990, and a bare majority is willing to pay more taxes to increase funding levels.[4] Contrary to the claims of some policymakers and researchers, however, Americans do not believe that AIDS has hampered efforts to respond to other diseases in this country. In two different 1990 surveys, 75 percent said they did not believe responding to AIDS had taken funding away from other diseases, and 78 percent said AIDS should continue to be a top priority and we should not reduce the time and money spent on this problem so that they could be put to address other health problems.[4,24]

Attitudes toward AIDS prevention. Americans want more information about AIDS. They want the government to provide it to them and the schools to provide it to their children. The vast majority support education about condoms, and nearly seven in ten Americans would find condom advertisements acceptable on television.

Early on in the AIDS epidemic, some researchers feared that AIDS education efforts would be hampered by the same objections that have long made public sex education efforts controversial. But it appears that concern about AIDS is significant enough in our society that Americans believe their best defense is information. Seven in ten Americans want the government to provide them with more information about AIDS.[14] An overwhelming majority of Americans, 94 percent, support education about AIDS in the schools, and approximately 80 percent want that education to include information about condoms as a preventive measure. A similar proportion think AIDS instruction should begin in grade school, and about 40 percent think it is acceptable to teach about condoms at that age.[4] Virtually all respondents say instruction about condom use should have been discussed by the time a student completes junior high school or middle school. Approximately seven in ten among parents of school-age children say their children have received some instruction about AIDS in school to date.[2,4]

The public is divided over the question about the actual distribution of condoms in schools, however. Surveys conducted in 1988 and 1990 showed that about four in ten Americans favored this practice and that black and Hispanic respondents (57 percent and 52 percent, respectively) were more likely to favor it than white Americans.[4,25]

Although Americans acknowledge that, other than abstinence, condoms are the most effective prevention method available for avoiding AIDS, discussion of condoms on television has been limited to occasional public service announcements. It has been the policy of the three major commercial television networks (ABC, NBC, CBS) not to air paid advertisements for condoms, usually citing the objections of viewers and pressures on advertisers. Surveys conducted by different organizations show that the proportion of Americans who think condoms should be advertised on television increased from 63 percent in 1990 to 70 percent in 1991.[4,10]

Duty to treat. Americans strongly support the notion that physicians and hospitals have an obligation to care for AIDS patients. However, they recognize the risks health professionals might face from treating an infected patient and are concerned about certain procedures that might put them at risk of infection as patients. There has been consistent support throughout the epidemic for mandatory testing of health care providers and all patients admitted to hospitals or undergoing routine medical examinations.

As early as 1985, 87 percent of Americans said that all hospitals should be required to care for AIDS patients. In 1983, at the beginning of the epidemic, a majority supported a physician's right to choose whether to treat a person with AIDS[26]; by 1990, 75 percent said physicians should not refuse care to such a patient.[14] However, worry over HIV transmission in both directions—from patient to caregiver and vice versa—translates into very strong public support for testing and disclosure on both sides. Nearly all Americans (97 percent) say persons who are HIV positive should be required to tell that information to their health providers, but nine in 10 favor testing all physicians, nurses, and other health workers for HIV and requiring these groups to reveal their HIV status to patients.[3,6,27]

In the event that a health care worker tests positive for HIV, 49 percent of Americans think the worker should be forbidden to practice. The public is even more concerned about those who perform invasive procedures. Sixty-three percent would forbid surgeons; 60 percent, dentists; and 51 percent, all physicians from continuing to practice if infected.[27] In 1991, about 80 percent of Americans favored routine HIV screening of patients at the time of routine medical examinations and hospital admissions.[3,6] When public concerns about HIV transmission from both blood donation and transfusion are taken into account, it is clear that the public is quite concerned about the risks of spreading the virus in health care settings, even though it wants those settings accessible to patients. What may surprise some observers is that, despite their perceptions of being at low personal risk for contracting HIV, Americans are as willing to be tested for the virus as they are willing to recommend that others be tested. Over 90 percent would be willing to have such a test performed by their health provider or on a routine basis during a hospital admission.[4]

Attitudes toward testing. The public's enthusiasm for HIV screening is strong. National data indicate that Americans are also concerned about the disposition of these test results and express greater willingness to make test results available to health agencies and sexual partners than to employers, insurance companies, or the federal government.

Polls reveal inconsistent attitudes toward the efficacy and desirability of HIV antibody testing as a preventive measure. Only 52 percent of Americans think mandatory testing programs will decrease the spread of AIDS, and 72 percent think education would be a more effective control measure than mandatory testing.[14] However, approximately 80 percent favor mandatory HIV screening for people in high-risk groups such as homosexuals and intravenous drug users, as well as for couples about to be married, inmates of federal prisons, immigrants applying for US residency, and health providers and patients. A much smaller proportion, but still about half of Americans (46 percent to 53 percent in surveys conducted in 1991), favor testing of all Americans.[3,6]

Most Americans (74 percent) place a higher priority on containing the spread of AIDS than on protecting individual privacy. There is a considerable measure of public support (89 percent) for tracing and informing the sexual contacts of persons who have tested positive for HIV.[14] Ninety percent say it should be illegal for a person who is HIV-infected to engage in sexual relations without informing his or her partner.[4] Although about seven in ten people favor making test results available to sexual partners of those who test positive and to state or local public health officials, in 1989 the majority (51 percent to 62 percent) opposed disclosure of this sensitive information to employers, insurance companies, and the federal government.[4,9]

Distribution of clean needles. Since 1988, the proportion of the public that favors the distribution of clean needles to drug addicts as a preventive measure has increased to the point where a slight majority now favor such a policy. Despite widespread fears of crimes related to illicit drug use in our society, more Americans view drug abuse as a disease than as criminal activity, and the vast majority are in favor of increasing drug treatment efforts in the United States.

Surveys conducted annually between 1988 and 1990 show that support for distributing free clean needles to drug addicts as a way to prevent the spread of AIDS increased from 40 percent to 51 percent. However, approximately even numbers of Americans say they strongly oppose or strongly favor such a measure, indicating the true division that has marked the consideration of this type of policy initiative from the outset.[4,9,16] Recognition that drug treatment programs are important to the control of this epidemic is reflected in the considerable measure of support among 73 percent of the public to increase spending on treatment efforts.[19]

In several 1989 studies, a majority of Americans consistently supported treatment and education as being more effective ways to reduce the use of illegal drugs than punishing drug users,[28,29,30] although the public strongly supports increased criminal punishment of persons who sell illegal drugs.[31] Sixty-eight percent express confidence in the ability of drug treatment centers to help drug users,[29] and 65 percent think we are spending too little as a nation on drug rehabilitation.[32]

Attitudes toward testing of immigrants and travelers. There is considerable public support for screening new immigrants and even tourists for HIV. If they are found to be positive, Americans support excluding them from admission to the United States.

Eighty percent to 90 percent of Americans believe that all immigrants to the United States should be required to undergo mandatory HIV screening,[3,6] and nearly six in ten believe that HIV-positive immigrants should be prohibited from entering this country.[4] The public expresses fewer reservations about screening and barring tourists, but two thirds say all should be tested,[3] and Americans are sharply divided on the issue of preventing HIV-positive tourists from entering the country (49 percent favor, 42 percent oppose).[4]

The national debate about this issue has focused on the concern that banning HIV-positive tourists and immigrants will send a message to the public that there is a threat of casual transmission of HIV. However, most Americans (80 percent) now clearly recognize that AIDS cannot be spread by casual personal contact, so the fear of contagion through these means is not likely to be a determining factor in the public's views on immigration.[2] Rather, one of the most recent national surveys of attitudes toward immigrants suggests that about six in ten Americans are concerned that these people may become dependent on public assistance or a burden on government services.[33] In this instance, public antipathy toward immigrants appears to relate primarily to anxiety that HIV-positive individuals will require public medical care and divert resources from other priority activities.

Comment

What lessons can be learned from public opinion as our nation confronts the second decade of the AIDS epidemic?

First, the public perceives the severity of potential health risks differently than scientists. Researchers have attempted to understand how the public responds to the risk of hazardous activities. When experts judge the risk of a hazard, their response generally corresponds to their best judgment about the magnitude of potential fatalities or morbidities growing from the taking of that risk. On the other hand, public behavior is more complex and does not respond well to the concept of statistical risk. Individuals' attitudes about what constitutes a serious health risk have been shown to be related

to people's assessment of three factors: (1) how catastrophic the consequences of taking risk could be for the individual, (2) whether a person
derives personal benefit by taking the risk (i.e., skiing or mountain climb-
ing), and (3) whether the risk is taken voluntarily (i.e., not wearing a helmet
when on a motorcycle) or involuntarily (i.e., the location of a nuclear power
plant in the community).[34,35,36]

The dilemma of what to do about HIV-positive health workers highlights
these differences between public and expert perceptions. Scientists see the
risk of patients contracting HIV from a health worker as an exceedingly
rare event that is costly to prevent.[37] The public sees the risk as a personally
dreadful event, with no individual benefit to be accrued from taking the
risk, and believes that, lacking disclosure by health professionals, it would
be taking this risk involuntarily. Public support for proposals to require
HIV tests of health workers and to penalize those who would conceal
positive test results underscores this concern about reducing the potential
for the accidental transmission of HIV to people who perceive themselves
to be at low risk.

Second, although discrimination against persons with HIV infection is
now illegal in the United States, people whose disease is associated with
their real or perceived sexual behavior or drug use practices continue to
face substantial public intolerance and a general lack of compassion about
their illness. As a result, maintaining confidentiality about diagnosis and
treatment remains an important protection for many HIV-infected persons
trying to live active lives in our workplaces and communities.

It is likely that American intolerance will also be observed as the nation
seeks to clarify federal policies about HIV-infected tourists and immigrants.
Despite reassurances from the public health and scientific communities that
persons in these groups do not present a public health threat to Americans,
about two-thirds of the public do not support admitting HIV-positive immigrants to this country. Their sentiments appear to be driven by concerns
that such persons would be a burden on government services. Countering
this concern will require confronting it with facts about the likely costs and
comparisons to current policies on how immigrants with other costly diseases are treated.

Third, the public wants to avoid a greater national crisis and is worried
enough about the potential spread of HIV that it strongly supports many
preventive measures to control the epidemic, especially education about
condoms. Despite a traditional unease about public sex education, the vast
majority of Americans want children to be taught about condoms in school
by the time they have completed junior high. The majority (70 percent)
think the major television networks should end their ban on condom advertising.[10]

Evaluative data from Switzerland emphasize the potential value of this
type of educational effort. In 1986, the Swiss made a decision to allow
television advertising of condoms in conjunction with a major public health

media campaign. Between 1986 and 1990, the number of 17- to 30-year-olds who had never used condoms declined from 69 percent to 13 percent. Those who reported they always used them increased from 8 percent to 29 percent.[38]

Beyond education about condoms, there is considerable support for other prevention efforts to control the spread of HIV in the United States. Three in four think measures to control the disease are a higher priority than the protection of personal privacy, and nearly the same proportion want to make HIV test results available to sexual partners of infected persons as well as to public health officials.

(Finally, in the years ahead, the intensity of the public's attention to the AIDS epidemic is likely to be cyclical. Major events in the epidemic—a new scientific discovery, a controversial policy proposal, the death of a prominent person from AIDS—will precipitate increased media and public attention, but it is unlikely that the level of that attention will be sustained over time. This phenomenon is not unique to the AIDS epidemic. Research on the waxing and waning of public attention to serious national problems has demonstrated that these cycles are generally caused by major events that trigger concern and then fade from the public's mind.[39]

For example, following President Reagan's diagnosis of colo-rectal cancer and the subsequent media focus on that disease, there was a sharp increase in telephone calls to the National Cancer Institute's information service, as well as in public demand for screening tests. Over time the level of interest in this problem has declined but has still remained higher than it was prior to reports of the President's diagnosis.[40]

The course of the AIDS epidemic has also been marked by reports of the diagnoses of prominent persons or persons with AIDS in our workplaces and schools that raise policy issues that touch all parts of our society. Most recently, on November 7, 1991, Earvin "Magic" Johnson reported that he would retire from his distinguished professional basketball career because he had been diagnosed with HIV. By the following week, 98 percent of Americans reported they had heard about his decision, and three surveys reflect the impact that his decision has had, at least in the short term, on American attitudes about AIDS.[10,22,41]

These surveys, conducted within two weeks of Magic Johnson's announcement of his retirement, showed increased public interest in AIDS screening prevention and educational practices and reported increased concern about the epidemic. They demonstrate three basic points about the impact of Johnson's announcement on the public's attitudes about AIDS. First, the announcement heightened public awareness about the overall threat of the epidemic. Forty-one percent of Americans reported that as a result of Johnson's announcement they are more concerned about the threat of AIDS in our society.[41] Second, it increased the proportion of people who recognize that they should be taking preventive measures to avoid contracting the disease. Third, we note that despite this increased awareness of a national threat, the proportion of Americans who see themselves as being at personal risk for contracting AIDS has not changed substantially.

Throughout the first decade of the AIDS epidemic, Americans have responded to stories of individual struggles with this disease. The experiences of Rock Hudson, Ryan White, and Kimberly Bergalis have led to philanthropic efforts, legislative action, and increased interest in public education. However, over time, in each case, the intensity of this interest has declined. It is clear that the Magic Johnson story has once again triggered increased public concern about AIDS. In the month since his disclosure, more than one million calls flooded a national AIDS hotline, six times the usual volume, according to federal health officials (Centers for Disease Control, unpublished data, December 1991). Policymakers and health professional should see this interval as a window of opportunity in this second decade of the AIDS epidemic—a time to increase public awareness and to enact public health measures that will help to control the spread of this disease.

Notes

1. Blendon RJ, Donelan K. Discrimination against people with AIDS: the public's perspective. *N Engl J Med.* 1988; 319:1022-1026.

2. Adams PF, Hardy AM. AIDS knowledge and attitudes for July-September 1990: provisional data from the National Health Interview Survey. In: *Advance Data From Vital and Health Statistics*, No. 198. Hyattsville, Md: National Center for Health Statistics; 1991:1-12. Dept of Health and Human Services publication (PHS) 91-1250).

3. Louis Harris and Associates. The Harris Poll, April 21, 1991. Storrs, Conn: Roper Center for Public Opinion Research.

4. KRC Communications Research and the *Boston Globe*. National attitudes towards AIDS, June 1990.

5. Authors' review of data on nation's most important problem, as measured by the Gallup Organization, 1980-1991. Storrs, Conn: Roper Center for Public Opinion Research.

6. The Gallup Poll. Gallup Polls News Service, May 15, 1991. Storrs, Conn: Roper Center for Public Opinion Research.

7. AIDS: America's most important health problem. *Gallup Rep.* January/February 1988 (No. 268/269).

8. ABC News/*Washington Post*. June 1983. Storrs, Conn: Roper Center for Public Opinion Research.

9. Media General/Associated Press. May 1989. Storrs, Conn: Roper Center for Public Opinion Research.

10. The Gallup Poll. November 14-18, 1991. Storrs, Conn: Roper Center for Public Opinion Research.

11. The Gallup Organization. October 1988. Storrs, Conn: Roper Center for Public Opinion Research.

12. The Gallup Organization. November 1989. Storrs, Conn: Roper Center for Public Opinion Research.

13. Dawson DA, Thornberry OT. AIDS knowledge and attitudes for December 1987: provisional data from the National Health Interview Survey. In: *Advance Data From Vital and Health Statistics*, No. 153. Hyattsville, Md: National Center for Health Statistics; 1988:1-12. Dept of Health and Human Services publication (PHS) 88-1250.

14. ABC News. June 1990. Storrs, Conn: Roper Center for Public Opinion Research.

15. Louis Harris and Associates. September 1985. Storrs, Conn: Roper Center for Public Opinion Research.

16. CBS/*New York Times*. September 1988. Storrs, Conn: Roper Center for Public Opinion Research.

17. Daniel Yankelovich Group. *Public Attitudes Toward People With Mental Illness: A Report to the Robert Wood Johnson Foundation*. Princeton, NJ: Robert Wood Johnson Foundation; 1990.

18. *General Social Survey Trends Tape Marginals, 1972-1989*. Chicago, Ill: National Opinion Research center; 1990.

19. National Opinion Research Center. General Social Survey 1990. Storrs, Conn: Roper Center for Public Opinion Research.

20. The Gallup Poll. October 1977. Storrs, Conn: Roper Center for Public Opinion Research.

21. The Gallup Poll. August 29-September 3, 1991. Storrs, Conn: Roper Center for Public Opinion Research.

22. Louis Harris and Associates. November 13-18, 1991. Storrs, Conn: Roper Center for Public Opinion Research.

23. The Gallup Organization/Times Mirror Publishing. *The People, the Press and Politics*. Storrs, Conn: Roper Center for Public Opinion Research; 1987.

24. NBC News/*Wall Street Journal*/Teeter and Hart. July 1990. Storrs, Conn: Roper Center for Public Opinion Research.

25. Kane Parsons. January 1988. Storrs, Conn: Roper Center for Public Opinion Research.

26. Audits and Surveys. August 1983. Storrs, Conn: Roper Center for Public Opinion Research.

27. Gallup/*Newsweek*. June 1991. Storrs, Conn: Roper Center for Public Opinion Research.

28. CBS News/*New York Times*. October 1990. Storrs, Conn: Roper Center for Public Opinion Research.

29. *Washington Post*, January 1990. Storrs, Conn: Roper Center for Public Opinion Research.

30. Associated Press/Media General. May 1990. Storrs, Conn: Roper Center for Public Opinion Research.

31. Princeton Survey Research Associates/*Times Mirror*. May 1990. Storrs, Conn: Roper Center for Public Opinion Research.

32. The Gallup Organization. January 1990. Storrs, Conn: Roper Center for Public Opinion Research.

33. The Gallup Organization/*Newsweek*. June 1984. Storrs, Conn: Roper Center for Public Opinion Research.

34. Slovic P. Perception of risk. *Science*. 1987; 236:280-285.

35. Storr C. Social benefit versus technological risk. *Science*. 1969; 165:1232-1238.

36. Slovic P, Fischoff B, Lichenstein S. Facts and fears: understanding perceived risk. In: Schuring RC, Albers WA Jr, eds. *Societal Risk Assessment: How Safe Is Safe Enough?* New York, NY: Peanum Press; 1980:181-213.

37. Roger DE, Gillin BG. AIDS and doctors: the real dangers. *New York Times.* July 16, 1991:A19.

38. *Boston Globe.* July 22, 1991. Baltimore, Md: Johns Hopkins Population Information Program and Population Services International.

39. Downs A. Up and down with ecology—the "issue-attention cycle." *Public Interest.* 1974; 4(2):38-50.

40. Brown M, Potosky A. The presidential effect: the public health response to media coverage about Ronald Reagan's colon cancer episode. *Public Opinion Q.* Fall 1990; 54:317-329.

41. *Los Angeles Times.* November 21-24, 1991. Storrs, CT: Roper Center for Public Opinion Research.

Chapter 17

No Time for an AIDS Backlash

Timothy F. Murphy

Writing in *Time*, Charles Krauthammer described the May 1990 protests by AIDS activists at the National Institutes of Health as a most misdirected demonstration: "The idea that American government or American society has been inattentive or unresponsive to AIDS is quite simply absurd." On the contrary, "AIDS has become the most privileged disease in America," this since Congress continues to allocate an enormous amount of money for research and for the treatment of people with HIV-related conditions.[1] Except cancer research, HIV-related disease now receives more research funding than any other illness in the United States, a priority Krauthammer maintains is all out of proportion to its significance since AIDS kills fewer people each year than many other diseases. The privilege of AIDS even extends to access to certain experimental drugs — access others do not share.

Chicago Tribune columnist Mike Royko has also challenged the view that there is government indifference regarding AIDS. "That might have been true at one time. But it no longer is. Vast sums are being spent on AIDS research. Far more per victim than on cancer, heart disease and other diseases that kill far more people."[2] In his view, some AIDS education posters have far more to do with the "promotion" of homosexuality than with the prevention of disease. Views of this kind reflect a movement that would assign AIDS a lesser standing in the social and medical priorities of the nation.

This view is not new in the epidemic; the sentiment that homosexuals with AIDS were being treated as a privileged class had surfaced as early

"No Time for an AIDS Blacklash," *Hastings Center Report* 21 (2), March-April 1991, pp. 7-11. Timothy F. Murphy, Ph.D., is assistant professor in the Department of Medical Education, University of Illinois College of Medicine at Chicago. Copyright © The Hastings Center.

as 1983.[3] What is new, though, is the increasing prominence of this view in public discourse and the extent to which the view is defended. In *The Myth of Heterosexual AIDS*, Michael Fumento mounts a full-scale defense of the proposition that the AIDS epidemic has achieved national and medical priority all out of proportion to its dangers, especially since the disease will make few inroads against white, middle-class heterosexuals.[4] Fumento writes in self-conscious sound-bites: "Other than fairly spectacular rare occurrences, such as shark attacks and maulings by wild animals, it is difficult to name any broad category of death that will take fewer lives than heterosexually transmitted AIDS." He also says that the mass mailing of the Surgeon General's report on AIDS to every household "makes every bit as much sense as sending a booklet warning against the dangers of frostbite to every home in the nation, from Key West, Florida, to San Diego, California." Because there is no looming heterosexual epidemic and because the nation has neglected other medical priorities by siphoning off talent and money for AIDS research, Fumento concludes that "the ratio of AIDS research and development spending to federal patients costs is vastly out of proportion to other deadly diseases." Fumento also believes that the priority assigned to AIDS will endanger the lives of other people: "The blunt fact is that people will die of these other diseases because of the overemphasis on AIDS. We will never know their names, and those names will never be sewn into a giant quilt. We will never know their exact numbers. But they will die nonetheless."

Not only the priority of AIDS on the national agenda but also the tactics used to put it there and keep it there have found their critics. Krauthammer concedes that the gains made by AIDS activists are a tribute to their passion and commitment, but he believes that such gains have been won by ingenious strategy. He charges that the "homosexual community," to advance its own interests, first claimed that AIDS was everyone's problem because everyone was at risk and its solution required universal social urgency. As it became clear that people would not fall at random to the disease, he says activists changed their tactics and began to prey on social guilt: how dare a society let its gay men, needle-users, their partners and their children get sick and die? But this guilt is unwarranted, Krauthammer believes, since for the most part HIV-related disease is the consequence of individual choices that ignore clear warnings.

Also objecting to activist tactics, the *New York Times* criticized the ACT-UP disruption that made it impossible for the Secretary for Health and Human Services to be heard during his remarks at the 1990 international AIDS conference in San Francisco.[5] "It is hard," that paper of record wrote, "to think of a surer way for people with AIDS to alienate their best supporters." The action was characterized as a pointless breakdown in sense and civility. "ACT-UP's members had no justification for turning a research conference into a political circus," especially since, in the standard refrain, society has not only not turned its back but has committed extravagant effort and resources to the HIV epidemic. The disruption, moreover, was all out of proportion to the matters protested: immigration restrictions (since lifted) for people with HIV infection and President Bush's absence from the conference by reason of an event important to the reelection of North Carolina Senator Jesse Helms.

In a different vein, Bruce Fleming suggests in *The Nation* that Americans have come to hype AIDS because of a distorted sense of what it means to be sick and dying.[6] Westerners, he says, assume that absence of disease is the normal state of human being, and that disease thereby becomes a divergence to be named, isolated, and eliminated. Thus can there be the fury and anger he found in a presentation at a Modern Language Association convention, an AIDS address full of Susan Sontag, Harvey Fierstein, and laments about the lost golden age of free sex. Accepting sickness and death as an integral part of life, he thinks, would free us from the frenetic feeling that AIDS and all disease was unfair treatment amenable to moral and medical control—control it is in any case impossible to achieve.

For all the good intentions here, intentions to remember people sick and dying with other conditions, intentions to keep priorities and discourse rational, intentions to recall the inevitable mortality of human beings as an antidote to their hubris, there is little good reason to shift the priority now devoted to the HIV epidemic, to smear the tactics that have made that priority possible, or to alter the view that sickness and dying with HIV-related disease are evils to be resisted.

Fumento's book makes the most direct claim that people are dying from neglect because the nation has chosen to worry about people with HIV-related conditions. For this reason he thinks AIDS needs to be put into perspective, but he offers not a word about what priority an infectious, communicable lethal disease should receive as against, for example, diabetes or certain heart conditions, which are noncommunicable and can be successfully managed by medicine throughout life. There is not a word, indeed, on how priorities ought to be set at all. Surely an infectious, communicable, lethal disease ought to receive priority over diseases that can currently be medically managed in a way that permits people to live into old age, a prospect not enjoyed by people with HIV-related disease. It is not even clear that funding should be allocated according to the number of persons affected by a particular disease, since such allocation would effectively orphan certain diseases altogether. Moreover, many of the diseases that do now kill people in numbers greater than AIDS have a *long* history of funding, and the expenditures made on behalf of AIDS research and treatment should be measured against that history, not against current annual budget allocations. It may be that AIDS is only now catching up with comparable past expenditures.

Perhaps it is the seemingly voluntary nature of infection that invites the notion that enough has been done for HIV-related conditions. After all, if only people refrained from behavior known to be associated with HIV infection, they wouldn't be at any risk of sickness and death. But HIV-related disease is not simply a matter of individual failure to heed clear warnings. Many cases of AIDS were contracted *before any public identification* of the syndrome. Even after the identification of the syndrome, there was no clear identification of its cause or how to avoid it altogether. Early on, there were no efforts to protect blood used in transfusions even when certain screening tests were available.[7] Even after the discovery of the presumptive causal virus and development of blood-screening tests, educational efforts to reach persons most at risk were inadequate and in any case no one knew what forms of education were capable of effecting behavioral change. What educational programs there were failed, then and now, to reach drug-users, their sexual partners, and persons in rural areas. Some persons were infected by means altogether beyond their control: by rape, by transfusion, by Factor VIII used in control of hemophilia, through birth to an infected mother, by accidental needle infection while providing health care or using drugs, through artificial insemination. Because of ambiguities and delays (culpable or not) in biomedicine, education, and public policy, it is not evident for the majority of people with AIDS that there were "clear warnings" that went unheeded.

Even now, when HIV-related disease is well known, it does not follow automatically that those people who contract an HIV infection do so in any morally culpable sense. Over ten years will soon have passed since the CDC first reported the occurrence of rare diseases in gay men and drug-using persons. Since that time, ten years of new gay men and drug-users have come along, persons who may not have been educated about the dangers of HIV, young persons who will not yet have maturity of judgment in sexual and drug matters, persons who may not have access to clean needles or drug rehabilitation programs, who may not have the personal and social skills necessary to avoid risk behavior altogether. In some cases there may be cultural and social barriers to protection from risk as well, such as resistance to condom use.[8] It is important to remember, too, that as regards the enticements of sex and drugs, people are weak and not always capable of protecting themselves even from those risks they know and fear. It is not surprising then that a considerable portion of *all* human illness is self-incurred, brought about through one's life choices. This is to vary the principle of double effect: what is chosen is not illness but sex, food, alcohol, drugs, and so on. Their aftermath, unchosen if inevitable, may be illness. But it is telling in this society that those whose heart or lung disease, for example, is related to their life choices are not asked to wait for research and treatment while those whose disease is accidental or genetic are served first.

It is odd that critics see misplaced privilege in the priority and attention AIDS has won where they might instead see a paradigm for other successes. Should the priority accorded to AIDS research and care be seen as an indictment of the wiles of AIDS activists or should it be required study in schools of public health? AIDS activists are not trying to bleed the government dry, and neither are they blind to the nation's other needs. They are merely trying to insure that government and medicine work together to achieve important goals. If other disease research and care is being neglected, the question is not whether activists have bullied the Congress or the American Medical Association into questionable priorities. The relevant question is why other health care research services cannot be delivered with the urgency and high profile that the HIV epidemic has received. In this sense, the HIV epidemic is an opportunity for critical thinking about the nature of health care in the United States: is it the nature of the disease itself or the design of the health care system that makes the HIV epidemic so formidable? Is it the transmissibility of the disease or social attitudes toward sexuality and drug use that make prevention so difficult?

But all this talk of the priority given to the HIV epidemic is likely to be misleading. It is important to remember that AIDS is no privilege. A diagnosis of AIDS amounts to a virtually unlimited onslaught against an individual's physical, emotional, familial, and economic resources. In addition, there is the burden of stigmatization, given that the disease has sometimes been seen as a punishment or deserved consequence of immoral behavior.[9] For example, a 1988 report showed that, depending on the social category of the respondent, some 8 to 60 percent of persons surveyed considered AIDS to be God's punishment for immoral sexual behavior.[10] A minority of Americans is prepared to tolerate considerable discrimination against people with HIV-related conditions.[11] Varying but significant numbers of persons surveyed report that they would refuse to work alongside people with AIDS, would take their children out of school if a child with AIDS were in attendance, would favor the right of landlords to evict people with AIDS, and so on. Perhaps most tellingly, the majority of people in one survey believed health professionals should be warned if patients have an HIV infection, and a third would allow physicians to decide whether to treat such patients.[12]

This last observation would be benign by itself except that medical students and faculty express a great deal of apprehension in working with people with AIDS and there is some evidence that some of them are choosing specialties and geographies that will keep them at a distance from such patients.[13] Some physicians have even taken to the pages of the *New York Times* to announce that they will refuse to treat any patients with an HIV infection.[14] Nursing recruitment has become difficult for hospitals that care for large numbers of people with HIV-related disorders. There are still places in the United States where hospital food trays are left at the doors of people with AIDS because the nutrition staff will not go into the rooms.

All the money thus far spent in the HIV epidemic has not by itself insured adequate medical care for all people with HIV-related conditions. This is most especially true for the homeless who have HIV-related illness.[15] Neither have the dollars spent on HIV research produced any medical panacea. Treatment with zidovudine (AZT) has proved important for some people but not for all, and there are still many unresolved questions about its long-term ability to extend the lives of all people with HIV infection or to guarantee the quality of life.[16] Zidovudine notwithstanding, as Larry Kramer has pointed out, there continues to be one HIV-related death every twelve minutes in the United States.[17] Is it therefore surprising that ACT-UP now chants, "One billion dollars . . . one drug . . . big deal"?

As Charles Perrow and Mauro F. Guillén point out in *The AIDS Disaster*, it is of course hard to "prove" that funding for AIDS research and care has been inadequate. But as they also point out, a broad array of highly credible reports have each drawn attention to government and philanthropic failures to respond to the epidemic. These reports have come from the Office of Technology Assessment, the Congressional Research Service, the General Accounting Office, the Institute of Medicine, and the Presidential Commission on the Human Immunodeficiency Virus Epidemic.[18] Whatever funding has occurred, it is hard to see that one can object to the amounts per se that need yet to be spent. The money called for by, for example, the Presidential Commission on the Human Immunodeficiency Virus Epidemic or the Institute of Medicine and the National Academy of Sciences[19] is not an invented figure pulled out of the air as a way of keeping scientists and bureaucrats in fat salaries. The figures represent estimates made in good faith about the extent of funding needed. It was clear early on that billions would be required, and that estimation has not changed merely because headlines have moved on to other subjects.

Perhaps the public is used to thinking in terms of billions only for military budgets, but the medical expenditures of the nation are measured in billions as well. The research carried out by the National Institutes of Health has always been enormously expensive, as has been the provision of medical benefits to veterans, the elderly, and the poor. The federal funding of dialysis for end-stage renal disease alone, for example, provides life-saving therapy for only some seventy thousand people, yet its costs have been measured in the billions since Congress decided to pick up the bill for such services.[20] If this kind of funding is any precedent, neither high cost nor small number of affected persons serve as a convincing rationale for limiting the funding now accorded to AIDS research and treatment.

Budget requests based on what should be done are one thing, of course, and budgets actually produced in government legislatures are another. The question at issue in discussions about the "privilege" of AIDS is the question of what priority should be assigned to AIDS funding given all the other funding needs that face the nation. Richard D. Mohr has argued that AIDS funding exerts a moral claim insofar as the disease is associated with gay men; in many of its most significant aspects, the HIV epidemic is the consequence of prejudicial social choices and arrangements.[21] Because its rituals, laws, educational system, and prevailing opinion fail to offer gay men any clear or supportive pathway to self-esteem or any incentives to the rewards of durable relationships, society has effectively forced some gay men into promiscuous behavior. Neither does society permit gay men the opportunity to form families that could shoulder at least part of the care their sick need. Patricia Illingworth has fleshed out this argument and extended it to drug users as well.[22] These are powerful arguments; it is hard to think, for example, of a single public ritual in family life, education, the media, religion, or the law that dignifies the love of one man for another, that supports any abiding union there. It is also hard to see that society has protected its needle-users where it cannot prevent drug use or offer successful drug rehabilitation programs. American society's enthusiasm for wars on drugs has not, after all, been translated into action capable of helping any but a fortunate few stop their drug use. Needle-exchange programs have been rejected out of fear that such action will appear to "condone" drug use — a fear that is odd given the de facto acceptance of drug use at every stratum of American culture from Supreme Court justice nominees on down.

It is not surprising then, that left to their own devices, many gay men, drug users, their sexual partners and children find themselves at the mercy of an indifferent virus as they try to lead what lives they can. Victims of disease rarely "just happen." More often than not society's choices permit them to happen, indeed make them inevitable. Robert M. Veatch has observed that it is fair to permit inequality of outcome where opportunities have been equal, but such a conclusion as regards health care would "not apply to persons who are truly not equal in their opportunity because of their social or psychological conditions. It would not apply to those who are forced into their health-risky behavior because of social oppression or stress in the mode of production."[23] Because many of the persons who have contracted HIV-related conditions have done so under circumstances implicating prejudicial social arrangements, there is a substantial claim that priority for HIV research and care is required for reasons of compensation.

But it is not compensation alone that frames the moral imperative about how a society should act here. Moral philosophy also avails itself of the supererogatory, those burdens we undertake beyond the call of formal obligation. Seen from this perspective, the society worth praising, the society worth *having* is the one that will find ways to care and to research, even though there is no formal obligation to do so and for no other reason than that its citizens are ill and dying. The care of those who contracted HIV infection through blood transfusions would be relevant in this regard, as would be women whose HIV risk was a secretly sexually active husband. The morally admirable society would do what it could to protect such persons from infection and care for them when they are sick whether or not society specifically *owes* them this concern and care as a form of compensation.

Cost alone should not be any obstacle for keeping AIDS research and care a national priority. The research is as important as any other research being conducted in the United States today. Delaying this research will not only impede therapy and vaccine development, but it will also subject the eventual costs to inflation; AIDS research will only get more expensive the longer it is delayed. Delays in researching treatments and vaccines will also increase the number of people who may be potentially at risk of HIV-related disease. It is worth remembering that only one disease (smallpox) has ever been entirely eliminated.[24] HIV-related disease is a problem for our time, and it will be a problem for future generations. It is not something that one can throw a fixed sum of money at before moving on. Even when fully effective vaccines and treatment become available, there will be people who will fail to benefit from either by reason of social deprivation, geography, choice, and chance. HIV-related disease therefore needs to be treated as a disease that is here to stay and not one that has already had its share of the limelight and public coffers.

Objections to ACT-UP disruptions of traffic and speech seem to share the view that quiet discourse, argued in mannerly fashion by legislators consulting with medical boards, is enough to insure that the nation will set appropriate medical goals. But this view of rationally framed public policy is not entirely true to history. There are few important social reforms that did not require the abandonment of polite discourse and the disruption of business as usual. It is important to remember that government and policy in this country are as much a product of protests, strikes, and civil disobedience as of reasoned debate. It is wrong to pretend that civil disobedience and social disruption are not part and parcel of this nation's political techniques, and it is wrong to blame AIDS activists for using these techniques as others have used them. Perhaps we have forgotten that the United States owes its very origin to acts of rebellion that the *New York Times* might have found easy to condemn as breakdowns in sense and civility.

Without protests, moreover, it is hard to see how the battle against AIDS would ever have gotten off the ground.[25] In the early years of the epidemic, the sickness and death of small numbers of gay men did not lend itself to the advocacy of important legislators and medical commissions. It was necessary then that impolite discourse be used in order to be heard. That need continues to this day. Most of the many recommendations of the 1988 Presidential Commission Report on the Human Immunodeficiency Virus Epidemic, for example, are already collecting dust. If an analysis with the stature of a presidential commission report cannot spur action on important goals, what other recourse is there than the tried and true methods of protest that are as much a part of American democracy as its parliamentary rules of order?[26] It is odd that where people do not see conspiracy behind AIDS activism, they see irrationality and impropriety when what they might see is a standard of urgency and passion by which to evaluate and improve the entire health care system in the United States.

It is hard to see moreover that an acceptance of disease and dying, in the way Fleming has urged, is anything but an invitation to quietism. If disease and dying are inevitable, what incentive is there to resist their damages? Granted, some Americans may have lost the sense of their mortality, but it is hard to see that much is gained by restoring it. On the contrary, it may be the perception of disease as "excrescence" that is the very spur to its control and eradication. There is no point in glorifying disease and dying; the lessons they teach are easily learned and do not require advanced instruction. There is a point at which sickness and dying cease to offer insights into the human condition or opportunities for strength and become instead unbearable, unredeemable absurdity. This is most often how AIDS appears to those who know it. To his credit, Fleming does say that hesitation by the U.S. government to carry out necessary HIV research would be criminal. But if this is so, then it's unclear that the change in the perception of death he counsels would make any practical difference in regard to the responsibility of government and medicine to resist the epidemic as much as it can with all the resources it can muster.

The sentiment nevertheless grows that AIDS is getting more than its share of media attention, resources, and social indulgence. But there really hasn't been any change in the status of the epidemic to warrant a change in the scope or intensity of research and treatment programs. HIV remains a highly lethal, communicable virus. Despite better medical management, the number of HIV-related deaths continues to increase. More and more hospital resources have to be directed to the care of people with HIV-related conditions. What accounts for the sentiment, then, that AIDS has gotten more than its share? From the onset of the epidemic, there have been many dire prophecies about the toll of the epidemic, predictions that millions to billions would die.[27] Is it possible that critics can say that AIDS has gotten more than its share because it has not yet killed *enough* people? Is the same indifference that first kept the epidemic at the margins of national attention now inspiring the claim that enough has been done? The sentiment that enough has been done for AIDS has primarily been argued in the press or journalistic accounts and not in professional journals of medicine, bioethics, or public policy. Could it be that this sentiment belongs to those who do not know the epidemic at first hand?

If HIV research and therapy are relegated to a lesser rank in the nation's priorities, it will be gay men, needle users, their sexual partners and their children who will continue to pay the price of neglect, and the epidemic will become again the shadow killer that it was in the beginning. In view of the people who are still sick, who are dying, who bear the costs of this epidemic, it is too early and shameful to say that enough has been done. In an epidemic not yet ten years old, it is too early for a backlash.

Notes

1. Charles Krauthammer, "AIDS: Getting More Than Its Share," *Time*, 25 June 1990, p. 80.

2. Mike Royko, "Message on AIDS Gets Lost in Poster," *Chicago Tribune*, 12 July 1990.

3. Randy Shilts, *And the Band Played On* (New York: St. Martin's Press, 1987), p. 295.

4. Michael Fumento, *The Myth of Heterosexual AIDS* (New York: Basic Books, 1990).

5. "AIDS and Misdirected Rage," *New York Times*, 26 June 1990.

6. Bruce Fleming, "A Different Way of Dying," *The Nation* 50 (1990): 446-50.

7. Shilts, *And the Band Played On*, pp. 221, 308.

8. Dooley Worth, "Sexual Decision-Making and AIDS: Why Condom Promotion among Vulnerable Women Is Likely to Fail," *Studies in Family Planning* 20 (1989): 297-307.

9. Some of the versions of the "punishment thesis" of the HIV epidemic are presented and critiqued in Timothy F. Murphy, "Is AIDS a Just Punishment?" *Journal of Medical Ethics* 14 (1988): 154-60.

10. "AIDS and the Real Electorate," *New York Times*, 24 January 1988.

11. Robert J. Blendon and Karen Donelan, "Discrimination against People with AIDS: The Public's Perspective," *NEJM* 319 (1988): 1022-26.

12. Robert J. Blendon and Karen Donelan, "AIDS, the Public, and the 'NIMBY' Syndrome" in *Public and Professional Attitudes toward AIDS Patients*, ed. David E. Rogers and Eli Ginzberg (Boulder, Col.: Westview Press, 1990), pp. 19-30.

13. Theodore B. Feldman et al., "Attitudes of Medical School Faculty and Students toward Acquired Immunodeficiency Syndrome," *Academic Medicine* 65 (1990): 464-66. See also Charles J. Currey, Michael Johnson, and Barbara Ogden, "Willingness of Health-Professions Students to Treat Patients with AIDS," *Academic Medicine* 65 (1990): 472-74. See also Thomas J. Ficarrotto et al., "Predictors of Medical and Nursing Students' Levels of HIV-AIDS Knowledge and Their Resistance to Working with AIDS Patients," *Academic Medicine* 65 (1990): 470-71. On the choice of specialty, see Molly Cooke and Merle Sande, "The HIV Epidemic and Training in Internal Medicine," *NEJM* 321 (1990): 1334-38.

14. Bruce Lambert, "AIDS War Shunned by Many Doctors," *New York Times*, 16 July 1990.

15. Charles Perrow and Mauro F. Guillén, *The AIDS Disaster: The Failure of Organizations in New York and the Nation* (New Haven: Yale University Press, 1990), pp. 166-69.

16. J. Ruedy, M. Schecter, and J.S.G. Montaner, "Zidovudine for Early Human Immunodeficiency Virus (HIV) Infection: Who, When, and How?" *Annals of Internal Medicine* 112 (1990): 1000-1002.

17. Larry Kramer, "A 'Manhattan Project' for AIDS," *New York Times*, 16 July 1990.

18. Perrow and Guillén, *AIDS Disaster*, p. 16ff.

19. *The Presidential Commission Report on the Human Immunodeficiency Virus Epidemic* (Washington, DC, 1988); Institute of Medicine, *Confronting AIDS: Update 1988* (Washington, DC: National Academy Press, 1988).

20. See John K. Iglehart, "Funding the End Stage Renal Disease Program," *NEJM* 306 (1982): 492-96. See also James E. Chapman, Ronald A. Sinicrope, and Douglas M. Clark, "Angio and Peritoneal Access for Endstage Renal Disease in the Community Hospital: A Cost Analysis," *American Surgeon* 52 (1986): 315-29.

21. Richard D. Mohr, *Gays/Justice: A Study in Society, Ethics, and Law* (New York: Columbia University Press, 1988).

22. Patricia Illingworth, *AIDS and the Good Society* (London: Routledge, 1990).

23. Robert M. Veatch, "Voluntary Risks to Health: The Ethical Issues," *JAMA* 243 (1980): 50-55.

24. World Health Organization, *The Global Eradication of Smallpox* (Geneva: WHO, 1980).

25. Herbert R. Spiers, "AIDS and Civil Disobedience," *Hastings Center Report* 19, no. 6 (1989): 34-35.

26. Alvin Novick, "Civil Disobedience in Time of AIDS," *Hastings Center Report* 19, no. 6 (1989): 35-36.

27. See Ronald Bayer, *Private Acts, Social Consequences: AIDS and the Politics of Public Health* (New York: Free Press, 1989), pp. 3-4

Chapter 18

Public Health Policy and the AIDS Epidemic: An End to HIV Exceptionalism?

Ronald Bayer

In the early and mid-1980s, when democratic nations were forced to confront the public health challenge posed by the epidemic of the acquired immunodeficiency syndrome (AIDS), it was necessary to face a set of fundamental questions: Did the history of responses to lethal infectious diseases provide lessons about how best to contain the spread of human immunodeficiency virus (HIV) infection? Should the policies developed to control sexually transmitted diseases or other communicable conditions be applied to AIDS? If AIDS were not to be so treated, what would justify such differential policies?

To understand the importance of these questions, it is necessary to recall that conventional approaches to public health threats were typically codified in the latter part of the nineteenth or the early part of the twentieth century. Even when public health laws were revised in subsequent decades, they tended to reflect the imprint of their genesis. They provided a warrant for mandating compulsory examination and screening, breaching the confidentiality of the clinical relationship by reporting to public health registries the names of those with diagnoses of "dangerous diseases," imposing treatment, and in the most extreme cases, confining persons through the power of quarantine.

As the century progressed, the most coercive elements of this tradition were rarely brought to bear, because of changing patterns of morbidity and mortality and the development of effective clinical alternatives. Neverthe-

"Public Health Policy and the AIDS Epidemic: An End to HIV Exceptionalism?" *The New England Journal of Medicine* 324 (21), May 23, 1991, pp. 1500-1504. Ronald Bayer, Ph.D., is at the School of Public Health, Columbia University, New York. Reprinted with permission.

169

less, it was the specter of these elements that most concerned proponents of civil liberties and advocates of gay rights as they considered the potential direction of public health policy in the presence of AIDS.[1] Would there be widespread compulsory testing? Would the names of the infected be recorded in central registries? Would such registries be used to restrict those with HIV infection? Would the power of quarantine be used, if not against all infected persons, then at least against those whose behavior could result in the further transmission of infection?

Although there were public health traditionalists in the United States and abroad who pressed to have AIDS and HIV infection brought under the broad statutory provisions established to control the spread of sexually transmitted and other communicable diseases, they were in the distinct minority. Typically, it was those identified with conservative political parties or movements who endorsed such efforts—e.g., the Christian Social Union of Bavaria—although not all conservatives pursued such a course.[2] Liberals and those identified with the democratic left tended to oppose such efforts. There were striking exceptions, such as the Swedish Social Democrats,[3] but in the end it was those who called for "HIV exceptionalism" who came to dominate public discourse.

In the first decade of the AIDS epidemic, an alliance of gay leaders, civil libertarians, physicians, and public health officials began to shape a policy for dealing with AIDS that reflected the exceptionalist perspective. As the second decade of the epidemic begins, it is clear that the potency of this alliance has begun to wane. The evidence of this change with regard to HIV testing, reporting, partner notification, and even quarantine is most visible in the United States, but it may begin to appear in other democratic nations as well. What follows is drawn from the American experience, but it most certainly has parallels in other countries.

Testing and Screening

The HIV-antibody test, first made widely available in 1985, was the subject of great controversy from the outset. Out of the confrontations emerged a broad consensus that, except in a few well-defined circumstances, people should be tested only with their informed voluntary and specific consent. When the clinical importance of identifying those with asymptomatic HIV infection became clear in mid-1989, the political context of the debate over testing underwent a fundamental change. Gay organizations began to urge homosexual and bisexual men to have their antibody status determined under confidential or anonymous conditions. Physicians pressed for AIDS to be returned to the medical mainstream and for the HIV-antibody test to be treated like other blood tests—that is, given with the presumed consent of the patient.

Thus, four clinical societies in New York State, including the New York

Medical Society, unsuccessfully sued the commissioner of health in 1989 to compel him to define AIDS and HIV infection as sexually transmitted and communicable diseases.[4] Among the goals of the suit was the liberalization of the stringent consent requirements for HIV testing. In December 1990 the House of Delegates of the American Medical Association called for HIV infection to be classified as a sexually transmitted disease. Although the delegates chose not to act on a resolution that would have permitted testing without consent, their decision on classification had clear implications for a more routine approach to HIV screening, one in which the standard of specific informed consent would no longer prevail.[5]

The movement toward routine or mandatory testing has been especially marked in the case of pregnant women and newborns. Pregnant women are already tested in this way for syphilis and hepatitis B. The screening of newborns for phenylketonuria and other congenital conditions is standard. Although as of this writing a deeply divided AIDS task force of the American Academy of Pediatrics had not recommended mandatory HIV screening of newborns, that decision was a function of the lack of specificity of the test and the lack of a definitive clinical regimen for seropositive newborns. The publication in the *Morbidity and Mortality Weekly Report* on March 15, 1991,[6] of recommendations for the prophylaxis of *Pneumocystis carinii* pneumonia in newborns will undoubtedly affect future discussion of the importance of identifying infants born to mothers with HIV infection.

Reporting of Names

Clinical AIDS has been a reportable condition in every state since 1983. But since the inception of HIV testing, there has been a sharp debate about whether the names of all infected persons should be reported to confidential registries of public health departments. Gay groups and their allies have opposed HIV reporting because of concern about privacy and confidentiality. Many public health officials opposed such a move because of the potential effect on the willingness of people to seek HIV testing and counseling voluntarily. By 1991 only a few states, typically those with relatively few AIDS cases, had required such reporting.[7]

Divisions have begun to appear in the alliance against the reporting of names in states where the prevalence of HIV infection is high and where gay communities are well organized. In New York State, as noted above, four medical societies have demanded that HIV infection be made a reportable condition.[4] In 1989, Stephen Joseph, then commissioner of health in New York City, stated that the prospects of early clinical intervention warranted "a shift toward a disease-control approach to HIV infection along the lines of classic tuberculosis practices," including the "reporting of seropositives."[8] Although political factors thwarted the commissioner, it is clear that his call represented part of a national trend.

At the end of November 1990, the Centers for Disease Control declared its support for reporting. In a carefully crafted editorial note in the *Morbidity and Mortality Weekly Report,* the agency stated that by using measures to maintain confidentiality, the implementation of a standardized system for HIV reporting to state health departments can enhance the ability of local, state, and national agencies to project the levels of required resources [and aid] in the establishment of a framework for providing partner notification and treatment services.[9]

Within a week, the House of Delegates of the American Medical Association endorsed the reporting of names as well.

Notification of Partners

Most important in the move toward the reporting of names has been the belief on the part of public health officials that effective programs of partner notification require reporting the names of persons with HIV infection as well as the names of those with a diagnosis of AIDS. Despite its long-established, though recently contested, role in the control of other venereal diseases, notification of the sexual and needle-sharing partners of patients with HIV infection or AIDS has been the exception rather than the rule. Opponents of such notification or contact tracing have denounced it as a coercive measure, even though it has always depended on cooperation with the index patient and protection of that patient's anonymity.

The early opposition to partner notification by gay and civil-liberties groups has begun to yield, as a better understanding of the practice has developed. Since 1988 the Centers for Disease Control has made the existence of partner-notification programs in states a condition for the granting of funds from its HIV-prevention program.[10] Such programs have also been endorsed by the Institute of Medicine, the National Academy of Sciences,[11] the Presidential Commission on the HIV Epidemic,[12] the American Bar Association,[13] and the American Medical Association.[14]

Many of the early strict-confidentiality statutes relating to HIV infection and AIDS appeared to prevent physicians from acting when confronted with infected patients who indicated that they would neither inform their partners nor alter their sexual practices. More recent acknowledgment of clinicians' ethical responsibilities under such circumstances has led to modifications of the stringent prohibitions on breaches of confidentiality. Both the American Medical Association[15] and the Association of State and Territorial Health Officials[16] have endorsed legislative provisions that would permit disclosure to people placed at risk by the HIV infection of a partner.

As of 1990, only two states had imposed on physicians a legal duty to warn spouses that they were at risk for HIV infection. Approximately a dozen states had passed legislation granting physicians a "privilege to warn or inform" sexual and needle-sharing partners, thus freeing clinicians from liability whether or not they issued such warnings.[17] In a remarkable acknowledgment of the extreme sensitivity of the issues involved, some of the legislation stipulated that the warnings could not involve revealing the identity of the source of the threat to the person being warned.[18]

Quarantine and Criminalization

On epidemiologic, pragmatic, and ethical grounds, there has been virtually no support for extending the power to quarantine to apply to all HIV-infected persons. There has, however, been periodic discussion of whether the tradition of restricting liberty in the name of the public health should be invoked when a person's behavior poses a risk of HIV transmission.[1] Although bitter opposition has greeted all attempts to bring such behavior within the scope of existing quarantine statutes, more than a dozen states did so from 1987 through 1990. When such measures have been enacted, they have generally provided an occasion to revise state disease-control laws to reflect contemporary constitutional standards of due process (Intergovernmental Health Policy Project: unpublished data). There have been a few well-reported instances of efforts to impose control over recalcitrant persons for reasons of public health. Almost always, states have used the existence of the authority to quarantine to warn those who persist in unsafe sexual practices and to counsel them aggressively about the need for a change in behavior.

More common, though still relatively rare, has been the use of the criminal law under such circumstances. From 1987 through 1989, 20 states enacted statutes permitting the prosecution of persons whose behavior posed a risk of HIV transmission (Intergovernmental Health Policy Project: unpublished data), a move broadly endorsed by the Presidential Commission on the HIV Epidemic.[19] The 1990 Ryan White Comprehensive AIDS Resources Emergency (CARE) Act requires that all states receiving funds have the statutory capacity to prosecute those who engage in behavior linked to the transmission of HIV infection to unknowing partners. Perhaps more crucial, aggressive local prosecutors have relied on the general criminal law to bring indictments against some people for HIV-related behavior, even in the absence of statutes specifically defining such behavior as criminal.

In the vast majority of instances, such prosecutions have resulted either in acquittal or in a decision to drop the case. When there have been guilty verdicts, the penalties have at times been unusually harsh.[20]

The Roots of the Challenge to HIV Exceptionalism

What accounts for the pattern of changes described above? When the communal welfare is threatened, public health policy always requires more than the application of a repertoire of standard professional practices. Inevitably, public health officials must contend with a range of extraprofessional considerations, including the prevailing political climate and the unique social forces brought into play by a particular public health challenge. In the first years of the AIDS epidemic, U.S. officials had no alternative but to negotiate the course of AIDS policy with representatives of a well-organized gay community and their allies in the medical and political establishments. In this process, many of the traditional practices of public health that might have been brought to bear were dismissed as inappropriate. As the first decade of the epidemic came to an end, public health officials began to reassert their professional dominance over the policy-making process and in so doing began to rediscover the relevance of their own professional traditions to the control of AIDS.

This process has been fostered by changing perceptions of the dimensions of the threat posed by AIDS. Early fears that HIV infection might spread broadly in the population have proved unfounded. The epidemic has been largely confined to the groups first identified as being at increased risk. As the focus of public health concern has shifted from homosexual men, among whom the incidence of HIV infection has remained low for the past several years, to poor black and Hispanic drug users and their sexual partners, the influence of those who have spoken on behalf of the gay community has begun to wane. Not only do black and Hispanic drug users lack the capacity to influence policy in the way that homosexual men have done, but also those who speak on their behalf often lack the singular commitment to privacy and consent that so characterized the posture of gay organizations. Furthermore, policy directed toward the poor is often characterized by authoritarian tendencies. It is precisely such authoritarianism that evokes the traditions of public health. Finally, in the United States as in virtually every Western democracy, the estimates of the level of infection put forth several years ago have proved to be too high.[21] As AIDS has become less threatening, the claims of those who argued that the exceptional threat would require exceptional policies have begun to lose their force.

The most important factor in accounting for the changing contours of public health policy, however, has been the notable advances in therapeutic prospects. The possibility of managing HIV-related opportunistic infections better and the hopes of slowing the course of HIV progression itself have increased the importance of early identification of those with HIV infection. That, in turn, has produced a willingness to consider traditional public health approaches to screening, reporting, and partner notification.

Conclusions

As of the end of 1990, eleven states had classified AIDS and HIV infection as sexually transmitted or venereal diseases. Twenty-two states had classified them as communicable diseases, infectious diseases, or both. Strikingly absent from this group are New York, California, and New Jersey, the three states that have borne the heaviest burdens during the epidemic (Intergovernmental Health Policy Project: unpublished data). Whether they and other states will follow will depend on epidemiologic and clinical developments. But more important will be the balance of political forces.

The pattern that has begun to emerge so clearly in the United States may not be replicated in every respect in other democratic nations where HIV exceptionalism has held sway in the first years of the epidemic. Much will depend on the tradition of public health practice with regard to sexually transmitted and communicable diseases and on the relative strength and viability of the alliances forged in the phase of the epidemic marked by therapeutic impotence. But what is clear is that the effort to sustain a set of policies treating HIV infection as fundamentally different from all other public health threats will be increasingly difficult. Inevitably, HIV exceptionalism will be viewed as a relic of the epidemic's first years.

Finally, the broad political context within which decisions will be made about the availability of resources for prevention, research, and the provision of care will be affected by the changing perspective on AIDS. The availability of such resources has always been the outcome of a competitive process, however implicit. In the beginning, the desperate effort to wrest needed resources from an unresponsive political system in the context of a health care system that failed to provide universal protection against the cost of illness compelled AIDS activists and their allies to argue that AIDS was different and required funding commitments of a special kind. However late these funds were in coming, and however grudgingly they were provided, it was inevitable that in a resource-constrained climate there would be challenges to the allocations that were made. Thus, in 1990 the Office of Technology Assessment was compelled to address the question of whether the resources made available for AIDS research had distorted the funding allocated for other medical conditions.[22] Winkenwerder et al. argued in 1989 that further increases in federal expenditures for AIDS would be disproportionate to the burden of disease in the population.[23] Such concern has begun to find expression in the popular media as well.[24] The erosion of the exceptionalist perspective on HIV infection will inevitably foster the further expression of such doubt, precisely when greater resources are required to treat those with HIV disease.

That the difference between the public health response to the HIV epidemic and the response to other conditions has been eroding does not necessarily mean that public health traditionalists will inevitably win out over those who have argued for a new public health practice. In Denmark, for example, the experience with AIDS has led to a reconsideration of the traditional approach to venereal disease.[25] Indeed, there are many reasons, both pragmatic and ethical, that some of the practices that have emerged over the past decade in response to AIDS should inform the practice of public health more generally. There are good reasons, for example, to argue that the principle of requiring informed consent for HIV testing ought to apply to all clinical tests to which competent adults may be subject. Furthermore, the lessons learned — about mobilizing an effective campaign of public health education, about the central importance of involving in the process of fashioning such efforts those who speak on behalf of those most at risk, and about the very limited and potentially counterproductive consequences of recourse to coercion in seeking to effect a radical modification of private behavior — could be applied profitably to the patterns of morbidity and mortality that represent so much of the contemporary threat to the public health.

Were the end of HIV exceptionalism to mean a reflexive return to the practices of the past, it would represent the loss of a great opportunity to revitalize the tradition of public health so that it might best be adapted to face the inevitable challenges posed not only by the continuing threat of AIDS but also by threats to the communal health that will inevitably present themselves in the future.[26]

Notes

1. Bayer R. Private acts, social consequences: AIDS and the politics of public health. New Brunswick, NJ: Rutgers University Press, 1991.

2. Frankenberg G. In the beginning of the world there was America: AIDS policy in West Germany. In: Bayer R, Kirp D, eds. Passions, politics and policy: AIDS in eleven democratic nations. New Brunswick, NJ: Rutgers University Press (in press).

3. Henriksson B, Ytterberg H. Swedish AIDS policy: a question of contradictions. In: Bayer R, Kirp D, eds. Passion, politics and policy: AIDS in eleven democratic nations. New Brunswick, NJ: Rutgers University Press (in press).

4. New York State Society of Surgeons et al. v. Axelrod, 1989.

5. Jones L. HIV infection labeled as STD; board to clarify testing policy. *American Medical News*. December 14, 1990:3, 28.

6. Working Group on PCP Prophylaxis in Children. Guidelines for prophylaxis against *Pneumocystis carinii* pneumonia for children infected with human immunodeficiency virus. *MMWR* 1991; 40 (RR-2):1-13.

7. Intergovernmental Health Policy Project. HIV reporting in the states. Intergovernmental AIDS Reports. November-December 1989:1-3.

8. Joseph SC. Remarks at the Fifth International Conference on AIDS, Montreal, June 4-9, 1989.

9. Update: public health surveillance for HIV infection — United States, 1989 and 1990. *MMWR* 1990; 39:861.

10. Fed Regist 1988; 53:3554.

11. Altering the course of the epidemic. In: Institute of Medicine, National Academy of Sciences. Confronting AIDS: update 1988. Washington, DC: National Academy Press, 1988:82.

12. Report of the Presidential Commission on the Human Immunodeficiency Virus Epidemic: submitted to the President of the United States. Washington, DC:

Presidential Commission on the Human Immunodeficiency Virus Epidemic, 1988:76.

13. American Bar Association, House of Delegates. Report from the House of Delegates, August 1989: annual meeting. Chicago: American Bar Association, 1989:23-5.

14. Abraham L. AIDS contact tracing, prison test stir debate. *American Medical News.* July 8-15, 1988:4.

15. American Medical Association Board of Trustees. Report X: AMA HIV policy update. In: AMA Proceedings of the House of Delegates, December 3-6, 1989, 43rd interim meeting. Chicago: American Medical Association, 1989:76-95.

16. Association of State and Territorial Health Officials, National Association of County Health Officials, Conference of Local Health Officers. Guide to public health practice: HIV partner notification strategies. Washington, DC: Public Health Foundation, 1988.

17. Intergovernmental Health Policy Project. 1989 legislative overview. Intergovernmental AIDS Reports. January 1990:3.

18. New York State Public Health Law, Article 27-F.

19. Report of the Presidential Commission on the Human Immunodeficiency Virus Epidemic: submitted to the President of the United States. Washington, DC: Presidential Commission on the Human Immunodeficiency Virus Epidemic, 1988:130-31.

20. Gostin LO. The AIDS litigation project: a national review of courts and human rights commission decisions, part 1: the social impact of AIDS. *JAMA* 1990; 263:1961-70.

21. Estimates of HIV prevalence and projected AIDS cases: summary of a workshop, October 31-November 1, 1989. *MMWR* 1990; 39:110-19.

22. Office of Technology Assessment. How has federal research on AIDS/HIV disease contributed to other fields? Washington, DC: Government Printing Office, 1990.

23. Winkenwerder W, Kessler AR, Stolec RM. Federal spending for illness caused by the human immunodeficiency virus. *N Engl J Med* 1989; 320:1598-603.

24. Krauthammer C. AIDS getting more than its share? *Time.* June 25, 1990:80.

25. Albaek E. AIDS: the evolution of a non-controversial issue in Denmark. In: Bayer R, Kirp D, eds. Passions, politics and policy: AIDS in eleven democratic nations. New Brunswick, NJ: Rutgers University Press (in press).

26. Supported by the American Foundation for AIDS Research, the Conanima Foundation, and the Josiah Macy Jr. Foundation.

Chapter 19

A Dual Approach to the AIDS Epidemic

Marcia Angell

Ten years ago five homosexual men in Los Angeles were reported to have acquired a mysterious and profound immune deficiency associated with pneumocystis pneumonia and other opportunistic infections. The report on these men, published in the *Morbidity and Mortality Weekly Report* on June 5, 1981, marked the beginning of the AIDS epidemic.[1] Within weeks, similar cases were being described elsewhere.[2-5] Even before the isolation of the causative virus in 1983 and the introduction of serologic testing in 1985, it was clear that a major epidemic had begun.

Now, a decade later, well over 100,000 Americans have died of AIDS and an estimated one million are currently infected with the virus, of whom more than 125,000 are thought to have clinical AIDS.[6] Women and children are affected, as well as both heterosexual and homosexual men. Although the rate of spread in the homosexual community has slowed, the reservoir is now huge, and we can therefore expect to see the number of cases continue to grow. Thus, AIDS is no longer an obscure disease known only to the medical and homosexual communities; it is now a household word, of concern to most Americans and frightening to many. Not since the polio outbreaks of the early 1950s have we been faced with so threatening an epidemic. Furthermore, with the advent of expensive treatments that extend the lives of persons infected with the human immunodeficiency virus (HIV) for many years, the cost of this epidemic has become a troubling issue in a time of shrinking resources.

In addition to the medical and economic issues surrounding AIDS, there are social issues unique to this epidemic that have greatly complicated our

"A Dual Approach to the AIDS Epidemic," *The New England Journal of Medicine* 324 (21), May 23, 1991, pp. 1498-1500. Marcia Angell, M.D., is executive editor of this journal. Reprinted with permission.

response to it. Unlike the polio epidemic of the 1950s or the influenza pandemic of 1918, AIDS tends to afflict people who are for one reason or another the objects of discrimination. Although increasingly a disease of inner-city black and Hispanic intravenous drug abusers of both sexes and their sexual partners, AIDS was at first almost exclusively a disease of homosexual men. It therefore carried the stigma of any sexually transmitted disease, but unlike syphilis or gonorrhea, it also carried the stigma of homo-sexuality—a double burden. Members of the homosexual community, artic-ulate and well educated and accustomed to injustice, mobilized to protect themselves from a discriminatory backlash more effectively than the polit-ically powerless drug abusers could possibly have done. Concerned that identification of those with AIDS would lead to loss of employment, hous-ing, and medical insurance, as well as to social ostracism, they and others sensitive to civil rights issues argued successfully for confidentiality and against screening and efforts to trace sexual partners. Thus, although AIDS is reportable in all states, HIV infection is not, nor are contacts systemat-ically traced. Instead, testing for infection is by and large voluntary, as is the notification of sexual partners.

We are now seeing growing opposition to this policy of strict confiden-tiality, as described by Bayer in this issue of the *Journal*.[7] With recent reports of the transmission of AIDS from patients to health care providers and, more recently, from a provider to patients,[8] we hear calls for the routine screening of both groups—all patients admitted to hospitals and all doctors and nurses. There are also calls for the routine screening of preg-nant women and newborns in response to the growing number of infants who contract AIDS from their mothers perinatally. Requiring the notifi-cation of sexual partners is less emphasized, perhaps because it is so dif-ficult, but it, too, is receiving renewed attention.

Debates about these issues, it seems to me, too often confuse the social with the epidemiologic problems. To be sure, both sets of issues are closely enmeshed, but there seems to have been little effort to sort them out. Many of those who believe that controlling the epidemic should be our most important priority recommend draconian methods for doing so, including not only widespread screening, but also the removal of infected children from their schools, infected adults from their jobs, and both from the neigh-borhood. On the other hand, those moved primarily by compassion for AIDS sufferers and concern for civil rights are likely to resist the usual methods for monitoring and containing an epidemic—methods that might spare more people suffering.

I believe we need a dual approach that attempts to distinguish social from epidemiologic problems and that deals with both, simultaneously but separately. Clearly, HIV-infected persons need to be protected against dis-crimination and hysteria, but doing so requires social and political meas-ures, not epidemiologic ones. Jobs, housing, and insurance benefits, for example, should be protected by statute. The economic consequences of

HIV infection require additional attention, since they go far beyond the possible loss of employment and ordinary insurance benefits. Treating AIDS is expensive, and the disease lasts for the rest of a patient's life, during much of which he or she may be unable to work. Even the most generous medical insurance is unlikely to cover all the health care needs of a patient with AIDS; thus, as patients grow sicker they also stand to become destitute.

We as a society should deal more systematically with the devastating economic consequences of HIV infection. I suggest we establish a nationally funded program, analogous to the end-stage renal disease program, for the medical care of HIV-infected persons. The end-stage renal disease program, established by Congress in 1972, extends Medicare coverage to all patients with kidney failure.[9] This was a response to the development of effective but extremely expensive treatments for end-stage renal disease — namely, long-term dialysis and renal transplantation. Handling the AIDS epidemic in the same way would probably cost society no more than it spends on HIV infection now. Increases in costs due to expanded access would probably be offset by the elimination of the expensive practice of attempting to shift costs. Under the present patchwork system, each potential payer (employers as well as federal, state, municipal, and private insurers) naturally wishes to pass the costs to another. Thus, for example, a health care institution that finds itself possibly liable for the care of an employee who becomes infected with HIV takes an adversarial stance, asserting that there is no proof the infection was work-related. Whatever the outcome of any such dispute, some element in the system, often Medicaid, eventually must assume the costs. A nationally funded program would have the advantage of uniformity, simplicity, and efficiency. It would also give those at risk an incentive to be tested, thus allowing for earlier treatment and the protection of sexual partners. The present system, in contrast, is filled with disincentives for being tested.

If by such measures we can soften the social and economic burdens on people with HIV infection, perhaps we will be freer to address the epidemiologic problems more rigorously. Concern about social issues now creates a reluctance to deal effectively with the epidemiologic problems. For example, systematic tracing of the sexual partners of HIV-infected persons is generally resisted because of the threat to confidentiality, although contact tracing makes sense from an epidemiologic standpoint and is officially required for other sexually transmitted diseases. Similarly, there is resistance to a screening program for all pregnant women and newborns,[10-12] although such a program would be reasonable, given the accuracy of new confirmatory tests and the fact that perinatally acquired HIV infection is now more common than congenital syphilis or phenylketonuria, both of which are tested for routinely. Infected women could make more-informed choices about family planning, and infected newborns could be treated earlier.

Testing health care providers and hospitalized patients is also controversial,[13] although it makes sense from several standpoints. Screening patients on admission would identify those with whom health care providers must be most alert; it is unrealistic to expect them to maintain the highest level of vigilance continuously. Similarly, because it is remotely possible that there could be an exchange of blood during a medical procedure, patients have a right to know whether a doctor or nurse who performs invasive procedures is infected with HIV. If necessary, retraining in non-invasive areas or early retirement could be provided for by special insurance programs for health care professionals. Screening both patients and health care providers would also, of course, identify those for whom treatment could be begun early and whose sexual partners could be protected.

I believe that, on balance, systematic tracing and notification of the sexual partners of HIV-infected persons and screening of pregnant women, newborns, hospitalized patients, and health care professionals are warranted. These populations are, after all, relatively accessible to the health care system and at some special risk. Attempting to screen the entire population would simply be impractical; on the other hand, targeting only high-risk groups would be unworkable, in part because it would entail making distinctions that are often impossible as well as invidious. With any increase in screening, however, the specter of discrimination arises once a person is known to be infected. Only if such discrimination at least in its more tangible expressions, is countered by statute and if those with HIV infection are assured of receiving all the medical care they need, can we pursue the basic elements of infection control more resolutely and so spare others the tragedy of this disease.

Notes

1. Gottlieb MS, Schanker HM, Fan PT, Saxon A, Weisman JD. *Pneumocystis* pneumonia—Los Angeles. MMWR 1981; 30:250-2.

2. Friedman-Kien A, Laubenstein L, Marmor M, et al. Kaposi's sarcoma and *Pneumocystis* pneumonia among homosexual men—New York City and California. *MMWF* 1981; 30:305-8.

3. Gottlieb MS, Schroff R, Schanker HM, et al. Pneumocystis carinii pneumonia and mucosal candidiasis in previously healthy homosexual men: evidence of a new acquired cellular immunodeficiency. *N Engl J Med* 1981; 305:1425-31.

4. Masur H, Michelis MA, Greene JB, et al. An outbreak of community-acquired *Pneumocystis carinii* pneumonia: initial manifestation of cellular immune dysfunction. *N Engl J Med* 1981; 305:1431-8.

5. Siegal FP, Lopez C, Hammer GS, et al. Severe acquired immunodeficiency in male homosexuals, manifested by chronic perianal ulcerative herpes simplex lesions. *N Engl J Med* 1981; 305:1439-44.

6. Karon JM, Dondero TJ Jr. HIV prevalence estimates and AIDS case projections for the United States: report based upon a workshop. *MMWR* 1990; 39 (RR-16):1-31.

7. Bayer R. Public health policy and the AIDS epidemic—an end to HIV exceptionalism? *N Engl J Med* 1991; 324:1500-4.

8. Update: transmission of HIV infection during an invasive dental procedure—Florida. *JAMA* 1991; 265:563-8.

9. Levinsky N, Rettig RA. The Medicare end-stage renal disease program: a report from the Institute of Medicine. *N Engl J Med* 1991; 324:1143-8.

10. Hardy LM, ed. HIV screening of pregnant women and newborns. Washington, DC: National Academy Press, 1991.

11. Working Group on HIV Testing of Pregnant Women and Newborns. HIV infection, pregnant women, and newborns: a policy proposal for information and testing. *JAMA* 1990; 264:2416-20.

12. Nolan K. Ethical issues in caring for pregnant women and newborns at risk for human immunodeficiency virus infection. *Semin Perinatol* 1989; 13:55-65.

13. Brennan TA. Transmission of the human immunodeficiency virus in the health care setting—time for action. *N Engl J Med* 1991; 324:1504-9.

Chapter 20

Another Approach to the AIDS Epidemic

David E. Rogers
June E. Osborn

Over the past two years, the National Commission on AIDS has held hearings almost monthly to gain a better understanding of America's relentlessly advancing epidemic of human immunodeficiency virus (HIV) infection. We have issued four interim reports containing our findings and recommendations,[1-4] and a comprehensive two-year report will be published this fall [1991]. During this period, there has been measurable progress in treatment, in legislation to discourage discrimination, in the provision of federal emergency funding for the communities hardest hit by the epidemic, and in some lessening of public hostility toward people living with HIV infection or the acquired immunodeficiency syndrome (AIDS). These are causes for hope.

Recently, however, there have been disquieting signs that AIDS is being routinized — tossed onto a waste heap of social problems, such as homelessness, drug use, violence, and poverty, that we decry but seem unable to address decisively. Although the number of patients with AIDS will triple during the 1990s, many communities are reducing their AIDS funding. The decision of Dr. Louis W. Sullivan, Secretary of Health and Human Services, to remove HIV infection from the list of diseases that would bar immigration to the United States has come under attack as perpetuating the misperception that persons with this disease represent a threat to the rest of us. The recent tragedy in which five patients were infected by contact with one dentist or his instruments has prompted a series of reactions that

"Another Approach to the AIDS Epidemic," *The New England Journal of Medicine* 325 (11), September 12, 1991, pp. 806-808. David E. Rogers, M.D., and June E. Osborn, M.D., are vice-chair and chair, respectively, of the National Commission on AIDS. Reprinted with permission.

183

threaten to convert health care settings into battlegrounds full of fear and mistrust rather than sanctuaries for the sick.

Now, in a *Journal* editorial,[5] Dr. Marcia Angell has proposed a blueprint for the containment of the AIDS epidemic that seems to ignore many studies from the past decade. We will not contest all her assertions, but we will comment on three before addressing the main issues of concern to the National Commission.

First, Dr. Angell says she is hearing calls for the routine HIV-antibody testing of all patients admitted to hospitals and all doctors and nurses. It should be noted that these are calls from the members of the public, not from scientists working on AIDS. At a conference on this issue convened in February 1991 by the Centers for Disease Control (CDC), almost 100 experts overwhelmingly agreed that such a response would not solve the problem it purports to address—the need to protect patients and health care workers from HIV infection.[6]

Second, the editorial states that there is "resistance to a screening program for all pregnant women and newborns, although such a program would be reasonable." This "resistance" represents the conclusions of a two-year study by the Institute of Medicine, which decided that at present such routine screening would work against the desired outcome of finding and treating the maximal number of infected women and children.[7]

Third, Dr. Angell asserts that "screening patients on admission would identify those with whom health care providers must be most alert. . . ." She goes on to state that it is unrealistic to expect health professionals to maintain the highest levels of vigilance continuously. This statement worries us. For one thing, the reality of a "window" period of seronegativity in early HIV infection is well recognized. Thus, simple screening of patients would yield a false and dangerous sense of security. More important, failure to maintain the highest levels of vigilance continuously leads to the far greater hazard of contracting hepatitis B, a much more likely killer in health care settings. Each year 12,000 health professionals become infected with the hepatitis B virus, and 250 of them die.[8] The risk of HIV transmission should not be trivialized, but it should be addressed in the context of the true issue—safety.

But let us turn to our central points. Dr. Angell suggests a "dual approach" that would distinguish social from epidemiologic problems and deal with them simultaneously but separately. She argues that worries about discrimination and access to treatment should not affect our medical response to the epidemic, which should proceed along traditional public health lines. Her proposed strategy to meet the cost of care for patients with HIV infection would use the financing of treatment for end-stage renal disease as a model. She would implement systematic testing of all hospital patients, health care professionals performing invasive procedures, pregnant women, and newborns. HIV-infected health care professionals would be retrained or retired early.

At first blush all this sounds reasonable. But alas, it fails to consider the unwanted ripple effects of many of these actions and flies in the face of many insights painfully acquired over the past decade.

First, the fact that HIV infection has prominent social trappings is a major part of the problem, as Dr. Angell points out. Social perceptions, attitudes, and prejudices are inextricably interwoven with the disease itself. The powerful punitive and discriminatory reactions of society to those with HIV infection contribute deeply and fundamentally to the suffering of HIV-infected patients. Where we disagree with Dr. Angell is in her suggestion that tough laws could eliminate the enormous destructiveness of discrimination. Although the need for such laws is absolutely fundamental, experience has shown that they alone cannot suffice. The civil-rights legislation of 1866 and 1964 did not abolish discrimination on the basis of color. The Americans with Disabilities Act of 1990 was a major step forward, but it will not even begin to take effect until 1992. All the laws in the world will not by themselves rectify the loss of home, family, friends, jobs, and insurance or the denial of care that now so commonly befalls those who are HIV-infected. This will come only with fundamental change in the attitudes of the larger society.

Second, suggesting that the problems of financing care for those with HIV infection should be solved by imitating the model of legislation for end-stage renal disease seems the wrong way to go. The *Journal* has carried a number of articles pointing out the inequities and problems posed by this particular law.[9,10] Clearly, those with HIV infection need immediate help. The 1990 Ryan White Comprehensive Care Act passed by Congress to provide emergency financial assistance is an attempt to address this shortfall. But over the longer haul, adopting a disease-specific model of financing that ignores at least 37 million other Americans unable to pay for their care is an invitation to public discord. Now seems the time to fight for solutions that are more broadly applicable, and many groups share the Commission's view.

Third, for reasons already set forth, it seems unlikely that routine, systematic testing of people in health care settings would do much to prevent further HIV infection. More important, it would divert precious resources from the central goal of primary prevention, at which we are failing badly. Testing principally those coming to hospitals while not making stronger efforts to reach hard-to-get-at groups with high-risk behavior seems like looking for a lost wallet under the street lamp because the light is brighter there.

Finally come the tormenting and controversial problems of what to do about HIV-positive health professionals. The editorial proposes HIV testing for all doctors and nurses who perform invasive procedures and retraining or early retirement for those who are found to be HIV-infected. An alarmed public would largely agree. The flurry of recent disclosures of infected doctors and dentists has left many Americans frightened and distrustful of the medical establishment. These fears must be swiftly addressed. But in this minefield we must make the most careful, science-based decisions if we are to fulfill our sacred trust to do no harm.

Here we do have data to help us. Except for the unusual cluster of heart-rending cases in the Florida dental practice, for which the mode of transmission is completely unknown, to date there is not one documented instance of an HIV-positive physician infecting a patient, despite hundreds of thousands of invasive encounters. Moreover, the three retrospective studies of patients operated on by HIV-infected surgeons have not uncovered a single instance of transmission of HIV in the 753 patients examined.[11-13]

Thus, it would seem that we should plan our strategies very carefully. Although intuitively the testing of health professionals seems sensible and the emotional push is all in this direction, the idea may not be so sensible after all. The reason? Such testing fails to address the central question: How can we best protect patients from being infected by HIV-infected professionals? With the question framed this way, the answer is easier. Data from two decades of experience with hepatitis B, a blood-borne virus that is one hundred times more infectious than HIV, ten times more prevalent among health professionals, and similarly transmitted, give us some guidelines. After the institution of rigorous universal precautions in 1987, the transmission of hepatitis B dropped dramatically to nearly zero.[14,15] Stricter adherence to newer precautions and better design of sharp instruments and protective equipment should allow us to do even better.

To suggest that HIV-infected health care professionals should be diverted to professional pursuits other than those for which they have been trained seems draconian and expensive, and it fans fear in the presence of a risk that so far is incalculably small. Health care professionals represent talent that is in all-too-short supply, particularly that used to care for HIV-infected persons. Furthermore, a policy that removes HIV-positive professionals from duty without strong justification sends a dreadful message to doctors: "Don't take care of HIV-infected people — to do so you run the risk of losing your professional life."

What, then, should we do to deal with this somber public health crisis? First, let us continue to plead for moral leadership at the highest level. If taken to heart, President George Bush's words of March 29, 1990, would do much to counter the discrimination so sadly apparent almost everywhere:

We are in a fight against disease — not a fight against people, and we will not tolerate discrimination. . . . In this nation in this decade there is only one way to deal with an individual who is sick — with dignity, compassion, care, confidentiality and without discrimination. . . . Once disease strikes, we don't blame those who are suffering. We don't spurn the accident victim who didn't wear a seat belt; we don't reject the cancer patient who didn't quit smoking. We try to love them and care for them and comfort them. We don't fire them, evict them or cancel their health insurance.[16]

Second, we must move swiftly to improve the financing that will make basic health care services available to all who now lack them. There are many voices calling for such change besides that of our commission. It is time to push hard for universal coverage.

Third, we must do far better at delivering explicit, culturally appropriate education so that all will know how AIDS is transmitted and, equally important, how it is not. It is now clear that those who believe that casual contact may transmit HIV infection are the most willing to buy into harsh discriminatory measures[17,18] — thus our concern about mixed or overreactive messages. We must achieve behavioral change and make protection available to more people.[19]

Fourth, we should extend voluntary testing aggressively, particularly to pregnant women, their newborns, drug users, and others potentially at high risk. Thoughtful counseling is a key ingredient in this effort, as is swift access to health care. It is cruel and irresponsible to test people without having services in place to deal with the consequences of the test. Recent evidence suggests that most people (even intravenous drug users) will, in fact, seek testing if both counseling and health care services are available.[20]

In a world where discrimination did not exist, where medical care was more readily available, and where sound science held greater sway over national policy, we would have less panic and fewer arguments. Most Americans would step forward for HIV testing. The dimensions and directions of the epidemic would be clearer. We could provide better care, educate Americans better, and protect them better from HIV infection. We are all working toward these goals. But it is our belief that to achieve them, we need at present to go in directions quite different from those suggested in the recent editorial.

Notes

1. National Commission on Acquired Immune Deficiency Syndrome. Failure of the U.S. health care system to deal with the HIV epidemic. Report no. 1. Washington, DC: National Commission on Acquired Immune Deficiency Syndrome, 1989.

2. *Idem*. Leadership, legislation and regulation. Report no. 2. Washington, DC: National Commission on Acquired Immune Deficiency Syndrome, 1990.

3. *Idem*. Research, the workforce, and the HIV epidemic. Report no. 3. Washington, DC: National Commission on Acquired Immune Deficiency Syndrome, 1990.

4. *Idem*. HIV disease in correctional facilities. Report no. 4. Washington, DC: National Commission on Acquired Immune Deficiency Syndrome, 1991.

5. Angell M. A dual approach to the AIDS epidemic. *N Engl J Med* 1991; 324:1498-500.

6. CDC Open Meeting on the Risks of Transmission of Blood Borne Pathogens to Patients during Invasive Procedures, February 21-22, 1991. Atlanta: Centers for Disease Control, 1991. (HIV/ODD (HIV) 3-91 #002.)

7. Hardy LM, ed. HIV screening of pregnant women and newborns. Washington, DC: National Academy Press, 1991.

8. Department of Labor, Occupational Safety and Health Administration. Occupational exposure to bloodborne pathogens. *Fed Regist* 1989; 54:23042-139.

9. Relman AS, Rennie D. Treatment of end-stage renal disease: free but not equal. *N Engl J Med* 1980; 303:996-8.

10. Eggers PW. Effect of transplantation on the Medicare end-stage renal disease program. *N Engl J Med* 1988; 318:223-9.

11. Mishu B, Schaffner W, Horan JM, Wood LH, Hutcheson RH, McNabb PC. A surgeon with AIDS: lack of evidence of transmission to patients. *JAMA* 1990; 264:467-70.

12. Porter JD, Cruickshank JG, Gentle PH, Robinson RG, Gill ON. Management of patients treated by surgeon with HIV infection. *Lancet* 1990; 335:113-4.

13. Armstrong FP, Miner, JC, Wolfe WH. Investigation of a health care worker with symptomatic human immunodeficiency virus infection: an epidemiologic approach. *Milit Med* 1987; 152:414-8.

14. Working Group Convened by the New York Academy of Medicine. The risk of contracting HIV infection in the course of health care. *JAMA* 1991; 265:1872-3.

15. Estimates of the risk of endemic transmission of hepatitis B virus (HBV) and human immunodeficiency virus (HIV) to patients by the percutaneous route during invasive surgical and dental procedures. Atlanta: Centers for Disease Control, 1991.

16. Presidential address—March 29, 1990, before the National Business Leadership Conference, the White House, Washington, DC.

17. Rogers DE, Gellin BG. The bright spot about AIDS: it is very tough to catch. *AIDS* 1990; 4:695-6.

18. Friedland G, Kahl P, Saltzman B, et al. Additional evidence for lack of transmission of HIV infection by close interpersonal (casual) contact. *AIDS* 1990; 4:639-44.

19. National Commission on Acquired Immune Deficiency Syndrome. Report of Working Group on Social/Human Issues to the National Commission on AIDS. Washington, DC: National Commission on Acquired Immune Deficiency Syndrome, 1991.

20. Sittitrai W, Brown T, Sterns J. Opportunities for overcoming the continuing restraints to behavioral change and HIV risk reduction. *AIDS* 1990; 4:Suppl 1: 5269-76.

Chapter 21

AIDS Prevention for Women: A Community-based Approach

Kathleen F. Norr
Beverly J. McElmurry
Matshidiso Moeti
Sheila D. Tlou

The AIDS pandemic threatens women everywhere. This threat is especially severe for women in developing countries. According to the World Health Organization's 1991 estimates, there are about 3 million HIV-positive women in the world today, most of whom are in their childbearing years.[1] A third of the world's HIV-positive individuals are women; by the year 2000, women will account for half of the HIV-positive population.[2]

Women in developing countries are at greater risk of contracting AIDS than are women in developed countries. Of the 3 million HIV-infected women worldwide, 2.5 million are from sub-Saharan Africa.[3] Latin America and the Caribbean are the regions with the second greatest number of women who have AIDS or are HIV positive. The incidence of AIDS was relatively low in Asia throughout the early 1980s, but from 1985 there has been a rapid rise in the rate of transmission.[1] There are now at least 200,000 HIV-positive women in Asia, mainly in Thailand, India, and China, and

"AIDS Prevention for Women: A Community-based Approach," *Nursing Outlook* 40 (6), November/December 1992, pp. 250-256. Kathleen F. Norr, Ph.D., is assistant professor of sociology at The University of Illinois at Chicago; Beverly J. McElmurry, Ed.D., R.N., is professor of education at The University of Illinois at Chicago; Matshidiso Moeti, M.Sc., is the Botswana National AIDS Program Coordinator in the Ministry of Health, Gaborone, Botswana; Sheila D. Tlou, Ph.D., R.N., is a member of the faculty in Nursing Education at the University of Botswana, Gaborone. Reproduced with permission from Mosby-Year Book, Inc.

this region has the potential for rapid spread of the AIDS virus in the 1990s.[3] The only developing regions where the rate of infection remains low for both women and men are northern Africa and the Middle East.

The routes of transmission for HIV infection differ for women in different regions of the developing world, but sexual contact is the most important route. In sub-Saharan Africa, heterosexual transmission is the predominate cause of HIV transmission, with women accounting for approximately half of all cases.[4] In Latin America, the Caribbean, and Asia both intravenous drug use and sexual transmission are important routes of transmission. In these regions sexual transmission is both homosexual and heterosexual, with transmission from bisexual males being an important route in Latin America. Intravenous drug use is less common for women than for men, but women partners of intravenous drug users are at risk for HIV infection through sexual contact.

AIDS affects women directly, as sufferers of HIV infection and AIDS. HIV-infected women also face the physical and emotional burden of bearing potentially infected infants. The indirect effects of AIDS on women are also great. In their roles as the providers of family health care, women assume much of the caregiving burden for AIDS victims. Their lower earning capacities and economic dependency on men means that women who lose their partners, sons, and other family members to AIDS are often impoverished as well as burdened with the care of AIDS orphans. For women in developing countries, the AIDS epidemic will also decrease the financial and human resources available to address their other urgent health and welfare needs, such as fighting maternal mortality.[2]

Epidemiologic and Medical Models of AIDS Prevention

Approaches to AIDS prevention have largely followed two basic models, the epidemiologic and the medical. The epidemiologic model approaches AIDS prevention from the perspective of population-level reduction of transmission. For the AIDS pandemic, this has meant identifying groups or categories of persons at highest risk and targeting interventions specifically to those groups. There is much that may be said in favor of this approach, especially when the prevalence of an infection is substantially higher in some groups than in others. This approach allocates the greatest prevention effort to the groups with the greatest prevention needs.

From the perspective of women's AIDS prevention needs, however, there are several problems with this approach. Targeting of especially high-risk groups for prevention efforts may have the unintended effect of supporting the stigmatization of AIDS sufferers and the definition of AIDS as a problem of "other people," not of the community as a whole. In the United States and other developed countries, AIDS has come to be defined as a problem of homosexuals and intravenous drug users. In developing countries, higher risk groups identified include commercial sex workers and their clients, and transients such as migrant workers and truck drivers. As the epidemic spreads beyond these boundaries, this stigmatization has worked against recognition of the very real threat of AIDS to all people. This is especially true for women, who are often put at risk by the unknown or unacknowledged behaviors of their partners. Focusing AIDS prevention efforts on categories of people at higher risk may slow acceptance by the general public that it is people's *behaviors*, not their social categories, that put them at risk of HIV infection.

Another limitation of the epidemiologic model is that the highest risk groups are not necessarily the easiest groups to change. Commercial sex workers, for example, may not find it feasible to use condoms in every transaction. Community-wide AIDS prevention efforts may achieve substantial risk reduction at lower cost than efforts focused on the highest risk groups. This is not a rationale for decreasing efforts at AIDS prevention for high-risk groups. Rather, it is a plea for equal attention to the AIDS-prevention needs of the community as a whole.

The second widespread model for AIDS prevention is the medical one. The medical model focuses on the individual—that is, each individual should identify his or her own risky behaviors and then change those behaviors; health professionals should provide education and support for change for individuals. This emphasis on the individual is inappropriate for addressing behaviors that are inherently social in nature. Obviously, heterosexual transmission of AIDS occurs in the context of a social, rather than an individual, behavior. A focus on individual change does not deal with the social causes of risky behaviors, and the changes in group norms and patterns of behavior that need to occur to support change.

While the "medical model" theoretically supports both prevention and treatment, there is a strong tendency to focus more on diagnosis and treatment when AIDS is defined as a medical problem. Now that drug therapy is available to slow seroconversion, early identification of HIV-positive status is increasingly relevant in developed countries. In developing countries, however, these treatments are usually unaffordable. Slowing the AIDS pandemic will require intensive prevention efforts. Allocating too large a proportion of AIDS efforts to treatment, rather than prevention, and its focus on individuals makes the medical model a limited approach to AIDS prevention.

The epidemiologic and the medical models are top-down approaches to change. The health professionals and government officials decide on a plan at the top and then implement it in the community. Opportunities for community input into the setting of priorities and determining the basic approaches to AIDS prevention are few.

The Botswana Project

Our community-based approach to AIDS prevention for women grew out of a model project at the University of Illinois headed by Dr. Beverly

McElmurry. Community-based teams of trained residents and a nurse work to promote health in two low-income inner-city communities in Chicago. Key elements of this program, which has been described elsewhere,[5] include: recognition of women as key health promoters for families and communities; acceptance of primary health care as a global strategy for providing the minimum essential health care needs; recognition of the interaction between health and social conditions, stressing self-care and community competency in maintaining basic health; and development of collaboration among health professionals, universities, and community members to define health problems and work toward their resolution. This collaboration of health professionals and residents provides an appropriate strategy for AIDS prevention in many countries.

We are implementing and evaluating this model for women in Botswana. A brief description of the country, its health resources, and its AIDS-prevention needs follows.

Botswana and Its Health System

The Republic of Botswana, about the size of Texas, lies at the center of the southern African plateau, bounded by South Africa, Namibia, Zambia, and Zimbabwe. The Botswana government reports that its per capita income of U.S. $1,600 is one of the highest in sub-Saharan Africa.[6] Nevertheless, the country remains predominately rural, and wealth remains unequally distributed, with more than half of the total number of cattle (about 4 million) owned by only 5 percent of the households.[7] The population of Botswana is about 1.5 million, small relative to the size of the country but growing rapidly. Most of the population belong to the eight major tribes of Botswana who share a common heritage and speak the same language.[6]

The government of Botswana is committed to a strategy of providing primary health care as the best way of improving people's health and promoting development. Since becoming independent in 1966, Botswana has worked to implement a primary health care delivery system, and approximately 90 percent of the population now live within walking distance (15 km) of a health facility. Nurses are the backbone of the country's health care delivery system. Most of the time they are the only professionals in health care facilities because of the scarcity of medical doctors. They are thus responsible for the provision of promotive, preventive, curative, and rehabilitative health care to the whole population. This includes supervision of primary health care workers and mobilization of communities, especially women, for self-care.

The primary health care system has made substantial gains in overall health. Tuberculosis remains the most serious health problem, followed by acute respiratory disease and diarrheal diseases. Sexually transmitted diseases also occur in large numbers; gonorrhea alone accounts for 3 percent of all outpatient treatments. The fertility rate is 5.0 percent, and approximately 40 percent of the women use some form of contraceptives. The overall mortality rate is now 9.7 per 1000, and life expectancy is 60.2 years. In the 25 years since independence, the infant mortality rate has fallen from over 100 per 1,000 to 37.[8]

AIDS in Botswana

The first case of AIDS in Botswana was identified in 1985, and the number of AIDS cases identified in Botswana is still relatively small. As of January 1991, 180 cases had been identified and there have been 59 AIDS-related deaths.[8] Among diagnosed cases, there are more females than males. Heterosexual transmission is the major route of AIDS transmission. Routine testing of blood donors has found HIV-seropositivity rates of 5 percent to 7 percent among donors in urban areas and 1 percent to 2 percent in rural areas (M.M., personal communication, August 15, 1991). There are 20,000 to 47,000 HIV-positive individuals in Botswana now.[8] Several of Botswana's near neighbors have high rates of HIV seropositivity,[9] and many workers from neighboring countries are drawn to Botswana in search of jobs each year. All these facts document that AIDS infection is a serious public health problem in Botswana. A widespread AIDS epidemic would have a devastating impact on the nation's health, economy, and social life.

Women's AIDS Prevention Needs

Women in Botswana, like women throughout the world, are key to family and community health because of their vital roles as mothers, health care providers, and decision makers in the home environment and related health areas.[10,11,12] Women in Botswana are traditionally the custodians of health care in their communities. As mothers-in-law and grandmothers, they are the major decision makers and educators on matters pertaining to the health of the family. Most women, even those in rural areas, belong to women's organizations such as YWCA, Girl Guides, Emang Basadi, and Botswana Council of Women. These organizations are an important source for positive change in Botswana society and the overall improvement in the quality of life.

Women in Botswana are an especially relevant group for the prevention of AIDS transmission. There have been more women than men among reported AIDS cases in Botswana, and the women identified have been young. Unlike other African countries, Botswana has almost no commercial sex industry. Relatively weak partner ties, frequent break-ups, and occasional multiple partners put most women in their childbearing years at moderate risk of HIV infection from their own and their partners' behavior. Urban women who frequent bars in search of casual sex are especially vulnerable, as are widows and separated women, wives of migrant workers, partners of immigrants from countries with higher rates of HIV infection, and women with untreated sexually transmitted diseases. The increasing sexual activity rates of unmarried teens makes them another high-risk group. Reducing AIDS transmission for women will also reduce perinatal transmission.

As a group, Botswana women have strong motivation to prevent AIDS transmission. Women as the caretakers of family health will bear a heavy burden if they, their children, or any of their relatives contract HIV infection. Women will still need strong support for behavioral change. The generally greater power of men over women in relationships makes it difficult for many women to ascertain the risky behaviors their partners may engage in outside of their own relationship. This same relative lack of power may make it difficult for women to bargain for safer sex practices with their partners. Strong support from other women may be an important strategy for empowering women to protect themselves and their children from HIV infection. The many women's groups that are very important to women's social lives are a potential mechanism for peer-based prevention of AIDS transmission among women. In Botswana, women have groups and leaders that may be mobilized to implement a peer education model for prevention of AIDS transmission.

The intervention. A two-stage study of the effectiveness of nurse-managed peer education/support groups for AIDS prevention for women is in its second year of operation. In the first phase qualitative interviews with more than 50 urban women explored their current risk of HIV infection and the risk-reduction strategies likely to be helpful for them. Simultaneously, our networking with the Botswana Council of Women and other women's groups identified groups interested in taking on the issue of AIDS prevention. They will provide leadership for the project, and they have collaborated to develop ways of implementing the intervention they feel would be effective. Based on this information, a culturally specific peer education intervention for AIDS prevention, including a training workshop for peer leaders, has been developed.

The pilot will be initiated in several sites in Gaborone, the largest city, and its effectiveness will be evaluated through preintervention and postintervention comparisons with similar control groups of women. If effective, the project will expand in three stages to other cities and rural areas. Gradually, full leadership and control of the project will be assumed by the women's groups who are providing the leaders for the peer groups.

The Botswana team is centered in the Ministry of Health, with substantial collaboration with the University of Botswana and with the many community-based women's groups established there. This means that the initial creation of the project team has already begun the process of building collaborative relationships between the community and health professionals. This collaboration is compatible with the primary health care model.

Our community-based approach to AIDS prevention for women also differs from the medical and epidemiologic models in its strategy for change, the target group focus, and the content or message. In developing each of these components, we have considered the explicit needs of women and the resources available to them in Botswana.

Strategy for change. This model uses peer education/support groups led by trained community women coordinated by a nurse. The peer education model focuses specifically on the supports needed to achieve lasting behavioral changes that promote health. The peer group model is congruent with the primary health care model, and grew out of the general self-help movement to empower people to take control of their own health. Successful examples of this approach in the United States include Alcoholics Anonymous and Weight Watchers. Well-organized women's groups that already exist in Botswana will provide a source of natural leaders that may be tapped to initiate peer education.

The peer education model is strengthened considerably by linking the peer education leaders with an experienced health professional. In the United States our demonstration project and research has shown that a professional nurse may be an effective leader of trained community residents at a reasonable cost.[5] When difficult behaviors with serious health risks to individuals are the target of intervention, nonprofessional group leaders can encounter problems that their training and background do not equip them to handle appropriately. Peer group leaders need a mechanism to continuously update their own knowledge base and to make sure they convey correct and current information. More important, specific individuals in the group may periodically require more intensive counseling and referral to health services than the peer group leader can provide. Linking the peer education leaders to a nurse will ensure that the more costly counseling and medical referral services are available when needed but are not wasted in broad screening efforts. This link will also ensure that peer group leaders know where to refer group members and that the relevant referral groups are prepared to deal with increased demand for condoms, blood tests, and treatment of sexually transmitted diseases. A team of a professional nurse and trained community residents integrates complementary strengths to support risk-reducing behavioral changes.

The peer education model explicitly recognizes that achieving health-promoting behavioral change is not just a matter of education. Many behaviors that put individuals at risk for health problems are complex patterns of behavior that give those individuals specific gratifications and frequently involve not just the individual but that person's whole network of social relationships and value systems. Accomplishing lasting change of such complex patterns of behavior requires a difficult and lengthy process of change.

First, individuals must recognize their personal behaviors that put them at risk for negative consequences. Then they can identify what they wish to change and recognize barriers to change in their own lives as well as internal and external resources they can use to help themselves achieve desired changes. Where complex behaviors are involved, change is rarely a single transition. Rather, people make a series of small steps toward their desired goals, with false starts, reversions to old habits or relapses, and new beginnings. The peer education model uses the group process to provide continuing education and support through the challenging process of behavioral change and to gradually establish new group norms about the importance and acceptability of AIDS prevention behaviors.

This model is especially appropriate for AIDS prevention, where decreasing risk involves adopting safer sex practices. There is probably no area of human behavior more difficult to change. Sexual practices are intertwined with ongoing social relationships, and are intimately connected to social and personal values, and self-identity. In most societies, sexual practices also involve an unequal relationship between the sexes that may make it especially difficult for women to adopt safer sexual practices without support. In addition, sexual practices are usually considered highly personal, and are very difficult for people to discuss. All these factors make the peer education approach a particularly strong strategy for reducing the risk of heterosexual transmission of AIDS. Peer group support for behavioral change has been effective in increasing condom use among homosexual and bisexual men in the United States,[13] and among Nairobi prostitutes.[14] This important prevention strategy has not, however, been implemented for ordinary women in a community.

Target group. This community-based approach will include all women in the community. In both developed and developing countries, women in their childbearing years are most likely to become infected with AIDS, and women who are commercial sex workers, intravenous drug users, or who have multiple sex partners are at especially high risk. Still, all women are potential victims of the direct or indirect effects of AIDS. Women often cannot accurately assess their full risk of HIV infection because their partner's undisclosed behaviors may put them at risk. In addition, a woman who is at low risk at one point in time may increase her level of risk if her life circumstances change. The grandmother who loses an adult son or daughter to AIDS and must care for her orphaned grandchildren has as great an interest in AIDS prevention as anyone in the community. All women need to recognize the threat of AIDS and work to support AIDS prevention for the entire community, not just for themselves. Women at different ages, in different life circumstances, and from different ethnic, religious, and regional groups may needs AIDS preventions tailored to their special needs and resources. The need for culturally sensitive and individualized AIDS prevention programs, should not be minimized. Nevertheless, there is an urgent need to reach *all* women, not just those who may belong to a high-risk group.

Content. Heterosexual transmission is the most important route of HIV infection for women worldwide, especially in developing countries. Therefore promotion of safer sex is the focus of the Botswana intervention. In countries where other routes of infection are also important, these would, of course, need to be added.

The promotion of safer sex as a strategy for AIDS prevention has many advantages. Promoting safer sex has minimal dollar costs and does not require expensive laboratory tests or health care services. Behavioral changes to promote safer sex have no physical risks to participants. If safer sex practices are introduced, this will substantially reduce the transmission of HIV infection directly by reducing sexual transmission, the most prevalent source of HIV transmission, and indirectly reduce perinatal transmission. In a society where children are highly valued and more women than men have been currently diagnosed with AIDS, the need to prevent perinatal transmission should have strong support. Many women and their partners who might find behavioral change difficult when considering only themselves will be highly motivated to make changes to protect their children. Promotion of safer sex practices among teenagers is also important because young people face the highest lifetime potential risk because of the longer years of exposure ahead of them.

Promotion of safer sexual practices offers multiple health benefits in addition to AIDS prevention. The same practices that prevent AIDS transmission also protect against other sexually transmitted diseases. These other sexually transmitted diseases, including gonorrhea, syphilis, and chlamydiosis, have high prevalence rates in Botswana, are costly to treat, and represent an important health problem. Safer sex practices will also reduce unintended pregnancies. Unintended pregnancies disrupt the educational attainments of young mothers and have high social and economic costs for the individual families involved and for the society as a whole. Their reduction, especially among unmarried teens, is an important goal. Safer sex practices will also promote child spacing, which is beneficial to the health of the mother and infant.

The message promoting safer sex needs to be sensitive to the context of women's lives. Having children is an important goal for many women. In many AIDS-prevention campaigns, the major behavioral change promoted is the use of condoms. Condom use is effective and avoids the issues of partner trust and moral judgments that emerge in promotion of sexually exclusive relationships. Condom promotion will not be acceptable to women at the time in their lives when they wish to bear a child, and condom use requires a cooperative male partner. Women need to learn how to reduce the risk of HIV infection throughout their lives. Other strategies for reducing the risk of sexual transmission of HIV infection include abstinence or postponement of sexual activity until young people are mature enough to act responsibly; having sexually exclusive relationships or reducing the number of sexual partners; avoiding sexual behaviors such as anal intercourse that are more likely to transmit HIV infection; and maintaining general health, especially by avoiding and treating promptly other sexually transmitted diseases. Women need to know about all of these risk-reducing strategies, their relative risks and limitations, and their appropriateness at different times and for different women.

Implementation for Women Cross-Culturally

This community-based AIDS prevention program, unlike programs based on the epidemiologic or medical model, is consistent with the philosophy of primary health care. Supporting AIDS prevention for all women in the community is compatible with the primary health care goal of access to essential elements of health care for all. This approach also avoids stigmatizing AIDS as a problem of "other people," and helps to define it as a community-wide problem. Rather than being designed top-down, the content and organization of the intervention is developed through collaboration with community leaders and existing groups right from the beginning. Early collaboration enhances the likelihood that this program will be sustainable by building the commitment and experience of community leaders and groups. The participatory process also builds ties for future collaboration around community health issues. Involving existing leaders and groups in project development, as well as through in-depth interviews with ordinary women, helps to ensure that the program's message and format is culturally sensitive and responsive to community needs and interests. Recognizing the wide variation in women's needs for AIDS prevention, and the behavioral changes they are willing and able to adopt, is especially important in developing culturally sensitive and individually appropriate education and behavior. The program is also affordable. It does not require costly and high-tech testing or treatment, requires only limited access to health professionals, and uses existing community resources and leaders. Promotion of safer sex practices will also address related community health needs by reducing other sexually transmitted diseases and unintended pregnancies.

This approach also explicitly recognizes that AIDS prevention is integrated into an economic and sociocultural context that must be taken into account. Specifically, women live in societies with gender inequalities in power, status, and independent control over resources. This is a major reason for focusing on women only, at least initially. Women are often in relationships where they feel little power or control over the terms of their sexual activities. Coming together with other women allows women to develop mutual support mechanisms to maximize their protection from AIDS in the context of their own lives. Eventually, women and men will need to address AIDS prevention issues together. Attempting to do this initially is not likely to succeed because the dialogue and the program will be dominated by men. An initial focus on women may be seen as exclusionary, but we feel it is compatible with the underlying philosophy of primary health care.

This research identifies a cost-effective and culturally sensitive strategy for community-based AIDS prevention among women that should have relevance for women in other developed and developing countries. If the model proves to be effective, it may be replicated widely at relatively little cost. Successful development of a peer group model of AIDS prevention for all women in Botswana and documentation of its effectiveness will be an important contribution to the prevention of heterosexual transmission of AIDS in Botswana and other developing countries. This study will also be highly relevant to the United States, where heterosexual transmission is the fastest growing route of HIV infection.

Notes

1. Palca J. The sobering geography of AIDS. *Science* 1991; 252:373-3.

2. Petros-Barvazian A, Merson MH. Women and AIDS, a challenge for humanity. *World Health* 1990; November-December:4-6.

3. Chin J. Challenge of the nineties. *World Health* 1990; November-December:4-6.

4. Piot P, Carael M. Epidemiological and sociological aspects of HIV-infection in developing countries. *Br Med Bull* 1988; 44:68-88.

5. McElmurry BJ, Swider SM, Norr KL. A community-based primary health care program for integration of research, practice, and education. In: Schaperow R, ed. *Curriculum revolution: community building and activism.* New York: National League for Nursing Press, 1991.

6. Botswana Government. *Country profile 1985.* Gaborone: Government Printer, 1986.

7. Staugard F. *Traditional medicine.* Gaborone: Ipelegeng Publishers, 1985.

8. Ministry of Finance and Development Planning. *National development plan 7, 1991-1997.* Gaborone: Government Printer, 1991.

9. Carswell JW. Impact of AIDS in the developing world. *Br Med Bull* 1988; 44:183-202.

10. World Federation of Public Health Associations. *Women and health.* Geneva: World Federation of Public Health Associations, 1986.

11. World Health Organization. Women as providers of health care. *WHO Chronicle* 1983; 37: 134-8.

12. World Health Organization. Women in health development: the view from the Americas. *WHO Chronicle* 1984; 38:249-55.

13. Valdiserri RO, Lyter DW, Leviton LC, Callahan CM, Kingsley LA, Rinaldo CR. AIDS prevention in homosexual and bisexual men: results of a randomized trial evaluating two risk reduction interventions. *AIDS* 1988; 3:21-6.

14. Ngugi EN, Simonsen JN, Plummer FA. Prevention of transmission of human immunodeficiency virus in Africa: effectiveness of condom promotion and health education among prostitutes. *Lancet* 1988; 2:887-90.

Chapter 22

Living Positively with AIDS

Janie Hampton

Introduction

The AIDS Support Organization (TASO) is the first organized community response to the AIDS epidemic in Uganda. Founded by a group of volunteers in late 1987, TASO now provides over 2,000 people with HIV or AIDS, and their families, with counseling, information, medical and nursing care, and material assistance.

Most TASO workers are themselves people with HIV or AIDS. They know that they may not have long to live. Yet TASO is not pervaded by gloom and despair. On the contrary, it is an organization in which there is an amazing amount of laughter, good humor, and infectious enthusiasm. There is always a sympathetic ear to listen to personal problems and a shoulder to weep on if necessary. But TASO's workers have an overwhelming positive approach to life. They embody the organization's commitment to "living positively with AIDS."

This [article] is about that commitment, and how it can be translated into practical action in the face of the prejudice, discrimination and fear that have been generated by the threat of AIDS.

AIDS in Uganda

The first cases of acquired immune deficiency syndrome (AIDS) in Uganda were reported in Rakai District, to the west of Lake Victoria, in

"Living Positively with AIDS," *Strategies for Hope* (2), February 1990, pp. 1-25. *Strategies for Hope* is a publication of The AIDS Support Organization (TASO), Uganda. Janie Hampton, who has written several books on health care in developing countries, is based in Oxford, England. Copyright © Janie Hampton and G & A Williams, 1990. Reprinted with permission.

1982. Since then the number of cases reported each month nationwide has doubled every six months. By December 1988 over 5,000 cases had been reported to the national AIDS Control Program, but these are only a small fraction of the total.[1]

The number of people infected with human immunodeficiency virus (HIV) — the virus which causes AIDS — is many times greater than the number of AIDS cases. Surveys in some urban areas of Uganda have found 15-25 percent of people in the sexually active age group to be infected.[2] At the Mulago Hospital in Kampala, the prevalence of HIV infection among patients admitted for medical treatment increased from 10 percent in late 1986 to 50 percent two years later.[3]

In Uganda, as elsewhere in Africa, transmission of HIV is mainly through heterosexual intercourse and from mother to unborn child. Men and women are affected in equal numbers. AIDS in Uganda affects all members of the family — either directly or indirectly. (In the industrialized world, by contrast, AIDS affects mainly single people.) The age of first being diagnosed HIV-positive ranges from around 18 to 30 years for women and from 17 to 37 years for men. The numbers of children born with HIV infection are increasing.

AIDS is an expensive disease. The medicines are costly, and patients are unable to work but need more food. Many Ugandans with AIDS never get to an AIDS clinic because they are too poor or too weak to travel and wait in a long hospital queue. Better-off patients tend to live longer and enjoy a better quality of life because they can afford to buy nutritious food and to pay for medical care and drugs.

For the people of Uganda, AIDS is part of a cumulative catastrophe. The country's economy and social infrastructure are only just beginning to recover from nearly 20 traumatic years of civil war and unrest. The damage has been enormous and recovery is painfully slow. Hospitals and health centers are run-down, and essential drugs and equipment in short supply or non-existent. Many health professionals have either left the country or taken other jobs because their salaries were so low. There are, for example, only five doctors for every 100,000 people.

The Ugandan health services, on their own, cannot possibly cope with the rapidly escalating numbers of people with AIDS who need medical and nursing care, as well as social, psychological, and material support. Government services need to join forces with community organizations in caring for people with AIDS and their families. That is why the emergence of an organization such as TASO is so important.

Origins of TASO

TASO has its origins in a small group of people who began meeting in one another's homes in Kampala in October 1986. The group consisted of a truck driver, two soldiers, a veterinarian's assistant, an office boy, an accountant, a physiotherapist, a nurse, a school teacher and a social scientist. All but one had HIV or AIDS. They met to exchange information, to give one another support and encouragement, and to pray.

In January 1987 one member of the group, Chris Kaleeba, died. His wife Noerine was devastated: "I just went to pieces. I knew that Chris was going to die, but when it happened it was just too much. I took my children and left Kampala to go and stay with my parents."

Three months later, when she returned to Kampala, Noerine Kaleeba was determined to do something practical to help people with AIDS and their families. The group which she and Chris had helped to start began meeting once more, and a few new members joined. When TASO was formally established in November 1987, the group consisted of seventeen people, including twelve who had HIV or AIDS (all of whom have since died).

The founding members of TASO had no training in counselling or experience of managing an AIDS support group. There were no precedents for such groups in Africa from which they could learn. They had no office, no transport and no funds. But what they did have was initiative, vision and a deep commitment to practical action on behalf of people with HIV and AIDS, who were being neglected by the health services and ostracized by the rest of society. It was this combination which persuaded two British organizations—ActionAid and World in Need—to provide TASO with the funds to get started. ActionAid also arranged for two founding members of TASO to participate in a one-week training course for AIDS counsellors in London.

All those involved in starting TASO were practicing Christians who regularly prayed together, but they made a conscious decision to make TASO a non-religious organization: "We want to be open to everyone," says founding Director Noerine Kaleeba. "Everyone should feel equally at home in TASO."

Although TASO is a non-governmental organization, another key factor in its establishment was the open and constructive attitude of the Ugandan Government. "One cannot rely on government funding, but the government's blessing is necessary," says Noerine Kaleeba. "We have been very fortunate. Uganda's National AIDS Control Program is run by creative and adaptable people, with a helpful attitude."

Language

At TASO the word "AIDS" is rarely used. People with HIV or AIDS are described as being "body positive." They are referred to as "clients," never as "AIDS victims" or "AIDS sufferers." The term "patient" is used only if a client is admitted to hospital. TASO is also sensitive to words like "catastrophe," "plague," and press statements such as "This person is going to die." "We are all going to die sometime, so why pick on a few of us?" said one TASO client. "I have already lived longer than my father, who died of malaria."

Some TASO clients are also annoyed by government slogans such as "I said NO to AIDS": "No one has ever said 'Yes to AIDS,'" says Susie, a TASO client and counsellor. "None of us have asked for it. Most of us who have it now had never even heard of it when we caught it. You cannot attach blame or assign guilt to anyone. It doesn't matter who was responsible—the husband or the wife or the blood transfusion. The important thing is to think and live positively."

Organization

TASO has two offices—one in Kampala and the other in Masaka, 80 miles to the southwest. These are open from Monday to Friday and clients can come without appointment. Most counsellors, however, work only part-time for TASO, so clients make an appointment if they want to see a particular counsellor. A file is kept on every client, with details of hospital admissions, medical treatment, material support, visits, and family conditions. Clients are allowed to read their own files.

TASO Kampala's office is a modest, unmarked room in Mulago Hospital, a collection of run-down buildings near the center of the city. A separate building, known as the "development unit," is used as a training center and a meeting place. Also in the hospital grounds is a day center where TASO clients and their families can meet. People come together at the center to make friends, share information and express their feelings in a safe, friendly atmosphere. Lunch is provided every day for clients, visitors, and any TASO workers who happen to be present. Taking meals together is an important part of demonstrating that HIV is not transmitted by sharing cups, plates and other eating utensils. Every Friday, all TASO workers come to the day center to share a meal with co-workers and clients, and to exchange ideas and discuss problems.

The day center is also equipped with four treadle sewing machines which clients use to make clothes and sheets for sale. One client, a talented artist, makes batik hangings which are sold to benefit both the client and TASO.

Places for rest are available for anyone who feels tired and needs to lie down for a short while. Young children are always welcome: their numbers are greatest on Fridays, when the AIDS clinic for children is held in the hospital.

Clients

TASO's clients are people with HIV or AIDS, and their families. In March 1989 there were 140 adult clients registered with TASO Kampala and 85 with TASO Masaka. Some male clients may have wives and families living in distant rural areas who may also be infected with HIV, but are not registered with TASO.

TASO Kampala works within ten miles of the city center, so their clients are urban and mostly of middle or low socio-economic status. Most are referred to TASO by the two AIDS clinics at Mulago Hospital, and some by other hospitals or private clinics.

TASO Masaka's clients are mostly rural, subsistence farmers referred from the AIDS clinic at Masaka Hospital. Some clients come straight to the TASO office after hearing about the organization from friends, and TASO then refers them to the AIDS clinic in the local government hospital for diagnosis.

Some clients want TASO to take over responsibility for everything — finances, food and housing, as well as emotional stress. TASO does not have the resources to do this, and in any case does not want to become simply a "hand-out" organization.

"The main objective," says TASO Director Noerine Kaleeba, "is to help people to come together and discuss things and feel accepted. The sense of belonging restores their dignity. It's much better if they can come out and have some activities and friends. Otherwise quite a few would just give up."

But not everyone who is offered counselling and other support from TASO takes up the offer. AIDS carries a powerful stigma, fuelled by fear and ignorance, and some people are afraid that TASO will tell their employers, or that their workmates or neighbors may learn that they are HIV-positive. Others fear they will be asked too many questions, or be blamed for contracting the disease. Some try to deny they have AIDS by moving house and changing their jobs, or even their names. (They may then continue to spread the virus through sexual activity.) Others reject the offer of counselling and medical care in the belief that it cannot help them. Some believe they have been bewitched or have not observed the correct rituals, and so seek treatment from "witch doctors" or traditional healers. Many ignore the problem until they are too ill to make plans for their families.

Confidentiality is of prime importance to all TASO clients. There is no sign outside the TASO office, and only one of the organization's four vehicles is identified as belonging to TASO. Several clients have specifically asked that this vehicle should not come near their homes. Some clients are able to work through the initial fear of being identified as a person with HIV or AIDS. Others, however, risk losing their jobs and homes, or being rejected by their spouses.

Noerine Kaleeba is well-known in Kampala as the Director of TASO, so she reassures new clients and counsellors that, for their own privacy, she will not greet them in public places: "Everyone knows what I do, so if someone sees me giving you a hug, they may start spreading rumors."

Staff

TASO Kampala employs seven full-time staff and seventeen part-time counsellors, trainers and advisors. The full-timers consist of the Director (Noerine Kaleeba), an accountant, a publicity officer, an administrator, a secretary, a driver, and a cook/cleaner. The part-time workers consist of a medical adviser, three counsellor/trainers, twelve counsellors and an honorary legal adviser.

TASO Masaka employs a part-time medical adviser and a full-time office messenger. The twelve part-time counsellors in Masaka include two nurses, a social worker, a medical assistant, a school teacher, and several unemployed people with HIV or AIDS.

TASO follows a policy of actively recruiting people who are HIV-positive, especially as counsellors. Many first come into contact with TASO as clients and then decide to become actively involved in the organization. They fall ill more often than healthy people and several have died since starting work with TASO. This causes a lack of continuity in TASO's work, but Noerine Kaleeba believes that the advantages of employing people with HIV far outweigh the disadvantages: "People with AIDS are a special asset to TASO as counsellors. They are closer to the clients and make them feel more normal. They can talk from personal experience of the emotions and problems caused by AIDS, and can help people overcome them."

Counsellors have about ten clients each, whom they visit at home once every week or fortnight. A counsellor remains with the same client from the diagnosis of HIV infection until death. Even when a client has died, the counsellor remains in touch with the family, which may contain other people with AIDS or orphaned children. Counsellors are accountable to their clients, but also report to the TASO doctors, their supervisors, and the office administration.

All counsellors first have to complete a four-day induction course run by TASO's own training staff. They are paid 1,200 Ugandan shillings (US$4.80) a day, and also receive a free lunch and transport to their clients' homes. Counsellors who are HIV-positive continue to receive material support such as eggs and school fees for their children.

Once a week all counsellors meet for a whole afternoon to discuss the progress of their clients as well as their own problems. The stress of working with terminally ill patients can lead to conflicts requiring quick resolution.

Medical Care

Medication is provided free to clients under medical supervision, as long as supplies (or funds to purchase them) are available. The drugs are given out at the TASO office, at the AIDS clinics in hospital, and on home visits.

TASO receives some drugs as donations and purchases others locally.

Drug supplies, however, are far from adequate. In 1988, for example, TASO budgeted $5,000 for expenditure on all drugs, but eventually had to spend $8,000 on supplies of a single product, *Nizoral* (for the treatment of oral thrush), which cost 500 Uganda shillings (US$2) per tablet on the open market.

Some TASO clients have reported relief from certain AIDS symptoms after taking herbal medicines, but these have not yet been tested scientifically. Research on certain herbal preparations, however, is now in progress.

Both TASO branches have a medical adviser, who is paid a token sum of 2,000 Shillings (US$8) a month for attending TASO clients one to three mornings a week, and whenever a TASO client needs urgent medical attention. They also run separate HIV/AIDS clinics for adults and children once a week in hospital, seeing up to 45 patients a day.

Dr. Elly Katabira, who is the medical adviser to TASO Kampala, also works as a physician at Mulago Hospital and as a Lecturer in Medicine at Makerere University. When he first set up an AIDS clinic at Mulago Hospital in late 1987, many of his colleagues were skeptical: "Health workers knew there was no cure for AIDS, so they assumed that people with AIDS didn't warrant any medical care. We started the AIDS clinic to show what could be done. We had to demonstrate to patients and health workers alike that people with AIDS who come in very sick can leave the hospital walking."

Dr. Katabira's AIDS clinic has been inundated with patients. By February 1989 he had seen a total of 850 adult patients—55 percent men and 45 percent women. The most common symptoms were weight loss, recurrent fevers and diarrhea.

Dr. Sam Kalibala is the medical adviser to TASO Masaka. Since his HIV/AIDS clinic opened in November 1988, the number of new clients has doubled every week. Working with TASO has changed his approach to treating people with HIV/AIDS: "I used to see people with AIDS, but before coming into contact with TASO I didn't know what to do. I didn't know what to tell them because I felt I couldn't do much for them. So we were hiding the diagnosis. It was too painful to tell them. But when I heard about positive living with AIDS, I saw there was something that could be done—for example, by counselling people before and after the HIV test."

Patients are usually referred to an AIDS clinic on the basis of their clinical history. The doctor at the clinic takes the patient's history and either makes a clinical diagnosis or offers the patient an HIV test. If the patient agrees to undergo the test—and providing HIV test kits are available at the time—a blood sample is taken. The result is usually available a week later. If the test is negative, a TASO counsellor explains how the patient can avoid becoming infected with HIV. If the patient asks for condoms the counsellor provides some free of charge and also explains how to use them correctly.

If the result is positive, the doctor explains the implications to the patient: "When I make an AIDS diagnosis," says Dr. Katabira, "I have to tell the patient that there is no cure for the virus, but there is a lot that can be done to treat the infections that may come along as a result of HIV infection. The period from HIV infection to death is usually less than two years, but it may be up to five years."

TASO counsellors are also on hand at the clinic to offer clients counselling and other support. Often, however, the clinics are packed and if only one or two counsellors are on hand it is impossible to meet and talk with all potential clients. At the time of the initial diagnosis clients are usually in such a state of shock that in-depth counselling is not possible. Counsellors concentrate on reassuring them that they are not about to die, and arrange to visit them at home within the next week.

Children's Clinic

An AIDS clinic for children is held every Friday morning at Mulago hospital in Kampala. Over 140 children with HIV/AIDS are registered with the clinic, and more than 30 are brought for diagnosis or treatment every week.

Most of the children are babies or toddlers. Babies infected with HIV develop AIDS more quickly than adults. Few survive beyond the age of two years, and many die before being diagnosed as having AIDS. Most die within a year of birth, often of dehydration or malnutrition due to repeated diarrhea and other infections. Many are not brought to the AIDS clinic until they are already close to death.

TASO counsellors talk with mothers as they sit on a low wall, suckling their babies before seeing the doctor. The nurse calls the mothers into a small room where Doctor Laura Guay sits close to them, clicking and smiling at the babies. She asks the mother how the baby is this week and examines the baby gently, feeling for swollen lymph nodes, listening to the chest, and looking in the mouth for thrush. Many babies require ampicillin for chest infections, others are given oral rehydration salts for diarrhea. Whenever the drugs run out TASO provides whatever it can until the hospital's supplies are replenished.

Blood tests are usually necessary to diagnose HIV infection in babies and young children because the symptoms of AIDS in young children are similar to many other children's diseases. But taking blood often involves a struggle. Doctors and nurses may have to take blood without the protection of rubber gloves simply because there are not enough gloves available. Inevitably, blood is spilled from time to time. Dr. Katabira insists that the safety risk is negligible: "It's quite safe as long as you wash your hands well with soap and water afterwards. The main danger of infection is not from HIV but from diseases such as TB, hepatitis or typhoid."

All the mothers of babies and young children with AIDS are themselves HIV-positive. They may discover this only when their babies are diagnosed.

Hospital Admissions

People with AIDS are admitted to the hospital whenever they require in-patient treatment, which is given free of charge. Severe dehydration after diarrhea or vomiting is the most common reason for admission. Most diseases associated with AIDS are treatable. Surgery, however, is used only very sparingly because of the risk of precipitating AIDS in a person with HIV infection by further weakening the body's immune system.

Mulago Hospital does not systematically test in-patients for HIV infection. However desirable it might be to do so, there are simply not enough AIDS testing kits available. Diagnosis is usually done on the basis of a physical examination. Many hospital patients are admitted, treated and discharged without the staff knowing that they are infected with HIV. Nurses are not issued gloves for general nursing care, but are taught to be careful and to wash their hands thoroughly after contact with patients.

The hospital does not have a special AIDS ward. Dr. Katabira believes that such a ward is not justifiable and could lead to other problems: "A special AIDS ward would increase the stigmatization of people with AIDS. These patients are no more of a risk in a general ward than other patients. We believe that all patients should be nursed and managed in the same way, as if they were all HIV-positive."

In any case the problem of AIDS is already too enormous to be dealt with by separating AIDS patients into a single hospital ward. In Kampala alone it would be necessary to allocate up to half of all hospital wards to AIDS patients, and there are no valid medical grounds for doing this. "Every AIDS patient," says Dr. Katabira, "is admitted with a different problem. They cannot all be lumped together."

Home Care

TASO counsellors try to visit clients once a week at home, unless clients prefer to come to the TASO office. Counselling is done in the local language whenever possible. TASO counsellors spend a great deal of time listening to clients and their families talk about their problems. Rather than prescribing solutions, they aim to provide their clients with information about how they can look after themselves and lead positive lives. Noerine Kaleeba is convinced that this approach is effective: "People with HIV can live positively by gaining morale, rather than giving up. They can choose to eat good nutritious foods, and not to smoke or drink alcohol. They can get immediate medical care for every infection. Through positive living, people with HIV can make the most of their remaining time and even extend it."

Home care has many advantages over hospital care. It enables the counsellor to assess the client's social and economic situation. It also helps to break down or prevent the sense of isolation experienced by many people with HIV and AIDS. Home care also brings the counsellor into contact with other members of the client's family.

Ugandan families have been caring for their sick relatives for generations. There is a great deal that family members can do to protect the health and prolong the lives of their loved ones with HIV/AIDS. By adopting a loving, positive attitude, they can help to maintain the person's morale. They can also make sure that the person eats well and gets prompt treatment for infections.

First, however, family members need to be reassured that they are not at risk of contracting AIDS through casual contact with the infected person. The TASO counsellor demonstrates this in practical ways—for example, by sharing cups, eating utensils and food with the client. Relatives may also be worried about bedding and clothes which become soiled with feces or blood. The counsellor demonstrates how to make these items safe by soaking them in a bleach solution or simply washing them with soap and hot water and drying them in the sun. Both methods kill the virus.

Material Assistance

Each TASO client receives free of charge thirty eggs a month and four kilos of milk powder. Other foods such as cocoa-mix, baby porridge and flavored drink powder are handed out as and when TASO receives them. This is not entirely satisfactory as the supply is erratic and the food is not all nutritionally sound.

Second-hand clothes, whenever available, are also given to families according to need. Condoms supplied by USAID are provided free. TASO has also produced a leaflet in Luganda (the main local language) about the use of condoms.[4]

School fees are paid for some children of TASO clients or deceased clients. Every effort is made to keep children at the same school, unless the cost is prohibitive or the child has to move to relatives in another area.

Orphans

One of the most agonizing worries of people with AIDS is the fate of their children after they die. In Uganda it is traditional for relatives to adopt children whose parents have both died. In recent years, however, some relatives have rejected children orphaned by AIDS because they do not understand how the disease is spread and are afraid of contracting it themselves. In some communities the traditional system of adoption has broken down because so many adults have died that the few surviving relatives are simply unable to bear the burden of caring for large numbers of young children.

TASO believes that orphaned children are best cared for within families rather than in orphanages. If no relatives are available, every effort should be made to place the child with friends of the deceased parents. In order to overcome prejudice against children whose parents have both died of AIDS, TASO helps clients to identify relatives or friends who can adopt their children after both parents have died. TASO counsellors also explain to potential foster parents how AIDS is spread in order to dispel misconceptions and overcome the powerful stigma associated with the disease. Together with the Save the Children Fund, TASO also provides foster parents with food, clothing and financial support to enable children orphaned by AIDS to attend school.

Training

All TASO workers — including drivers and cleaners — attend a four-day induction course which covers the basic facts about HIV and AIDS, explores the emotions of people diagnosed as being HIV-positive, and imparts basic counselling skills. Trainee counsellors start by watching experienced counsellors at work in the AIDS clinics for children and adults, and later are allocated their own clients.

This course is also open to health professionals, social workers, and religious leaders. (Twenty nuns, three Catholic priests, one Protestant pastor and one Islamic leader have so far completed the course.) Visiting journalists who wish to film or write about TASO's work are politely but firmly requested to participate in this course before interviewing TASO workers or clients.

TASO also offers a 20-week half-time certificate course in advanced AIDS counselling for counsellors who already have some training and experience. In addition, TASO organizes orientation AIDS workshops of one-to-three days duration for various types of health and social workers, as well as community and religious leaders. About 150 Catholic and Protestant leaders, for example, have so far taken part in these workshops.

Counselling the Counsellors

Counselling people with AIDS is very stressful and places the counsellors themselves under a great deal of strain. All have families of their own to care for and most have difficulties in making ends meet. However much they try to encourage their clients to live positively, the fact remains that everyone with AIDS is going to die prematurely. For those counsellors who are HIV-positive the strain is even greater. Yet the pressures on them — from clients and family members alike — are enormous and unrelenting. Inevitably there are times when the stress becomes too great. One sign of excess stress is when counsellors feel that no one appreciates their work and there is no point in carrying on. Stress may also come to the surface in arguments about management issues, or how supplies should be distributed. When everyone is under stress people do not notice when others are as well. Counsellors need to feel that their work is appreciated. They also need opportunities to share their feelings and frustrations.

When several counsellors were nearing the point of "burn-out" TASO organized a Quilt Day. Clients and workers (there is no distinction in the way they are treated) gathered at the TASO development unit with pieces of cloth and began to make a colorful patchwork quilt. Six feet long and three feet wide, the quilt was to be sent to "The Names Project," which commemorates people who have died of AIDS all over the United States. The TASO quilt is the first to be made in Africa, sewn by people with AIDS as their own memorial.

Funding

Since the establishment of TASO in November 1987, two British organizations — ActionAid and World in Need — have paid TASO's running costs (salaries, drugs, supplies, transport, office administration) and capital expenditure. In 1988, for example, the budget was $140,000, of which $40,000 was capital expenditure, mainly for the purchase of three four-wheel-drive vehicles. In 1989 TASO expects to spend approximately $300,000 on running costs and capital expenditure.

Two U.S. organizations — Experiment in International Living and USAID — have contributed funds for training and equipment. In addition, Voluntary Service Overseas (UK) has provided a trainer of counsellors for two years. The Danish Red Cross, the German Emergency Doctor Service, and the Pentecostal Church have also provided assistance, and local voluntary organizations have held fund-raising events for TASO.

The Future

In the immediate future TASO aims to train more counsellors to meet the rapidly growing needs in Kampala and Masaka. TASO also plans to help establish AIDS support groups in other parts of the country. Says Noerine Kaleeba: "These groups must be initiated by committed local people. We can show them what we have done and give them training, but it is up to each group to run itself independently. All you need is a willing doctor, counsellors and commitment."

Orientation workshops will also be organized for health professionals — from orderlies through to senior consultants — at all hospitals throughout the country, starting with Mulago Hospital in Kampala.

TASO workers are also writing a booklet on positive living with AIDS, based on their personal experiences. Also in preparation is a broadsheet explaining the aims and work of the organization, to be distributed at AIDS clinics throughout the country.

The growing demands on TASO's services also mean that there is a need for more vehicles, drugs, equipment, and physical facilities. The hired buildings currently used by TASO in Kampala are already totally inadequate, and ActionAid has pledged support for a new building which will have three offices and counselling rooms, a kitchen, toilets, a day center and a garage. This building will also be sited within the Mulago Hospital, which provides TASO's clients with a degree of anonymity and is easily accessible.

As TASO continues to expand in response to growing needs, it will inevitably encounter management and personnel problems. As in the past, the organization's staff and volunteers will identify and tackle each problem with ingenuity, commitment and good humor.

Conclusion

TASO has provided hundreds of people with HIV/AIDS, and their families, with invaluable information, medical care and material support. Perhaps even more importantly, it has helped people with HIV/AIDS regain their self-respect through playing socially useful lives within their families and communities. It has also helped change the attitudes of many health workers and community leaders towards people with HIV/AIDS.

But TASO is only one small organization within a vast sea of need. Uganda needs AIDS support groups in every town and rural district. Many other countries in Africa also need community organizations of this kind.

TASO has demonstrated that a small group of people, with some external assistance but with no previous experience, training, or institutional support, can establish an effective organization within a matter of months. What is needed, above all, is a combination of initiative, commitment, and a vision of a future in which people with HIV/AIDS will be treated with compassion and respect rather than prejudice, ignorance and fear.

Notes

1. Uganda AIDS Control Program, "Review of Uganda AIDS Control Program," December 1988.
2. Ibid.

3. Elly Katabira, "Two years experience in the AIDS Clinic in Uganda," paper presented at "Integrated AIDS Management: a Conference for Field Workers," Nairobi, 21-24 May 1989.

4. The text of this leaflet is based on *Body Positive*, a pamphlet published by the Terrence Higgins Trust in the United Kingdom.

Chapter 23

A Conference of Hope:
A New Beginning

Jonathan Mann

We come together at the start of a critical week in the history of our global confrontation with AIDS. Today, faced with an expanding pandemic, we can see — more clearly than ever before — the critical limits of our current national and global response. For the course of the pandemic within and through global society is not yet being influenced — in any substantial manner — by current efforts. We now recognize the painful reality that existing approaches to prevention — as remarkable as some of these efforts have been — will not be sufficient to stem the pandemic. The gap between the intensifying pace of the pandemic and the lagging national and global response is widening, rapidly and dangerously — and global vulnerability to AIDS is increasing.

At this critical moment — when the pandemic intensifies and complacency, lack of leadership, and loss of confidence all threaten — we must ask ourselves the most fundamental question: what will it take to prevent and control AIDS? This is the central issue — we cannot escape it.

Let us be clear: to recognize, with realism and unstinting honesty, the limits of our work thus far, and the dangers ahead, is not to yield to despair. For we know — intellectually and in our hearts — that we can control AIDS and we can care well for all those who are affected by the pandemic.

Therefore, this conference is a conference of hope — not despair. It is a summit — not of political leaders or organizations, but of people working in the front lines of every field — research, education, care, support — in coun-

"A Conference of Hope: A New Beginning," Opening Remarks to the VIII International Conference on AIDS/III STD World Congress, July 1992. Jonathan Mann, M.D., is at the Center for Health and Human Rights, Harvard School of Public Health, Boston. Reprinted with author's permission.

tries around the world. This assembly is our common meeting place. This conference is the forum in which we can see precisely where we stand — in research, prevention and care — these are the traditional goals of a conference. Yet this week, our need, our challenge, our responsibility — is greater. In order to move ahead against AIDS, with strength and confidence in the future, we must literally transform our understanding and approach to AIDS. This week is the historic opportunity to chart a new course, to change — perhaps forever — how we — and the world sees AIDS.

Why is this transformation necessary today — what does this new vision involve — and how can it be expressed — concretely and directly — in action?

It is necessary to change our current vision of AIDS because it is outdated, having been developed mainly during the early period of the pandemic, with then-available, quite limited knowledge and experience in research, prevention and care. At that time, AIDS was seen — and approached — as a separate, unique and isolated health problem. This led us, perhaps necessarily in order to mobilize effectively, to develop isolated AIDS programs, to focus prevention strategies on the behavior of individuals, to support isolated AIDS activism, and to consider research in isolation from its application.

This approach has had its successes.

- We have mobilized governments around the world — yet most national AIDS programs remain isolated from community efforts and from other health and social sectors; true national mobilizations against AIDS have not yet occurred.
- We have seen remarkable successes in HIV prevention, at the pilot project and community level — yet these successes have remained isolated and with minimal impact on the pandemic.
- We have seen activism successfully focus intense attention on inequities, inertia, and intolerance, and achieve concrete results, but we have not yet seen activism become sufficiently international, or connected with a broader view of health and society.
- We have seen important success in basic and applied research, yet that research in isolation from concern about access to its achievements has severely limited its impact on lives of people with HIV.

The basic issue before us is that — just like for any other problem — how we see AIDS, how we understand it, what we think it is really about — determines both what we do about it and also how successful we will be.

Thus, if we believe the entire problem of AIDS is really only about a virus, then we really need only a virucide or a vaccine. Yet if AIDS is deeply, fundamentally also about people and society — and if societal inequity and discrimination fuel the spread of the pandemic — then, to be effective against AIDS, we would have to address these issues.

The old vision of AIDS has now become a straitjacket. Having recognized — with realism and honesty — the critical limits of our current approach, we can start to define a new approach, taking into account the vital lessons we have learned about prevention and care—not as theory, but as lessons grounded in the experience, knowledge, and lives of people worldwide.

First, we have seen that HIV exploits societal weaknesses, and the major fault-lines in society along which it proceeds are those of inequity and discrimination: belonging to any marginalized or stigmatized social group creates an increased risk of HIV infection as well as an increased risk of receiving inadequate care and support. Therefore, to approach the individual as if her or his behavior was independent of economics, culture and politics—or independent of human rights and dignity—would be to deny the reality we know.

Second, we all realize—each in our particular fields—as scientists, care givers, educators, activists, program managers—that we share a common problem: we have learned that we cannot succeed alone—alone in our discipline, alone in our culture, alone in our country or region—yet we have difficulty finding a common language and working together. We have seen that isolation is inefficient and dangerous—and that exchange, dialogue, tolerance and solidarity are sources of strength and pathways to more effective control and care.

Third, we have discovered, or rather, uncovered and illuminated, a fundamental problem—the central modern paradox—in health. It is clear that people in all countries are deeply concerned about their health, the health of their families and children. For the first time in history, we understand a great deal about the underlying causes of ill health in the world and we have tools to address them. Despite all this, health has not become a central, defining principle of local, national and global purpose. Why has no government—and no society—been called to account for failures in health? Why do governments tremble when the inflation rate or the price of gasoline rises, yet no elections are lost over the infant mortality rate, low immunization levels, or violent deaths among adolescents; why does national shame over the homeless, or deaths from tobacco, not lead to demands for change in political leadership?

Paradoxically, we health workers have contributed to this problem. For we have accustomed ourselves to playing a secondary, reactive and minor role in community, national, and global life. We have trained ourselves to expect and to accept second-class political attention for health concerns.

Thus, a broad definition of health was pioneered by WHO, invoking the positive concept of physical, mental and social well-being, yet this vision has yet to be transformed into health policy or practice. The WHO constitution states that health is a fundamental human right—yet this principle is not championed.

The enormous disparity in health between what people seek and what they receive, the second-class political attention given to health and health aspirations, is not limited to AIDS. This is not a problem we can simply allow ourselves to blame on others, on the so-called decision-makers or on politicians. We must now take responsibility to help give voice to the basic desires of people for better health.

The environmental movement has created political movements — green parties — to bring forward an environmental agenda. Why is it that there are not political movements in health — to help health reach a higher level of social and political influence?

To date, we have not been confident enough — bold enough — to do what we know is needed to be more effective against AIDS: to confront — in concert with our colleagues and people concerned about health — the problems deeply embedded in the status quo of societies worldwide which fuel the spread of HIV, interfere with care for affected people, and underlie the major causes of ill health worldwide.

We must listen — as increasingly, a claim is being heard — that health is a human right, not a privilege. To control AIDS — and as citizens of the modern world — we must join together as a bold vision is proclaimed — that health — in its full, modern definition — take its rightful — central — place as a universal aspiration, a common good of humanity.

Now is the time for boldness and for confidence — for a creative renewal — a new approach to the prevention and control of AIDS which brings together what we have learned from science, global experience, and from our new understanding of the relationship between AIDS, human rights, health and society. A new understanding of AIDS will be nothing less than the key to future control of the pandemic.

But we are not satisfied with ideas — we want action and assurance that a new approach to AIDS will be more effective. In practice, how will a change from seeing AIDS as an isolated phenomenon to understanding AIDS within a larger vision of health and society help to strengthen our work?

- In prevention: Unequal access to care, to education, to employment and to a future with dignity makes societies vulnerable to HIV. Once we have understood that AIDS exploits the fundamental weaknesses in society — inequity and discrimination — is it not essential for us to confront these issues — as deeply rooted and difficult as they are? In addition to our education-based prevention, we need to identify — and join with others to change — the critical features of the social environment in a community or country which fuel the spread of HIV. Anything less would be to place — and accept — a severe limit on what we can hope to accomplish in HIV prevention.
- In national AIDS programs: once we recognize the inherent limits of an isolated approach, it is imperative to create practical and strategic linkages with other sectors — education, business, women's issues — and to forge clear links — on the basis of common values and interests — with other health programs and workers.
- Activism can expand to include both the societal conditions within

which AIDS flourishes, and the broader view of health of which AIDS is an integral, catalytic part.

• In research, the goal can be broadened from making a drug or vaccine to prevention of HIV infection and care of affected people.

The creative renewal of the global AIDS effort—upon which our collective future depends—starts within each of us. Regardless of where, in what setting or at what level we are, we can look into our own hearts, our own work, our own lives. We can—we must—ask ourselves: "Is what we are doing—is what I am doing—and how I am doing it—enough to make my own best contribution?" and then we may ask ourselves: "What then is needed—what would be needed?"

Information is not enough to change behavior: this insight also applies to us. At an intellectual and conceptual level, we are now fully aware of the limited scope and capacity of current work, the limited ability of any single discipline, individual or group working alone, and the dangers of isolation and fragmentation. We recognize that the potential for effective work against AIDS made possible within the old way of thinking about AIDS is rapidly becoming exhausted.

Thus, we are at a personal and collective threshold—the transitional moment when our knowledge and ideas are ready to lead to changes in our behavior—and to how we work against AIDS: as individuals, in our communities and nations, and for the entire world.

In preparing this conference, inclusiveness, dialogue and active participation have been central themes. We have tried to prepare a setting, an environment of tolerance, mutual respect, diversity and solidarity, in which it would be possible to go beyond traditional conference practice and goals. The fundamental technology of a meeting—whether around a single table or in an enormous conference center—is in some ways quite primitive: we move our bodies long distances to gather together. Yet the outcome is complex and powerful: meetings, conferences, gatherings can affect us deeply, can move us and change our thinking. The critical element is to be there, for face-to-face discussion, for a kind of learning which does not work through books, for looking at people we meet, touching and observing, and for feeling what we feel in a gathering of 8,000 people today: all qualities which fax machines cannot replace.

This is our collective opportunity to catalyze, to prepare the future of AIDS prevention and care. Then, returning to our clinics, laboratories, schools, communities, nations and homes, we can take concrete steps:

• Consider who, in the context of a broad and collaborative vision of AIDS, you might start talking to and working with; reach to those in your community and nation who are working in social issues, and on protection of human rights.

• Take the first step to make an alliance with those working against other health problems; catalyze the health movement in your community and country; call injustice, inequality and discrimination by their name.

We are not bound—we refuse to be bound—why should we be bound—by the limits of existing institutions, boundaries, and frontiers. We are thousands—but we represent millions: our local actions, informed by a global vision, will start an unstoppable movement towards the global health revolution so long in coming.

This is a time for exploration—for pioneers. We are discovering a new world. In contrast to the past 500 years, our explorations are not geographical, for to us geography holds few mysteries. The great new world which lies before us is human, and our exploration is for new ways of connecting individuals, communities and the world community; our discoveries will be of how best to protect human rights and promote human dignity.

This is a conference of hope—not of despair. Let us send forth to the world a message of hope and life—a message of our confidence despite the danger. This is in our power, for it has been given to us, at this turning point in the history of AIDS, to create, out of our knowledge and our realism, our experience, our unstinting honesty and our dreams, a new understanding of AIDS, as part of a new global vision of health. This may yet be the most precious contribution we make—a vision of health, solidarity, rights, and peace: let it become a vision strong enough, wise enough and humane enough to protect and ensure our global future.

IV

RELIGION AND AIDS

Compassion and Care

Chapter 24

Religion and Attitudes toward AIDS Policy

Andrew M. Greeley

In the modern world there is relatively little connection in ordinary circumstances between religion and public policy with regard to contagious diseases. The quarantine rules about leprosy (a much wider collection of diseases than what is now called Hansen's Disease) in the Mosaic law — rough and ready public health measures in retrospect — are now enforced by governmental agencies and not by religion.

Acquired Immune Deficiency Syndrome, however, is a special case both because of the inevitably fatal outcome of the disease and because it is normally transmitted through sexual contact, is especially likely to spread under conditions of sexual promiscuity, and in the United States has in fact spread in great part through homosexual contact. Since the traditional religions have disapproved of promiscuity and homosexuality, AIDS has become or seems to have become an issue of morality as well as of public health. Indeed some religious leaders have pronounced it a punishment of God on immorality and especially homosexual immorality.[1]

Thus the question arises as to whether religious affiliation and devotion might have an impact on AIDS policy issues and decisions. Will the more devout have more repressive attitudes toward those who are victims of AIDS?

The 1988 General Social Survey (GSS) (Davis and Smith 1988) contained two additional modules beyond the usual sets of GSS questions, the fortuitous combination of which makes it possible to address this question.[2] The first module was a battery of questions about AIDS funded by the

"Religion and Attitudes Toward AIDS Policy," *Sociology and Social Research*, April 1991, pp. 126-130. Rev. Andrew M. Greeley is professor of social science, The University of Chicago, NORC, Chicago. Reprinted with author's permission.

National Opinion Research Center (NORC),[3] the second was an extensive series of items about religion.

The eight AIDS policy items[4] were as follows (the percentage in parentheses indicates the proportion of respondents who took a position that indicated hostility toward AIDS victims):

Do you support or oppose the following measures to deal with AIDS:

A) Prohibit students with AIDS virus from attending public schools. (26 percent)

B) Develop a government information program to promote safe sex practices, such as the use of condoms. (14 percent)

C) Permit insurance companies to test applicants for the AIDS virus. (62 percent)

D) Have the government pay all of the health care costs of AIDS patients. (67 percent)

E) Conduct mandatory testing for the AIDS virus before marriage. (89 percent)

F) Require the teaching of safe sex practices, such as the use of condoms in sex education courses in public schools. (88 percent)

G) Require people with the AIDS virus to wear identification tags that look like those carried by people with allergies or diabetes. (63 percent)

H) Make victims with AIDS eligible for disability benefits. (40 percent)

The impact of denominational affiliation, frequent church attendance and religious imagery on responses to these items will be explored in the remainder of this note.

Denominational Affiliation

Statistically significant correlations were found between Protestant[5] affiliation and negative AIDS attitudes on three items — sex information (.10), sex education (.11), and identification tags (.16).

Seventy percent of the Protestants in the sample supported the imposition of identification tags on AIDS victims as opposed to 54 percent of the Catholics. Some of this difference was concentrated among members of fundamentalist denominations (Smith 1986), of whose members 73 percent supported the identification tags, and conservative denominations, of whose members 73 percent approved of the identity tags. However, 61 percent of Protestants in liberal denominations also supported identification tags for AIDS victims; the difference between them and Catholics is not statistically significant.

In an endeavor to explain the differences between Catholics and Protestants, this writer tried to reduce the .16 correlation (sixteen percentage points difference) to statistical insignificance through the use of multiple regression equations into which religious variables would be entered successively. My assumption was that variables associated with fundamentalist religious orientations would account for much of the differences between Protestants and Catholics.

When three items were inserted which measured attitudes toward the Bible,[6] the correlation (as measured by the beta in the regression equation) diminished to .11. Catholics, in other words, are less likely to support identification tags for AIDS victims than are conservative and fundamentalist Protestants because they are less likely to emphasize the Bible, as literally interpreted, than are Protestants.

The correlation was diminished to .09 when an attitude about formal church membership when growing up[7] is inserted in the equation and to .07 and statistical insignificance when the South as a region of the country is added.

Catholics are baptized into the church and usually do not consciously reaffiliate in their adolescent years. However, members of the more conservative Protestant denominations are more likely to go through such a process of formal reaffiliation. It would appear that those who do are somewhat more likely to have a repressive attitude toward AIDS. Finally, Protestants, being disproportionately Southern in comparison with Catholics, may share a cultural attitude toward morality which has an impact above and beyond biblical fundamentalism.

Thus one can account for differences between fundamentalist and conservative Protestants and Catholics in their attitudes toward identification tags for AIDS victims by a model which takes into account explicit beliefs about the Bible, early formal relationship to a church, and region of origin.

It should be noted that 38 percent of all Americans believe in the strict literal interpretation of the Bible and 26 percent both believe in this interpretation and support prayer and Bible reading in the public schools; 47 percent of Protestants believe in literal interpretation and 36 percent of Protestants believe in this interpretation and support prayer and Bible reading in public schools. The "fundamentalist" strain in American religion is thus large. Moreover, it is not a new phenomenon. According to a Gallup index composed of the experience of being "born again," belief in a literal interpretation of scripture, and an attempt to persuade others to "decide" for Christ, a fifth of the American population has been "fundamentalist" for the last several decades with neither increase nor decrease during that period of time (Greeley 1989). Fundamentalism is a major component of American religion which did not "emerge" during the 1980s; rather the national elites and the national media discovered (again) what has existed in the United States since the First Great Awakening—in 1744. In attempting to understand the relationship between fundamentalism and AIDS attitudes it is helpful to realize that half of the population of the South believe in the literal interpretation of the Bible as opposed to a quarter of the rest of the country.

There are also somewhat smaller relationships between Protestant affiliation and attitudes on AIDS education. Of Catholics 8 percent oppose sex

education about AIDS in public schools as opposed to 16 percent of Protestants. Of Catholics 10 percent as opposed to 17 percent of Protestants
oppose government information campaigns about "safe sex." Again there
are no statistically significant differences between Catholics and liberal
Protestants. Opposition among fundamentalist Protestants is higher — 20
percent against sex education in the public schools and 25 percent oppose
government information campaigns about "safe sex."

While there is, then, a correlation between Protestantism and especially
fundamentalist Protestant and opposition to information campaigns about
AIDS, it is nonetheless true that at least three quarters of the fundamentalists do NOT oppose such campaigns.

Regression models based on the three biblical items used to account for
differences between Protestants and Catholics on the issue of identification
tags for AIDS victims reduce to statistical insignificance the differences
between the two denominations in attitudes on information campaigns,
both in the schools and outside the schools. It is precisely rigid biblical
literalism which accounts for greater Protestant opposition to such campaigns.

Church Attendance

Church attendance does not correlate with attitudes toward identification tags for AIDS victims, but it does correlate negatively and powerfully
with attitudes on sex education in the public schools and government information campaigns — -.32 and -.24. Of those who attend church weekly or
more often 38 percent oppose sex education about AIDS in public schools
(as opposed to 6 percent) and 29 percent opposed government campaigns
about "safe sex."

Again the differences between frequent attenders and others can be
diminished substantially by use in multiple regression equations of models
based on biblical and moral rigidity. The -.24 relationship with opposition
to sex education in public schools is reduced to .13 by taking into account
belief in biblical literalism and frequent reading of the Bible. It diminishes
to -.08 (and statistical insignificance) when three attitudes on moral decision making are entered into the equation.[8] The difference in attitudes
toward government informational campaigns is reduced by half by the same
model: the correlation decreases from -.32 to -.165, though the difference
remains statistically significant.

Those who attend church frequently are more likely to be opposed to
AIDS education programs in substantial part because they accept a more
literal interpretation of the Bible and because they see moral decisions in
a more simplistic fashion than to those who do not attend church so frequently. Among those regular church-goers who do not have such rigid
religious orientations there is less difference (or no statistically significant

difference) from those who do not attend church weekly.

In one sense it is not such a striking series of findings that are reported here: The religious correlation with negative attitudes toward AIDS victims or AIDS education is the result of moral and religious narrowness among certain members of the more devout population. It is what one might have expected. Nonetheless this finding establishes that it is not religion as such but a certain highly specific type of religious orientation which tends to induce hostility on the subject of AIDS. While this religious orientation represents a strong component of American culture and society, it is not a majority orientation; and even among fundamentalists the majority support AIDS education programs.

The question remains, however, whether other kinds of religious orientation correlate positively with compassion on AIDS issues. Obviously more flexible attitudes on biblical inspiration and moral decision making produce greater tolerance and sympathy. But are there other indices of religious devotion which are likely to induce such positive attitudes?

Religious Images

Religion according to a theory developed elsewhere (Greeley 1982, 1988, 1990) finds its origins and its raw power in the imaginative dimension of the self. It begins with 1) *experiences* which renew hope, which experiences are encoded in (2) *images* (or symbols) stored in the imaginative memory, and share in 3) *stories* with members of a 4) *community* with a common narrative and symbolic tradition, and often acted out in community 5) *rituals*. This paradigm is pictured not as a line but as a circle so that symbols, stories, community, and rituals in their turn shape the hope-renewing experiences of those who are part of a tradition. The symbols, stories, and rituals constitute a (pre-rational) system which purports to explain what creation and human life mean.

It is suggested that a quick and crude measure of the religious imagination can be obtained by measuring a person's image of God, since it is this image which summarizes in an abbreviated fashion the stories and symbols in a person's imagination. For several years the National Opinion Research Center has been administering a battery of four items which attempt to measure a person's image and story of God and their relationship with Her/Him.[9]

A scale was constructed from these items in which one point was given for each response that picture God as mother, spouse, lover, and friend.[10] The scale is referred to in the literature dealing with this theory as the GRACE scale because it purports to measure a more gracious story of what life means and to predict a more graceful response to problems and concerns of life. A person with a higher score on the GRACE scale, it is theorized, will have experienced a more benign relationship with the powers (or Powers) which govern the cosmos and hence will be more benign in his or her attitudes toward and relationships with other human beings.

There are modest but statistically significant positive relationships between grace and tolerance questions on the AIDS questionaire—those who are more likely to have a gracious image of God are less likely to approve of identification tags for AIDS victims (-.13), of the exclusion of AIDS victims from public schools (-.14) and of premarital AIDS tests (-.09). They are also more likely to support education about "safe sex" in public schools (.11)

Thus religion measured not by affiliation nor by church attendance but by images of God correlates with tolerance and flexibility toward AIDS policy issues.

The four [measures] illustrate the nature of this relationship for Catholics and Protestants. For both groups tolerance increases with GRACE on all measures—save for attitudes toward premarital tests among Catholics. On two of the four measures—identification tags and attendance at public schools—the correlation is essentially the same for Protestants and Catholics, though on both Catholics are more tolerant than Protestants (only slightly more tolerant on the subject of public school attendance).

On the other two measures—premarital tests and AIDS education in the schools—there is essentially no difference between Catholics and Protestants at the higher end of the GRACE scale because the scale leads to an increase in tolerance for Protestants and no significant changes for Catholics.

Thus images of God's—codes which tell stories of a person's relationship with God and provide templates for relationships with other human beings—do correlate with AIDS policy attitudes. To understand the relationship between religion and AIDS policy attitudes, one needs to know not only about attitudes toward the Bible and moral decision making but also about the religious imagination which, according to the theory, underlies the formation and expression of such cognitive attitudes.[11]

Conclusion

Since 1988 Americans may have become more tolerant on such matters as identity tags for AIDS victims and premarital testing. Moreover, some religious denominations, especially liberal Protestant and Catholic, have insisted vigorously on the need for compassion for victims—though Catholic leaders have campaigned (with their usual success in such matters) against "safe sex" education campaigns. It would be useful to know whether these changes, should they have taken place, might also relate to religious convictions, practices, and images. One would predict that the greatest resistance to attitudinal change would come from those with rigid religious orientations and the highest likelihood of attitudinal change from those with the most gracious images of God.

It is to be hoped that a future research project would include both the religious measures and the policy attitudes discussed in this note.

Notes

1. It is perhaps appropriate that, as a cleric, at the beginning I note that the God I know doesn't work that way. Are children born with AIDS guilty of anything? However, it is also true that in a non-promiscuous population, the disease would spread much less rapidly. This is a fact of epidemiology and not of divine justice.

2. The General Social Survey is funded by the National Science Foundation, which of course is not responsible for this analysis.

3. Unfortunately there was no funding available for subsequent replications of the questions so there are no data on changes in these policy attitudes since 1988.

4. The first four items were asked of one-half of the sample and the other four of the second half.

5. The size of the sample permitted only comparisons between Protestants and Catholics. For the total sample $N = 1381$. Since the items on AIDS policy were administered to only half the sample, the number of cases on each of these questions does not exceed 700.

6. The wording of the three items:

—Which of these statements comes closest to describing your feelings about the Bible: a) The Bible is the actual word of God and is to be taken literally word for word; b) The Bible is the inspired word of God but not everything in it should be taken literally, word for word; c) The Bible is an ancient book of fables, legends, history and moral principles recorded by men.

—The United States Supreme Court has ruled that no state or local government may require the reading the Lord's Prayer or Bible verses in public schools. What are your views on this—do you approve or disapprove of the court ruling.

—How important is each of the following in helping you to make decisions about life—the Bible.

7. Did you ever join a church when you were growing up, that is become a member by confirmation or such?

8. The items:

—Morality is a personal matter and society should not force anyone to follow one standard.

—Immoral actions by one person can corrupt society in general.

—Right and wrong are not usually a simple matter of black and white; there are many shades of grey.

9. The question: There are many different ways of picturing God. We'd like to know the kinds of images you are most likely to associate with God. Here is a card with sets of contrasting images. On a scale of 1-7 where would you place your image of God between the two contrasting images: Mother, Father; Master, Spouse; Judge, Lover; Friend, King.

10. Or equally Mother and Father, etc.

11. The scale correlates negatively with ALL the variables in the models discussed in previous sections of this paper: Literalism -.22; Bible reading -.10; Bible

in public schools -.11; morality is personal not social .08; morality is a matter of black and white not gray -.15; immoral actions can corrupt society -.12.

References

Davis, James A. and Tom Smith. 1988. General Social Surveys 1972-1988. Cumulative Codebook. Chicago: The National Opinion Research Center.

Greeley, Andrew. 1982. Religion: A Secular Theory. New York: The Free Press.

———1988. "Evidence That A Maternal Image of God Correlates with Liberal Politics." *Sociology and Social Research.* 73:3-8.

———1989. *Religious Change in America.* Cambridge Mass: Harvard University Press.

———1990. *The Catholic Myth.* New York: Charles Scribner.

Smith, Tom. 1986. "Classifying Protestant Denominations," GSS Technical Report No. 67, Chicago: NORC.

Chapter 25

The Biblical and Theological Basis for Risking Compassion and Care for AIDS Patients

Newell J. Wert

Ralph C. Johnston wrote recently that while AIDS is "a disease syndrome whose parameters can be described and whose etiology is thought to be known, it is also a symbol upon which have been projected several of the cultural anxieties of the late twentieth century" (77). These include anxiety about sexuality in general and homosexuality in particular, anxiety about drug users, racial otherness, public health and, finally, death. AIDS is not just a disease of persons who have AIDS; it is, in a sense, an affliction of a society suddenly aware that there is a disease for which there is no known cure, the fear of which is projected onto the victims.

On the cover of a 1986 issue of *Hospital*, the illustration of the lead article on AIDS was a bomb with a burning fuse. In a 1985 end-of-the-year reader's survey, *U.S. News and World Report* posed the question: "Which of the following problems concern you most?" Readers were given four alternatives: crime, recession, nuclear war and AIDS. This list itself indicates the degree to which fear about AIDS has entered the consciousness of the American people. Unfortunately, it also indicates that the most common perceptions of AIDS involve despair, panic, even hysteria, rather than signs of genuine compassion for those who are suffering and dying from the illness (Altman, 23).

What is more, because AIDS is commonly seen as having a necessary

"The Biblical and Theological Basis for Risking Compassion and Care for AIDS Patients," *UTS Journal of Theology* 93, 1989, pp. 48-59. Newell J. Wert, Ph.D., is a professor at United Theological Seminary, Dayton, Ohio, and editor of the *UTS Journal of Theology*. Reprinted with author's permission.

connection with homosexuality, with some public recognition that other groups are affected, it is an illness defined by the group it most affects. It is, therefore, an illness of "The Other." The news media speak of "innocent victims" to characterize those affected who are not gay men and IV drug users. The implication is that if one is among these two groups, one is somehow guilty of the disease (Altman, 24). Many people fail to make the distinction between what causes a disease and how it is transmitted. Altman goes on to say: "This view persists despite the fact that over one-third of the AIDS cases in New York City, the epicenter of the disease in the United States, are not found among gay men, and this proportion is increasing" (24). Former Surgeon General C. Everett Koop recently predicted that by 1991 the majority of those infected will be in the heterosexual community.

My posture in coming to this topic is as a Christian ethicist concerned for the moral health of the human community and the grounding provided in Christian theological understandings and scriptural sources. I am concerned about moral values and moral relationships both as individual experiences and as social phenomena. There is a very close relationship between the way individuals relate to each other morally and the public policy that they tolerate or create. AIDS is a very clear example of this connection, but more than that it has revealed things about ourselves as a society that have the marks of illness.

I want to address the morality of the community as it responds to the AIDS crisis and its victims. I do not speak as a care giver, although I have had the benefit of discussing AIDS and the issues related to it over the last two years with nursing, medical and seminary students who have been in interprofessional ethics courses taught jointly by faculty of the Wright State University Schools of Medicine and Nursing and United Theological Seminary. In that context I have learned from the physicians, nurses and chaplains who are specialists and who have been brought in to help provide resources for the course. I have discovered that those who care deeply about this problem are eager to have allies in thinking about the issues as they do research, provide treatment and give care.

Professional Care Giving: Responsibilities and Risks

It has become common in the professions today to think of each practitioner as an entrepreneur. That is, each one is in practice for himself or herself. Even when a professional is paid a salary, there is some sense in which there is a kind of individual freedom granted the professional. The basis for this is the recognition that professionals have access to special knowledge that is acquired through long years of study, that there is a common link among the professionals in a particular field that sets them apart. It is also recognized that professionals have special responsibilities because they have special knowledge. But there is an individualism in the practice of the professions today in which the practitioner's rights and the contractual model of care giver/care receiver are dominant considerations.

The fact is, however, that the practice of professional care giving is rooted in community. The first code of the American Medical Association when it was formed in 1847 spoke of the duty of the physician to care for patients regardless of the risk, clearly a recognition of the reality of community and the professional's responsibility in and to it. Such references are, however, no longer to be found in the medical codes. Instead, the emphasis is on the individual right of the physician to choose his or her patients, which first appeared in the 1912 code. None of the codes now mention the physician's duty to accept personal risk in the care of patients. Only two classes of physicians are bound by a specific duty to provide care, those in emergency medicine and those employed by public hospitals. Principle VI in the 1980 AMA Guidelines reads, "A physician shall in the provision of appropriate patient care, except in emergencies, be free to choose whom to serve, with whom to associate, and the environment in which to provide medical services."

Don Browning in his very instructive book, *The Moral Context of Pastoral Care,* expresses a similar concern about the state of pastoral care as a profession. He says, "On the whole, recent theory and practice of pastoral care has been without an ecclesiology, without an interpretation of modern culture and institutional life, and without a social ethic" (21). The emphasis in Browning's work is that a chief role of pastoral care is to establish a community of care giving as a context for pastoral care. Browning notes that the role of the clinical pastoral care giver has been largely separated from the congregation that is the base of the church's life. As a consequence the religious care giver is often reduced to a practitioner of theories of religious psychotherapy as a kind of physician, counselor, nurse or social worker. At best this brings in a much needed dimension of meaning in the complex of health care. At worst it marginalizes the pastoral care giver.

AIDS, then, is raising the question of the nature of the professional responsibility of all care givers in new and acute ways. Recent articles in the *Journal of the American Medical Association* have questioned the current state of professional ethics in medicine, precipitated by the AIDS crisis. Edmund Pellegrino says that it has become clear that two opposing conceptions of medicine have emerged in medical ethics today: one entails self-effacement, the other rejects it. Self-effacement is clearly a concept that is based on the idea of the practitioner as a member of the community in a special way, and not free to withdraw from it for purely personal reasons (Pellegrino 1987, 1939-1940).

What is being said about the social responsibility of physicians can also be said of other health care professionals and even to some extent clergy who are pastoral care professionals. Professionals do not have their knowledge and privileges just as proprietary rights. Doctors, nurses, ministers and other care givers are part of the larger community that has not only made their profession possible, but has made the knowledge and the education possible. Entering a profession is itself a pledge to make its knowledge available. Furthermore, each profession is part of a professional community of which each is a representative and to whose tradition something is owed.

For pastoral care givers there is the added relationship to the church that calls, ordains, interprets and disciplines the clergy. This connection to the religious community is easy to forget when the religious care giver is functioning in the environment of another institution like a hospital. Here other communities are normative and the care giver must be part of both the health care community and the religious community. The possibility of being marginalized is great, but so is the possibility that the health care institution rather than the religious community will be the normative source of the religious care giver's identity. John Bohne's study (1986) of the attitudes of chaplains points to the need for models of care giving to AIDS patients and families that address the issue of sexuality and help chaplains deal with relationships with which they may be unfamiliar and for which the religious traditions are ill-equipped.

AIDS is causing all care givers to reexamine not only their obligations as professionals but also the risks. It is not uncommon to start the discussion about risk as it relates to AIDS by pointing to the plagues and epidemics of the past. The fact is, however, as many researchers have pointed out, that AIDS has very little in common with the other great, historic epidemics like smallpox, yellow fever or the bubonic plague. These were poorly understood, quite large and rapidly spread. The risk of AIDS, on the other hand, has been exhaustively evaluated, and infection control has made these risks manageable, unlike the epidemics of the past (Zuger and Miles, 1926).

The examples of professional responsibility in the past in facing risk are not encouraging. The literature reveals, for example, that many physicians fled past epidemics in fear. It was so serious in Venice in one period that the government threatened to revoke the citizenship of any physician who failed to treat victims. At another point citizens were moved to draw an analogy between physicians and soldiers and likened physicians who fled to deserters from the battlefield.

In 1847 the AMA drew up the first code of medical ethics. It reads in part: "and when pestilence prevails, it is their duty to face danger and to continue their labors for the alleviating of suffering, even to the jeopardy of their own lives." Zuger and Miles point out that this statement is unprecedented in the history of ethical codes for the medical profession. "The stories of the nineteenth century cholera pandemic, plagues in the Orient, influenza pandemic of 1918, polio in 1950, are largely of medical heroism" (1926-28). But despite this judgment, they say, it is difficult to ground a professional ethic for the care for HIV-infected persons in the tradition. It is too mixed.

Beyond that, the links to community values, meanings and connections that have undergirded health care professionals over the last century have been steadily eroded in favor of an individualistic philosophy. Health care also has changed as a result of the remarkable success of medical and biological science, so that the underlying assumption is that there is in principle a cure for everything. AIDS challenges both our individualism and our optimism as care givers, and it is causing us to reexamine what it means to be a professional.

The Morality of Care Giving

Our society has characteristically linked infectious disease to moral judgment. The 1832 cholera epidemic, for example, was said to be the scourge of the sinful. Successive episodes by the year 1866 saw the increase of charity and less tendency to blame the victim as more scientific explanations were found. Yet when AIDS struck more than a hundred years later, one religious leader said, "We have the Pill. We have conquered venereal disease with penicillin. But then along comes Herpes Simplex II. Nature itself lashes back when we go against God's will" (Schelp and Sunderland, 16).

On the other hand, the major denominational bodies have, by and large, adopted helpful resolutions and issued statements regarding the church's witness in the AIDS crisis. Recently, bishops of the United Methodist Church issued a statement on AIDS that says, in part, "We, the Council of Bishops, say as clearly as we can to our brothers and sisters that acquired immune deficiency syndrome is not a sin, as many claim. ... While the origin of the AIDS virus is still in question in the medical community, we in the religious community are certain that its origin is not sent as a curse from God on those whose life style is called into question." The Bishops call on church members to reach out compassionately to AIDS sufferers and their families and urge society to deal fairly and compassionately with sufferers in the public policies that are made and the support of effort to understand and treat victims (*United Methodist Reporter*, 1; for an "evangelical" view see Sider).

The archbishop of the Cincinnati diocese of the Roman Catholic church spoke in Dayton pastorally on behalf of a priest with AIDS as he comforted the congregation that rose up in unified support of the pastor who had given them dedicated pastoral care for some years. When asked how the priest got AIDS the Archbishop replied, "I don't know. That is between him and his doctor." That is perhaps one of the most significant statements on AIDS to be uttered by a religious leader, one that I applaud. Note, he did not say "between him and God." He refused to make it a matter of Divine judgment.

AIDS has struck the community as few diseases have because it is a community concern. It cannot be treated like any other disease as if it were a chance occurrence of a malady that may befall all of us at one time or another. Care giving in this context is more than ministry to sick people and their families. It now requires a social response because the moral health of the nation is at stake. People with AIDS, their family members and friends have a personal claim on the church, the synagogue and the community at large simply by virtue of their plight (Schelp and Sunderland, 122).

All care givers will soon encounter HIV-infected persons. A professional ethics that employs the right to decline to treat or minister to these patients will be terribly inadequate, to say the least. A 1987 article in the *Journal of the American Medical Association* asks,

> What then should be the attitude of physicians in taking on the responsibility of treating patients with HIV infection? Some would opt for avoiding even the smallest risk and transferring the responsibility to another physician. Others, realizing that the risk is minuscule, will take ordinary precautions and treat those patients no differently than anyone else with an infectious disease. And there are those who will take up the challenge of personal risk and, putting the patient's welfare ahead of their own, will reaffirm their vow to serve their fellowman. ... I will follow that method of treatment which, according to my ability and judgment, I consider for the benefit of my patients. (Dan, 1940)

The Council on Ethical and Judicial Affairs of the American Medical Association has recently come out with guidelines for dealing with AIDS patients (Pellegrino 1988, 1360-61). These include the following protocols:

> AIDS patients are entitled to competent medical service with compassion and respect for human dignity and to safeguard their confidences within the constraints of the law. ... [patients] have the right to be free from discrimination. ... A physician may not ethically refuse to treat a patient ... solely because the patient is seropositive.

The Religious Motivation for Compassion and Care

James Wharton asks the fundamental question that all religious care givers need to answer for themselves:

> Is there an understanding [of the relationship] of self and other within the biblical faith communities that is distinctive and not merely borrowed from the behavioral sciences? If so, is it sufficiently powerful to undergird professional ministry with a sense of its own authenticity that it is not merely borrowed from the other disciplines? (18)

These questions are especially important for persons who practice their pastoral care in institutions that are public and where religious language and practice is not normative, such as is the case in most health care facilities. Wharton goes on to say, "Even stout and clear convictions about what one does as a minister are difficult to maintain in the face of popular opinion that ministers are at best second-stringers in the scientifically grounded arts of helping people" (19).

Can pastoral care givers have the same authenticity as other professionals in the field of health care? They can only as they pay attention to their own unique sources of professional identity and practice. I take these to be the scriptures of their religion and the theological tradition to which they are committed, and the religious communities of which they are a part.

Wharton says,

In both Judaism and Christianity the quality of relationship between self and other lies near the heart of faith. How one relates to human others is the indispensable litmus by which the relationship to God as Other is tested. How one relates to God as other determines the framework within which the faithful community perceives and deals with human others. Ministry to human others is, in the ultimate sense, ministry to God. (20-21)

The Hebrew scriptures do not offer metaphysical speculation about the relationship between God and the human creation. Rather, they tell the story of a God who is involved with the people, who makes covenant with them, who cares for them, who makes God's own self vulnerable to the faithlessness of the people.

The images of God in the scriptures are active, relational images. God is always initiating and responding. These images were drawn from the experience of the people as they tried to understand God. Albert Outler, in speaking of the need to find new metaphors for God that reflect our experience, says that the shepherd image in Psalm 23 might well be replaced with the word, "therapist" (31 ff.). No longer in an agrarian society, perhaps people would understand that image better. I think that metaphor has some peculiar problems because of other images it invokes. I don't particularly want to say, "The Lord is my therapist." But there are aspects of the good therapist that may help us think about God: willing to give freedom, willing to be free for the patient, seeking to elicit the wholeness of the patient. Outler calls all of this "purposive love." Above all, the therapist makes himself or herself vulnerable to the patient. This is the way the story is told in the Hebrew scriptures. God is not just the one who does acts of mercy and provides comfort from a distance. God does not just intervene at crucial times in the life of the people. God involves God's self in the whole fabric of real relationships: the mutual disappointments, the times of separation and reunion, the times of sorrow and of joy.

If that is the model for the religiously motivated care giver, then it involves freely chosen vulnerability on the one hand and unflagging commitment to the freedom and wholeness of the other on the other hand. To follow this model is more than seeking to be a good care giver; it is to enter into a relationship with others.

The key to understanding the nature of God's relationship to Israel is the word *covenant*. God initiates a relationship of promise in which God is absolutely faithful and attests to this by God's own gift. For the Hebrews it was the gift of freedom from the slavery of Egypt. For Christians it is the covenant initiated in the gift of God's Son, Jesus Christ. Covenant is not contract. It is not some mutual understanding that legally binds and out of which one can negotiate. One can refuse to respond to God's covenantal love, but it will always be there. This is the model that is enjoined on those who believe this about God, and it is especially appropriate to the relationships that characterize the care giver and the care receiver. The care receiver does nothing to deserve care. The care receiver is simply in need. The giving is unconditional.

To care this deeply faces the care giver with the hard reality of the plight of the person who is ill and the question of its ultimate meaning. It is impossible to give care and not wonder why people suffer. In the case of AIDS there is a particular temptation to play God and to answer the question in terms of the fault of the victim. The linking of homophobia with the AIDS question is one of the most challenging problems in the AIDS issue. But care givers in the Judaic-Christian tradition, if they are authentic witnesses to the nature of God, will not fall into the temptation to blame the victim.

In any authentic care giving there is the need to be reassured that life is not ultimately absurd. The crisis of faith experienced by those who suffer is often matched by the crisis of those who give care. And part of the stress of giving care to AIDS victims is the intensification of the tragedy that accompanies the illness and its absurdity. Only confidence in the constant love and care of God will undergird victims, friends, families and care givers. That this confidence is not easy to come by is witnessed by Job. There were plenty of people around him who wanted to blame him for his misfortune.

Samuel Karff reminds us that "[w]hen Moses asked to be shown the ways of God, demanding evidence of God's presence, he was told, 'My presence will go with you.' The rabbis reminded Israel that the name, 'I am the Lord' ... means 'I am He who is present beside my neighbor' " (100).

The New Testament displays a God who is revealed through Jesus of Nazareth, one whose teaching and acts we believe tell us about God. His was a life of compassion and care that tells us about the nature of God and the difference between our understandings of life and God's understanding. Jesus refused to assign blame in the case of the man born blind. However, the real point of the New Testament is that Jesus himself underwent humility and death and in that respect is like all of us, especially those who suffer the most, the victims and outcasts. All that Jesus did and said is significant finally because in him God made visible God's care for humankind, a care dependent on God's grace and benevolence toward the creation.

But it was in the passion week culminating with the open and empty tomb that the meaning of Jesus became altogether clear. It changed the way humanity looks at itself and its future. Those who now follow the risen Christ know that whatever their fate and the fate of the world seem to be, in the end it will be transformed into the kingdom of a merciful God who gives us hope within and beyond the often tragic years of our human existence. Those who follow the risen Christ know that life is not finally a tragedy but joy and victory. This is the resource for pastoral care givers. God cannot be finally defeated, and this is the faith that is communicated by those who take the risk to provide care under the most trying circumstances. It is communicated in the care itself. In that role the care giver is not just an individual believer but a representative of the Christian community, past and present, that understands itself as the embodiment of Christ.

Models of Care Giving

If this is the essence of our biblical and theological grounding, three models of care giving are especially pertinent for care givers who deal with AIDS patients.

1. The first of these is *covenant*. Several years ago William May of the Kennedy Institute of Ethics at Georgetown University wrote an article entitled, "Code, Covenant, Contract, or Philanthropy" (1975). In it he contrasted these four models of physician-patient relationship. Code, contract and philanthropy are all inadequate, in his judgment. Code understands the responsibility with reference to law rather than to persons. Contract intervenes between the patient and the physician and makes them adversaries. Philanthropy he calls the physician's conceit, gratuitously giving care out of the giver's largess. Covenant is the most appropriate image of the four. Drawing on biblical material May develops the model as one that begins by recognizing the obligation that physicians have by virtue of the gifts that have been given them by society: their education, the physical facilities to practice medicine, the honor accorded them by society. I think this analysis applies to the minister and other professionals as well as to physicians.

Later May developed these ideas in a book entitled, *The Physician's Covenant,* in which he extended the idea of models in a very helpful way. The book is sub-titled, "Images of the Healer in Medical Ethics." Here May identifies additional models such as the parent, the fighter, the technician and the teacher, and he shows their applicability to the physician's own self-understanding. It would be instructive today if we were to ask what models inform the practice of our profession. Perhaps there are some that May has not included. However, he grounds the professional's art in covenant, and I think this is particularly important for the point of view suggested in this paper.

2. The second image that I want to suggest is *hospitality to strangers*. Of special significance in considering the religious basis of care giving is the constant theme in the Hebrew and the Christian scriptures of the centrality of the believer's responsibility to the stranger, the poor, the oppressed and the outcast. Many writers today point to the parallels between these figures and the victims of AIDS. The theme is everywhere in the Bible. Note Isaiah: "Shame on you! you who make unjust laws and publish burdensome decrees, depriving the poor of justice, robbing the weakest of my people of their rights, despoiling the widow and plundering the orphan" (10:1-2, NEB). Jesus said, "Inasmuch as ye have done it unto one of the least of these ye have done it unto me" (Matt 25:40 KJV).

The people of God are called to be a community that welcomes the stranger, the poor, the oppressed and the outcast and treats them as full members of the community. Those who are in the Jewish-Christian tradition do not have the option to avoid responding to those in need. Hospitality to strangers is itself the mark of religious commitment.

Hospitality is one of the pillars on which our society stands, and yet we are so loathe to exercise it. The AIDS crisis both threatens to undermine it even further and at the same time challenges us to fulfill the obligation of hospitality to strangers. This will call not only for attention to individual care giving but to institutional and public policy.

3. The final model I want to suggest is one for which we are indebted to Henri Nouwen. It is the *wounded healer*, which is the title of his well-known book. AIDS, in a significant way, affects the healer, as I have described earlier. Care givers who are faithful cannot escape the pain, the tragedy, the psychological toll of care giving. They can only be described as "wounded." That may be a much greater risk than getting AIDS. While they cannot heal this particular disease in the physical sense, it is their capacity for care and empathy, their willingness to be "wounded," that brings a special kind of healing to those who are afraid, alone and dying.

Nouwen tells an old legend from the Talmud. A rabbi came upon Elijah, the prophet, and asked him, "When will the Messiah come?" Elijah replied, "Go ask him yourself." "Where is he?" "Sitting at the gates of the city." "How shall I know him?" "He is sitting among the poor covered with wounds. The others unbind all their wounds at the same time and then bind them up again. But he unbinds one at a time and binds it up again, saying to himself, 'Perhaps I shall be needed: if so I must always be ready so as not to delay for a moment' " (83,84).

So it is with the care giver. One must look after one's own wounds but at the same time be prepared to tend the wounds of others. The figure of Jesus on the Cross is the ultimate image of the Wounded Healer.

Is Death the Enemy?

In a 1984 article Richard Landau and James Gustafson say that we are in danger of making death ultimate and thus an idol, replacing God. The pursuit of health is replacing the pursuit of salvation and the glorification of God (2458).

The AIDS crisis forces us to put death in perspective. St. Paul reminded his hearers that in Jesus Christ death has been conquered. Death is no longer the enemy.

John Snow in his book, *Mortal Fear: Meditations on Death and AIDS,* writes:

> If death is viewed merely as the end of life, a minor chemical event, and life as a kind of survival strategy ... then we are all going to be driven to irrationality or despair. Until we come to grips with our mortality, learning to accept it without denial or despair, until we can fit death into a larger pattern of trustworthy corporate life that provides continuity from one generation to the next, the human enterprise is doomed to the consequences of its own aimlessness. (Preface)

The final enemy is not death. It is hopelessness and despair. When the care giver is only intent on saving life and life is in principle savable, then a kind of victory over death is possible. But when death is inevitable and it is seen as the final enemy, then all is lost and life has no meaning.

The care giver of AIDS patients must declare that death is not the enemy. The true enemy is despair, hopelessness, and that can be overcome. And it will be overcome not by sheer mental will but by entering into the pain of others, by joining together as care givers to support each other, by searching out the roots of faith and by demonstrating the love of God in the care we give.

References

Altman, Dennis. 1987. "The Politics of AIDS." *AIDS: Public Policy Dimensions*. New York: United Hospital Fund.

Bohne, John. 1986. "AIDS: Ministry Issues for Chaplains." *Pastoral Psychology*. Volume 34, Number 3. Spring; pp. 173-192.

———. 1988. "AIDS and Action: Review of Schelp and Sunderland's *AIDS and the Church. Christianity and Crisis*. Volume 48. March 7; pp. 65-67.

Browning, Don. 1976. *The Moral Context of Pastoral Care*. Philadelphia: Westminster Press.

Dan, Bruce B. 1988. "Patients Without Physicians: The New Risk of AIDS." *Journal of the American Medical Association*. Volume 258, Number 14. October 9; p. 1940.

Johnston, Ralph C., Jr. 1987. "AIDS and 'Otherness.' " *AIDS: Public Policy Dimensions*. New York: United Hospital Fund.

Karff, Samuel. 1981. "Ministry in Judaism." In *A Biblical Basis for Ministry*, edited by Earl E. Schelp and Ronald Sunderland. Philadelphia: Westminster Press.

Kubler-Ross, Elizabeth. 1987. *AIDS, the Ultimate Challenge*. New York: Macmillan.

Landau, Richard L. and Gustafson, James M. 1984. "Death Is Not the Enemy." *Journal of the American Medical Association*. Volume 252, Number 2. November 2; p. 2458.

May, William F. 1975. "Code, Covenant, Contract, or Philanthropy." *Hastings Center Report*. Volume 5. December.

———. 1983. *The Physician's Covenant*. Philadelphia: Westminster Press.

Nouwen, Henri. 1972. *The Wounded Healer*. Garden City, New York: Doubleday and Company.

Outler, Albert. 1968. *Who Trusts in God: Musings on the Meaning of Providence*. New York: Oxford University Press.

Pellegrino, Edmund D. 1987. "Altruism, Self-Interest and Medical Ethics." *Journal of the American Medical Association*. Volume 258, Number 14. October 9; pp. 1939-1940.

———. 1988. "Ethical Issues Involved in the Growing AIDS Crisis." *Journal of the American Medical Association*. Volume 259, Number 9. March 4.

Schelp, Earl E. and Sunderland, Ronald H. 1987. *AIDS and the Church*. Philadelphia: Westminster Press.

Sider, Ronald J. 1988. "AIDS: An Evangelical Perspective." *Christian Century*. January 6-13; pp. 11-14.

Snow, John. 1987. *Mortal Fear*. Cambridge, Mass.: Cowley Publications.

United Methodist Reporter. 1988. "UM Leaders urge caution, say AIDS not 'sin.' " Volume 134, Number 48. April 29.

Wharton, James A. 1981. "Theology and Ministry in the Hebrew Scriptures." In *The Biblical Basis for Ministry*, edited by Earl E. Schelp and Ronald H. Sunderland. Philadelphia: Westminster Press.

Zuger, Abigail and Miles, Stephen H. 1987. "Physicians, AIDS, and Occupational Risk: Historic Traditions and Ethical Obligations." *Journal of the American Medical Association*. Volume 258, Number 14. October 9; pp. 1924-1928.

Chapter 26

The Orthodox Church and the AIDS Crisis

Basil Zion

Everything about the controversy surrounding AIDS is shocking to the mind of Orthodox Christians. It is not only a disease which is lethal in its progression, but it is a disease in which 70 percent of those infected in the United States are by homosexual contact, and another 20 percent by intravenous drug use. The disease threatens us like an avalanche; we see it coming and its effects are known to be inevitable and devastating. There are concerns about receiving Holy Communion by the common spoon, fears of infection, fears of contamination. But the most profound dismay would lie in the presence of the disease within the ranks of the holy church of God. Those who succumb to it are often thrust out into outer darkness, no longer recognized as the sons (and daughters) of the people of God. There are even some who have been refused Christian burial in Orthodox churches because of the deep suspicion that they were sinners who cloaked their sins behind a pretense of piety.

No one can responsibly deal with this crisis by denial, and that is what we are tempted to do. We are not immune as some would imagine. As one person is regarded to have said, "I could not have AIDS since I am an Orthodox Christian." But certain facts demand our attention. One is that a person can be infected with AIDS by accident, however rare that may be. There are also those who have received blood transfusions before they were closely monitored and have been infected in this way. There are babies born with AIDS from mothers who had been infected by husbands whom they did not know to be HIV positive. It is tempting to talk of such people as the innocent victims of AIDS, as indeed they are. However, we must be

---

"The Orthodox Church and the AIDS Crisis," *St. Vladimir's Theological Quarterly* 36 (1-2), 1992, pp. 152-158. Reverend Basil Zion is professor of religion, Queens University, Kingston, Ontario. Reprinted with permission.

extremely cautious in pointing our finger at the guilty ones. We are admonished by the Lord not to judge one another, and yet that is our perennial temptation. Moral theology would teach us that we can never know the extent to which a person has inwardly consented to a sin. Only God, and to a much lesser extent the person doing the deed, can have any knowledge of the degree of consent or the intention involved. The Orthodox tradition teaches us that there are sins which are voluntary and those that are involuntary. We are to acknowledge those sins which are involuntary and to repent of them, but the tradition treats them as light in their matter since the will is not involved in them. Our Lord cautioned us against throwing stones at sinners, most particularly as the Pharisees did in regard to the woman caught in adultery. In fact, the church has always known that judging others is more spiritually dangerous than sins of the flesh, since such judgment comes from a pride that manifests a lack of compassion and mercy on our part. Furthermore, it springs from a lack of humility, a desire to be superior and to deny the fact that we are all sinners.

It is the compassion of God which pervades the prayers of the church. Those preparing us for Holy Communion repeatedly appeal to this compassion. Only on the basis of God's compassion do we dare to approach the Holy Chalice. A fitting Christian response for those with AIDS is one of unconditional compassion. In fact, the Lord Jesus taught us again and again that we can't be forgiven by God if we forgive not those who trespass against us. The pretence by which we are morally superior to those who are branded with this new form of leprosy is itself a diabolical inspiration.

Furthermore, the claim made by many that AIDS is God's punishment for sinners is itself without foundation, since we can never know what is God's punishment and what is not when it comes to illness. It is possible to perceive that certain acts have consequences, such as the lung cancer and cardiovascular pathology that so frequently result from smoking, but few of us would want to say that these illnesses are God's punishment for sin. The notion that those with AIDS are any different from others suffering from any terminal illness is one that we must banish. The scandal of an illness which is contracted from sexual sin (and we must never draw that conclusion in regard to AIDS without knowing the facts) may have more to do with our distorted notions of the supreme gravity of sexual sin than with reality. We should be shocked at the greed, the indifference to poverty and the suffering of others, the pride of superiority, and other spiritual sins. To consider sexual sin as somehow more grave than any other is deeply contrary to the most fundamental insights of Orthodox spirituality.

It is important, nevertheless, that the Orthodox church remain constant in her rejection of sexual activity which is not blessed by God. The norm of that legitimate activity remains heterosexual marriage as celebrated and blessed by the church. Homosexuality, however, is rarely a condition that is chosen. The condition is akin to that of persons who are "color-blind." It has been compared also to those who are left-handed rather than right-handed. Since society has offered to homosexuals little more than condemnation, both for their impulses and for the acts that may flow from them, one may rightly as did Father Lev Gillet have a very special concern for the plight and suffering of homosexuals. Dr. Elizabeth Moberly has referred to them as "orphans" for whom Christians must have a very special care.[1] The church may indeed offer healing to homosexuals, but we can no more expect all persons with AIDS to be healed than those who suffer from cancer or a heart condition. Those who are afflicted with various pathological conditions such as autism, or a nervous temperament, or an inability to learn certain things, are not cursed by God. Such conditions, like homosexuality, are part of the limitations of our finite condition in the flesh. The causes of homosexuality remain opaque. It is true that St. Paul associates it with the consequences of idolatry in Hellenistic society and God surrendered the idolatrous Greeks to it as a "dishonorable passion." It would, however, be a mistake to conclude that all homosexuality is a punishment for idolatry. Theories of its etiology are manifold, from genetic to psychodynamic explanations. None has been proved at this point to be definitive.

Human perfection is not possible short of the Kingdom of God, and we come into that perfection by way of the Cross. The Cross is a way through the hatred of human beings, through pain and anguish in a very dark and confused world. That drug users and homosexuals have been those most afflicted with AIDS in North America tells us about ways of life resulting in the first case from poverty and despair, and in the second from self-hatred and promiscuity. The church has never accepted homosexual acts as moral, but a black and white assessment of them will provide little light. Homosexuals are not evil because they are homosexual. Rather, the *anomie* of the world in which they have lived, and the introjection of hatred reflected in attitudes toward them, have often led to the self-destructive promiscuity that has marked the gay world and resulted in conditions conducive to HIV infection. This is recognized by a multitude of homosexual observers today, and the way of sexual restraint is even preached by advocates like Dennis Altman who have no use for morality or Christianity.[2] Survival necessitates the termination of the activities which were so frequent in the anomic world of the gay ghetto.

One may rightly perceive the gay world as a milieu of a moral heresy. It is very important, however, that Orthodox Christians condemning heresies not fall into condemning persons who may, through no fault of their own, be trapped in heresy. Just as Judaism as a religious system is a heresy insofar as it is the rejection of Jesus as the Christ, so the gay movement is a heresy which legitimizes homosexual liaisons as normative. Few Jews have ever been presented with a setting where it would be possible to accept Jesus Christ and remain within their familial and ethnic setting. Similarly, homosexual persons have been so wounded by the rejection that they have received from society that they have defensively exalted their way as a good and legitimate use of their sexuality. The heresy must be rejected, but the heretic can well be understood as invincibly ignorant of the error in which he is involved. The anathemas originally hurled at the dissident community stand at the objective level, but subjectively they are inappropriate since a hardening of heart is the most likely consequence of the censures. What must remain foremost for Orthodox Christians must be the charity by which persons are affirmed, even when they have gone far astray in the error of their ways. If the persecution of Jews or homosexuals manifests a lack of charity, it is the persecutor rather than the persecuted who has fallen away from Christ. A Christian who seriously understands that God in Jesus Christ put Himself in the place of the victim must have the gravest misgivings about victimizing either heretics or sinners.

The fact remains that those with AIDS, and those living under the threat of AIDS because they are seropositive, are full human beings. They deserve our prayer and our support. They will die the most horrible of deaths if they perceive our rejection and our blame. It is not the homosexual condition as such but our easy judgments, our rejection of persons, and our indifference which fall under the severity of God's judgment. It is essential that we recognize that as human beings both drug users and homosexuals are lovable, and that they sometimes have lovers who are blessings to them. This in no way means that we are called to accept their sexual activities. Yet there is no need to condemn the relationships and friendships which they have established with other homosexuals. The homophobia that comes from the anxieties aroused by what is foreign to heterosexuals must not blind us to the fact that even in the darkest of conditions of life, in prisons, in the death camps, in scenes of utmost despair, God's light may shine through in the faces of those who love us. It is time that we made our evaluation of human sexual behavior not by codes and taboos, but by discerning whether that activity is a sign of the Kingdom of God. What is most indicative of immorality is the impersonality and the promiscuity which have been the marks of the gay world. It is out of that milieu, as well as that of heterosexual promiscuity, that AIDS has emerged. Love is the norm of Christian sexual ethics, and whenever there is a gesture of love, such a sign must not be cast to the swine as if it were worthless.

AIDS will test the Christianity of the church as nothing else in our age other than the holocaust itself. This ambivalent attitude of condemning the sin but loving the sinner is often experienced by persons with AIDS as condemnation and blame. As Mother Maria Skobtsova gave her life for the Jews being swallowed by the satanic ovens created by Nazism and anti-Semitism, so we are called to identify with those who suffer and die from AIDS. We are sinners like them, but in their suffering we often see very holy deaths. We see the presence of Christ in those who lie dying upon the cross of their pain and agony. We shall be judged by how we respond to the sick, the hungry, the naked, and the prisoner, for there we find the living presence of the crucified one. This is the teaching of the Lord in Matthew 25:36, "O blessed of my Father, inherit the kingdom prepared for you from the foundation of the world; for I was hungry and you gave me food, I was thirsty and you gave me to drink, I was a stranger and you welcomed me, I was naked and you clothed me, I was sick and you visited me, I was in prison and you came to me."

We may take comfort in the following conclusions:

1. AIDS cannot be passed on casually or by the spoon in Holy Communion. There is now sufficient evidence that the virus is passed only through the blood stream, and that means by sexual intercourse, by intravenous drug use, and by contaminated blood. It is not passed by saliva except in large quantities of fluid.[3]

2. AIDS is not a disease to which Orthodox Christians are automatically immune. We are as vulnerable as anyone else if we do certain things which may infect us. That some have fallen into sinful acts by which they have been infected should come as no surprise, any more than the greed, the pride, and the indifference that mark any of us. There will be few large urban parishes that will be spared persons with AIDS. Rather than excluding the person with AIDS and rejecting his or her presence in our midst (and ultimately their funeral), we must reach out to express our compassion, our love, and our support.

3. Just as AIDS brings into grave question the ways of the gay world and the drug use of many, we should not gloat over the fall of so many. It is so easy to unload our hatred on those who are not only different but broken in the consequences of their life-styles. The creation of specters in those whom we identify as heretics must be avoided so that we can see their humanity. This will help us to avoid distancing ourselves from those whom disease marks as outcasts from normal and healthy society. Those who have lost loved ones to lethal disease, many of them radiant in their holiness, know that this mentality must be resisted.

4. The very sensitive issue of education for safer sex is one that we cannot entirely ignore. The teaching of the church is that sexual abstinence before marriage is the Christian norm. The fact remains that many fall into sin and error on this point. There are many who cannot marry because of their sexual orientation or personal instability. They very much need intimate relationships of affection and love. Such love cannot be found in the never-ending liaisons of the gay world, but they can be found in friendships, which need to be respected and encouraged. The premise that with the use of condoms the promiscuous activities of the gay world can once more be safely pursued is entirely false. Certain acts must be avoided since the risk is too great. The use of condoms is not a secure and certain method of safety from infection, though condom use is safer than unprotected intercourse. It is not the church's task to enter into specific recommendations about condom use, but opposition to education about prevention of AIDS — whether by condoms or clean needles — would seem to be reactionary. The church must speak, however, about sexual morality. That is her task and her duty.

5. The AIDS pandemic speaks of moral decay, and the solution must lie in a moral renewal. But that renewal will not come by harshness or rigidity. Rather, it will come by a firm intention of taking responsibility to avoid infection and to abide by the moral teachings of the church. Doing that depends not only upon regular confession and Holy Communion, but upon support by a forgiving and accepting Christian community. The disaster which AIDS represents in the urban setting, and most particularly for the ethnic ghettos and the gay community, is one that we cannot greet with an attitude of "we told you so." Rather, it is an invitation to a spiritual renewal, whereby compassion, humility, and fervent prayer for those who suffer can become once more the primary note of Orthodox Christians. It bids us to come out of the ethnic ghettos which would give us such a false security that it could never happen to people like us. It calls us to come forth and recognize that we are all in this together, that we are all sinners and depend entirely upon the compassionate mercy of God. Only by sharing our sense that we are all in this together can we mobilize attitudes to promote research for a cure, educate people for prevention, and negate the tendency to push the disease aside as being a malady of perverts rather than a human dilemma.

The attitude that HIV infection happens only to degenerates is a false security which would put ourselves and our children at risk. Only by embracing the person with AIDS as one loved by God, and in whom the mystery of sin and salvation is being worked out, can we creatively cope with this challenge to our faith, our community, and our integrity as Orthodox Christians.

Notes

1. Elizabeth Moberly, *Homosexuality: A New Christian Ethic* (Cambridge: James Clarke, 1983).
2. Dennis Altman, *AIDS in the Mind of America* (Garden City, NY: Doubleday, 1986).
3. David Spurgeon, *Understanding AIDS: A Canadian Strategy* (Toronto: Key Porter Books, 1988), p. 15.

Chapter 27

AIDS: A Serious and Special Opportunity for Ministry

John Backe

Acquired Immune Deficiency Syndrome (AIDS) is serious and deadly. It is serious for those who contract it: at present there is no cure. It is serious for family members and friends of People With AIDS (PWAs) and People With AIDS Related Complex (PWARCs), who struggle to care for their loved ones, and grieve at their loss. It is serious for our health care system, where increased demand for care strains existing resources. It is serious for our society as we sort out issues of individual rights and the need for public health protection. Finally AIDS is a serious opportunity for the church to understand what it means to minister in the name of Christ to those who have been, are, and will be affected by it.

Information about AIDS has become increasingly available. The bulk of material produced thus far has focused on medical facts about transmission and prevention. This is important and necessary information. The medical implications are only one aspect of the effect of AIDS. There is also a growing need to consider the emotional, social, political, theological, and spiritual implications.

This paper will focus on issues and concerns involved in doing ministry in the context of AIDS. While this includes direct pastoral care to PWAs, there are many other aspects of our daily lives that are being affected by this disease.

This document is an attempt to examine how the context for such a ministry of pastoral care is shaped; who is involved; what some of the social

"AIDS: A Serious and Special Opportunity for Ministry," *Mission Discoveries*, July 1987, pp. 2-10. Pastor John Backe is hospice chaplain at St. Luke's-Roosevelt Hospital, New York. Copyright © 1987 The American Lutheran Church. Reprinted by permission of Augsburg Fortress.

and ethical questions are; and to explore some specific responses churches might make when considering their pastoral, educational, and liturgical ministries.

Public Awareness of AIDS

AIDS was initially portrayed in this country as a disease linked almost exclusively to homosexual and bisexual males and intravenous drug abusers. This perception created a false sense of security for persons who did not regard themselves to be in such a so-called "high risk" group. It is now apparent that this initial perception was shortsighted. The virus that causes AIDS (called the Human Immunodeficiency Virus—HIV) does not distinguish between men and women, adults and children, rich and poor, gay and nongay, Christian and non-Christian. The reported and projected pattern of the spread of AIDS to groups other than the first two identified does not mean the virus has "spread to the general population." AIDS has always been in the "general population" where it is now manifesting itself more noticeably.

This means most people will find themselves involved in or touched by the AIDS epidemic in a variety of ways. Having personal friends or family with AIDS will become a more common experience. Friends, co-workers, or church members may have family members with AIDS. There are also people whose professional involvement includes caring for PWAs or PWARCs. News reports and social conversation are increasingly permeated with the subject. Encounters with people who are worried or frightened by the prospect of "catching AIDS" are on the increase. Requests for support or opposition of public policy proposals related to AIDS will be a common experience. The health care and insurance industries already are affected. All such realities will in turn affect everyone in ways we can't yet foretell. Such circumstances might make us angry, defensive, or afraid. It is important to recognize and deal with legitimate concerns without becoming paralyzed by irrational fear or bigotry. Two things should be remembered:

- There is no one to blame but the virus.
- We are not powerless.

AIDS Brings Awareness of Death's Reality

Underlying any approach to ministry in the context of AIDS is the recognition that addressing people's fears and concerns will ultimately involve more than the disease itself. This disease brings people face to face with two of the most powerful and enduring forces in their lives: death and sexuality. The reality and power of death in our lives is unavoidable. Regardless of attempts to study, analyze, and understand death it remains incomprehensible. However much one tries to avoid or deny death, it remains inevitable. A great deal of energy, physical and psychic, is expended in attempting to manage or control death. Philosophers, theologians, and psychologists have helped define and understand the process of dying and people's feelings about it. Much is known about anger, denial, bargaining, grief, and acceptance as emotional elements in the dying process. AIDS confronts every facet of human understanding and fear.

PWAs experience the same feelings with greater intensity and even deeper concerns. They are often ostracized by church, society, and members of their own family, especially if they are gay, or even thought to be gay.

Consider the mixed emotions for a person with AIDS who knows that at present, from a medical standpoint, there is no treatment or cure. Life expectancy following diagnosis of AIDS may be less than two years. At the same time, that person also knows of the intense research being conducted, and the attention being paid to the problem. This raises hope for a scientific breakthrough. People with AIDS are often caught between despair and wishful optimism, which is emotionally wearing. Many people have a fear of dying alone, of being abandoned by friends and family in their last hours. People with AIDS know this is not vague psychological apprehension, but too often a painful reality.

Friends, lovers, and family members may have a difficult time accepting the diagnosis. Think of the trauma parents experience when they are told their son, in the prime of life, has a terminal disease, and then also come to realize that he is gay. Elements of past relationships may be exacerbated. Others may not feel emotionally equipped to deal with the pressure involved, the possible stigma, or the grief of watching a loved one die. This often results in guilt feelings or the abandonment of the person with AIDS, which adds anguish to anguish in this tragic cycle. Ministry here requires an awareness of such dynamics offering support both for patients and those around them. In one-to-one pastoral relationships, and as examples of compassionate concern, we need to be present to all who suffer and are in pain. Churches need to be perceived as places where people can bring their pain and grief and receive a comforting and caring reception. The organization of support groups for families and friends that provide physical and emotional help could be one small way to manifest such concern.

Traditionally, as church people, we find some measure of comfort or control in the face of death by assigning it to a place in the "natural order." This is true, but any temporary relief is limited by our fears. We are sad, but relatively comfortable with the death of an older person. This is especially true if the person "did not suffer," and if we have some specific cause, a disease or heart attack, as a convenient explanation. Disruption of this order in isolated events such as accidents, or the death of a young child, is more disturbing but is ultimately accepted on the grounds of being beyond our control and random enough to be nonthreatening. Large-scale manifestations of death, war or famine for example, are sufficiently removed from our personal experience (unless we know someone who dies in battle) that we are also able to cope with it as a minimal disruption in our personal routine.

AIDS intrudes on such scenarios. The majority of those afflicted are young (under 45), increasing numbers are children. Many would be considered "in the prime of their lives," full of potential for service and success. The numbers and projections are sufficiently large and alarming to make it impossible to write this disease off as statistically irrelevant. AIDS is not limited to some clearly defined "other" that we can conveniently disregard. One cannot avoid dealing with the reality of death as it so aggressively positions itself in the path of life.

The Church as Partner with Other Disciplines

AIDS has been a special challenge to the medical community. Here the church has a special relationship and opportunity. Forthright support and appreciation for the work of nurses, doctors, researchers, and volunteers who work in the medical disciplines and health care services are important. Such talent, compassion, and intelligence are gifts which God uses in service to those in need. God uses medical knowledge and skill as an important channel for health and healing. At the same time, people, in and out of medicine, often find it necessary to cope with the limits of medicine and technology. For some, acceptance of such limits is extremely difficult. At times, the death of a patient is perceived with a sense of personal failure by the health care professional. Given the nature of AIDS, such perceptions can be very discouraging and painful. As a gathered community of believers, the Christian church could well seek out, celebrate, and support such people and their work. Lifting up the holistic nature of God's concern for all can help people in their struggle with illness and death, be they the afflicted or the care-giver.

Confronting Issues of Sexuality

Ministry in the context of AIDS cannot avoid attitudes and feelings about sexuality. This subject has proven difficult enough under the best conditions.

If the people of a church are not accustomed to addressing issues of sexuality and relationships in the regular course of their life together, they are likely to have a difficult time doing so in this context.

Frank discussion of the facts involved is absolutely necessary, though many may feel it to be inappropriate in a church setting. In fact, there is no other agency or institution that should be as well-qualified. The church should have something to say regarding sex education in the home, churches, and schools, the destructive dynamics of homophobia, and intimacy and relationships. The discussion of sexuality and AIDS necessitates the use of the explicit language of sexuality. Responsible education for people about AIDS requires the use of words like "anal sex" and "condom" at some point. Many people may become disturbed or even angry if this is done. Some people may die of AIDS if it is not.

One major route of transmission for the AIDS virus is through sexual intercourse. Some people may be too embarrassed to discuss AIDS for this reason. A fearful response to the danger of AIDS has even created an atmosphere in which people have begun to equate sexual contact with death: "If you have sex, you will get AIDS and die, so don't have sex." To complicate the issue further, there is the multitude of fears and biases concerning homosexuality called homophobia; that is, fear, distress, and hostility toward gay and lesbian people. All together, this leaves a formidable tangle of emotions, fears, feelings, and facts for people to sort out. One doesn't have to approve of homosexuality to care for people who are ill. One doesn't have to be a homosexual to be concerned about the AIDS epidemic. One doesn't have to practice sexual abstinence in order to avoid AIDS.

Sexuality is a gift from God, meant to be enjoyed and used creatively. That will mean different things to different people. Like all gifts, it can be abused or damaged. When that happens, lives and relationships suffer. God's response to our brokenness and suffering is healing and wholeness, not punishment and disease. Sexual intercourse does not cause AIDS. Homosexuality does not cause AIDS. A virus causes AIDS.

Public Health and Human Rights

An issue of this magnitude also arouses strong feelings in the community at large. There are questions about public health and well-being that need to be discussed and debated. People need to be informed. Elected officials and government agencies need to develop policies to protect public health while also protecting individual rights. Churches can serve an important role in this process, providing information to members, joining community coalitions for education, developing opportunities for a variety of views to be included and discussed. In one small community in rural Minnesota, in response to the first reported AIDS case, a county-wide seminar was held by a coalition of clergy, social workers, and medical care providers. Presently, education is the only preventive we have against the virus.

But the educational task is not limited to facts about the disease. In discussions about public policy, there will be ethical and political considerations as well. Churches can help provide a voice for the voiceless by reminding people of their presence. People with any illness are often perceived as less than fully human. A terminal illness makes this even more true. Add to this the fact that many people with AIDS are gay or drug abusers or poor and you find more reasons their voices may be diminished in the public arena where decisions will be made about them. There are broad socioeconomic justice questions of AIDS as it relates to race and poverty—that is that black, Latino, and poor people are disproportionately affected by AIDS, and have fewest resources available to them. All the voices must be heard. Space limitations do not allow for discussion here of all aspects of the issues involved in public policy concerns, but a partial list of those issues would include:

- Should blood tests for AIDS be required? Of whom? When?
- Can the results be kept confidential?
- Should there be tests before issuing marriage licenses?
- Should employers or insurance companies be able to require negative test results?
- Should children with AIDS be allowed in school?
- Should condoms be distributed in prisons? In schools?
- Should drug users be given sterile needles?
- Should people with AIDS or ARC be quarantined?
- Should a person who tests positive be required to name his or her sexual partners?
- Should people with AIDS be barred from traveling between countries?
- How do we protect people with AIDS from discrimination?
- How will we pay the cost for the extensive medical treatment required?
- How will our government spending priorities have to change?

The list goes on.

An Opportunity To Be the Church

Christians historically and in the present are called to be the proclaimers of life in the face of the awesomeness of death. What life do Christians proclaim? Not the "false life" of cheery slogans, whistling past the grave-yard, assuring people that things will be better "someday," or retreating to the blasphemy of pronouncing a disease a specific punishment for someone's life. This "false life" does not recognize and confront the power of death. Death causes pain and suffering. This is not illusion. Christians proclaim life that is the Good News of Jesus Christ in whom God has taken the initiative to proclaim that the reality of death is not the final reality. The Christian faith seeks to offer healing, comfort, and life itself in a broken world. AIDS reminds us that we are mortal creatures living limited lives in an imperfect world. All suffer and are subject to death. All are loved by God. All are offered comfort and release from suffering through God's gracious action on our behalf through Jesus Christ. God's will is health and wholeness for all of God's creation.

Many opportunities exist to witness to God's love in the AIDS epidemic.

One is in regard to the effect on doctors, nurses, and health care professionals who witness the death of a large number of contemporaries. Another is the special grieving of a parent for a dying child. Such opportunities need to be understood and addressed in terms of personal as well as community response in the church. This is the context of the church's call to be a healing community in the midst of the hurts, fears, and griefs of people's lives affected by AIDS.

Ministry is opportunity. It is the opportunity to serve all of God's people without regard to race, color, creed, or sexual orientation. It is the opportunity to bring healing in the midst of brokenness. "The AIDS epidemic . . . may just be the church's latest best opportunity to show itself and the world what it is for the church to be the church" (Robert W. Lyon, Asbury Theological Seminary, *Engage/Social Action*, February 1986).

Consider what form a ministry in the context of AIDS might take. To begin with, such a ministry must be defined in terms of what the church is and not what AIDS represents. Secondly, an approach to such a ministry begins with a sense of repentance for past failures and an acknowledgment of one's own limitations and inabilities.

There is need to offer one's own self to God, allowing God to shape and lead, rather than relying on one's own judgments and predispositions. God does not call us to more than we can bear. The opportunity to experience God's unconditional love by sharing it with those in need, is both a tremendous gift and a tremendous responsibility.

Pastoral Care

Accepting the opportunity for ministry, and moving to implement specific plans, is not always an easy task. People involved in a ministry that deals with AIDS need to begin by examining their motivations, presuppositions, and limits. Too often, the attempt is to minister to people who are ill or grieving as though we have something to give them, rather than entering into and participating with them in their experience. Advocacy might well be considered an important pastoral role when ministering to PWAs and their loved ones. When working with patients who are considered terminally ill, as is now the case with AIDS patients, there can be a tendency, usually unintentional, to "bury them before they are dead." The tendency is to treat them as dying people whose life is, in effect, over rather than as living people like ourselves, with hopes, fears, problems, and joys.

In the case of AIDS-related illness, there is the danger of the unintentional response of feeling that in some way or other the patient deserves his or her illness; the feeling that he or she did something wrong and is somehow responsible for his/her situation. This is irrelevant at the point they are in need of concern and loving service. No one wants to contract a deadly disease; no one sets out to get AIDS.

Most people with AIDS today had little or no information about the virus at the time they contracted it. The fact that many people do get AIDS is a tragedy. Judgments on the part of the care giver about what should have been done or how they should have lived need to be put aside. The call, in the moment of need, is to be the presence and witness of God's unconditional love. The possibility of a minister's need for esteem, control, to demonstrate self-righteousness, to pass judgment, or place limits on grace, is a far cry from the faithful, Gospel based witness to which Christian ministers are called. One might anticipate that working with terminally ill patients would be a burden and depressing. People who actually do the work most often use the word "privilege" to describe their experience.

One is not called to do everything, nor is it possible. At first people may not be personally comfortable in dealing with a PWA, but may be willing to offer support to family members by running errands, or helping supply materials for parents of a child with AIDS. In that particular situation, there may be a variety of needs such as money, bleach, disposable diapers, or food. Whether we are working with adult men or adult women, children, families, the "worried well," drug abusers, or minority populations, we need to learn from them how they might best be served. Only by coming close to them, by entering into their lives, can we realistically expect them to enter into ours. When this happens it becomes all the more possible to bring a message of hope and healing that is more than words, but which God proclaims through the enfleshment of service and love.

Whatever the setting, pastoral ministry should be prepared to deal with a variety of manifestations of despair and depression. Many people adopt a fatalistic view (nothing matters, I'm probably already infected, I'm not worth much, and there is no hope). There will be issues of hopelessness, feelings of abandonment, guilt, anger, opportunities for reconciliation, and feelings of isolation. We should be prepared to recognize these, address them as best we can, and utilize other resources (counseling, support groups) to fully serve. The initial news of a positive HIV antibody test can be upsetting. Though it is not a guarantee that a person will develop AIDS, the fear has been planted. A diagnosis of ARC or AIDS can be especially devastating. For some people, telling their families that they have AIDS may be the first time they have told their family they are gay or used drugs. Everyone involved will need help in finding ways to cope together, and the church can play a major role in providing supportive care for all concerned.

One additional aspect of attempts at pastoral ministry in this regard needs to be considered. One may feel called to this work. One may feel good about this ability to respond to needs. But it's important to be prepared to face up to a hard reality that the minister may face as a symbol of the church. This is especially true if the people we seek to include in our ministry are gay, or are drug users, and to a lesser extent, if they are poor. Their initial reaction might be different than we expect. In some form or other, the AIDS patient may feel or say: "You didn't make me feel welcome when I was well. Now that I am dying, I've qualified for your concern. You didn't see me as a person before, I was just a cause. No thank you."

One may not agree with such perceptions. One might be uncomfortable examining the truth of what is being said. This may be an opportunity for us to grow as "church" — to understand more fully our call to be the inclusive body of Christ in the world. Such shouldn't be a matter for debate. It is not necessary to try to "convince" people of our purpose. We can recognize the truth that we have all, church and individual, been less than God intended. We start again, by God's grace, to be what we can.

Need for Education

It would be difficult to think of another disease in our history about which we have learned as much in as short a time. Medical research continues to reveal new information which may lead to a treatment or cure. A large volume of material has been produced in a variety of formats to inform the public of the dangers of AIDS, the means of transmission, and the measures which enhance prevention. We might think that there is now a well-informed public, and that there is little need for education. We would be wrong.

There continues to be a need for ongoing education for all sectors of the community about the medical facts. Safer sex information is important for everyone. Drug abusers need information about their special risk behaviors. This is only the beginning of what needs to be an extensive educational curriculum. Adolescents in particular need sex education information that includes understanding of relationships and intimacy. AIDS awareness education in this context would be appropriate for confirmation classes, along with consideration of the meaning of health and wellness. Adults should become aware of the public policy concerns being discussed and the variety of opinions on crucial questions. In addition, education within congregations on issues of death and dying, grief and loss, estate and funeral planning would help general awareness. The specific needs of PWAs and their loved ones can be shared, in turn leading to ministry options. For example, in many cases PWAs experience food emergencies that we otherwise associate with homelessness. They have specific nutritional needs, and often have to use limited funds for medical equipment and don't have enough for food. In response to this, some congregations have begun meal programs to provide a needed lunch or dinner, either in a pleasant, welcoming atmosphere in a church, or delivering food to those unable to leave home. An outright gift of money or time might be given to support already existing efforts. The caring human contact is as nourishing as the food. The development of support and discussion groups where people can share concerns and learn of resources available to them are vital. Groups may be formed around specific populations (e.g., women, "worried well," families, PWA) or concerns (e.g., grief). We all need to continue to learn more about AIDS and about one another.

The Question of Testing

The question of testing needs to be openly discussed. Testing by itself is not a solution to the problem we face, nor is it a substitute for changed behavior. Testing for HIV antibodies should be done with complete anonymity. Some suggest the only purposes for HIV testing are screening blood donations or to establish a diagnosis of illness. The question is raised about the value of testing when current estimates are that between 20 and 80 percent of seropositives later develop ARC or AIDS. Would knowing result in pointless anxiety or careless behavior? In lieu of testing, people should live their lives in general without being obsessed about illness or death. In terms of sexual practice they should assume that they or their partners have been exposed.

AIDS and the Worshiping Community

The church worships. Worship is intrinsic to its being. While we are always on guard to be faithful to whom we worship, we need to be aware of the importance of the specifics in our worship life that pertain in this discussion. We can begin with the weekly liturgy. We can ask ourselves how members of our congregation would react if they knew someone with AIDS was worshiping with them. Should they know? How should the issue be addressed? What is the issue? While we might hope that there would be no problem, we know that the family of God gathered at worship is made up of people like ourselves, fallen and forgiven, constantly struggling to be faithful, sometimes failing. People will be fearful, confused, welcoming, indifferent. Each place will be different. This is not to minimize the potential for good or ill in a given situation, but rather to suggest that pastors need to know their own particular situation. Pastors are in a position to take deliberate steps (through education, planning, and so on) to minimize negative responses, thereby maximizing the possibility of true worship.

There may be specific concerns about the use of the common cup in sharing the Eucharist. Evidence indicates that this is not a way of transmitting AIDS. Evidence does not always allay fears. Recognizing the emotional issues involved, there may be no easy solution. As there are specific resources available to deal with this question in the detail it deserves, we will not attempt to do that here.

The church at worship needs to appreciate and redevelop its important legacy of the healing power of prayer. Services of healing for persons with

AIDS, persons with ARC, families, lovers, and friends can be conducted by individual congregations or on a community basis. Regular intercession in the prayer of the church should include PWAs, lovers, family members, those who grieve, those who are afraid, volunteers, public policy makers, and professionals in the medical profession. We pray for all of our needs in anticipation of the total healing of all creation.

Funerals: Remembering the Dead in Worship

There is one final area of our worship life which is often overlooked but which has special significance for our discussion. Funerals are worship services of the whole church. We do not often consider them this way. There may be a variety of mitigating circumstances, but ideally we should gather as the whole family of God's people to mourn with those who mourn, but also to proclaim the hope and joy of new life that God in Jesus Christ gives us. Funerals serve a variety of cultural functions as well, and we can be sensitive to this without compromising what we feel to be important in our liturgy. Pastors and congregations would do well to consider funeral-related issues in order to better serve those in need. Preplanning of funerals can be a meaningful experience for both dying people and their loved ones. This is not always possible, but should be considered. Preparation of a last will and testament and establishing power of attorney can be important protection for designated heirs in order to retain the integrity of committed relationships. Pastors should be aware of the various options available and the legal requirements in a given location. Questions will arise about the need for embalming, for example, or how cremation can be arranged. The cost of funerals is often a burden; providing information beforehand on choices and charges is a real service. In doing so you will confront some societal taboos perhaps, as well as the psychological defense of pretending something won't happen if you don't plan it. There is no need to push people into anything, but to be available when needed is a real comfort. Choices about whether to conduct a funeral (body present) or a memorial service (no body present), as well as the location of the service should be considered. Are funerals only for church members? Are there restrictions? Fees? Discussion of these concerns and providing answers to these questions can be a real ministry.

All of the things we have said about funerals so far apply to everyone. In death, as in life, AIDS changes the context in which we minister. The fears and concerns that attended the life of an AIDS patient do not necessarily end with death. Pastors especially need to be aware of special problems that families, friends, or lovers may encounter in making funeral arrangements. Some funeral directors may be insensitive, or communicate their own disdain or prejudice. Others may be more compassionate. Directing families to the latter would be a service. Depending on location, there

will be different requirements by health departments or agencies regulating
funeral practice, for preparation or presentation of bodies of AIDS victims.
These should be known beforehand. Discrimination against PWAs or their
loved ones in regard to funeral practice should not be tolerated, and in
many places is illegal. Many local governments have an AIDS discrimination office which will advocate on behalf of families or friends if the need
arises.

Beyond the mechanics of the funeral arrangements, the funeral liturgy
and sermon provide a tremendous opportunity for proclamation of the
church's message of hope, forgiveness, and healing. The challenge for those
of us who claim to believe is to determine what it is, exactly, that we do
believe, and how we communicate that. The people attending the funeral
have suffered a great loss in their lives. They are angry, sad, confused, and
hurt. They may feel they have evidence that God does not love them, but
in fact, the opposite may be true. It is precisely in the midst of that hurt
and despair that we are called. We are not there to present dazzling arguments to convince people that their feelings are wrong or to impress them
with our theological acumen. Rather by our presence, our compassion, our
prayers, and our lives, we demonstrate that God has not abandoned them.
God has brought them into the fellowship of the rest of the community of
faith, where we all share the burden of loss as well as the hope and joy of
new life in Christ.

Ministry in the context of AIDS is a ministry in which we need to be
especially mindful of the setting, the specifics of the situation and the people we are called to serve. We proceed from there with the resources and
faith that God gives us. We represent the God of life. We are called, at all
times, to minister to a world and people in the grip of death. In the face
of the fears and concerns that people have, we can proclaim hope and
healing. Death is the end of dying, not the end of life. The God who made
us and cared for us does not abandon us in what we consider to be our last
moments, but as a caring friend sees us through and welcomes us at our
destination. Ministry in this context may require new images, and the ability
to deal with paradox or dichotomies.

In terms of death and dying, many of us need to unlearn our upbringing.
Instead we may want to help people see their illness and their dying in
terms of going home, or of claiming our name before God, or of healing,
or of a journey. People will need help to maintain a sense of hope rather
than one of optimism; to feel their lives can be fruitful even if they are not
judged to be productive. Lives have meaning even if one feels there is no
purpose.

In our ministry, we can offer theology over technique; understand people
rather than reassure them, remind people that we are called to believe, not
to be convinced.

In all of this, we discover that the issues of dying are not reserved for
people with AIDS or the terminally ill. Our ministry can lead us to discover

how much we have in common, how much God cares for us, what a precious gift life is, how important we are to one another. God calls us to be the church, our concern is redemption, not survival. God gives us new life and the opportunity to discover one another, through caring and service. Today AIDS presents a special and serious opportunity for ministry.

Chapter 28

A Measure of Our Humanity

Julian Filochowski

Introduction

The opening words of Vatican II's *Gaudium et Spes,* the Pastoral Constitution on the Church in the Modern World, read as follows: "The joys and hopes, the griefs and anxieties of the people of this age, especially those who are poor or in any way afflicted, these, too, are the joys and hopes, the griefs and anxieties of the followers of Christ" (*GS,* 1).

The aim of this article is to set the scene for church agencies and Catholic institutions and associations, to clarify motivation, indicate the wide range of possible ecclesial responses to the AIDS pandemic and to underline how crucial, indeed how imperative, such a response is if we are to live up to that inspiring commitment of the universal church at Vatican II.

It is necessary to begin by considering a few of the startling statistics relating to the worldwide spread of AIDS. The headlines for AIDS are these:

- By the end of 1990 more than 300,000 cases of AIDS from over 150 countries had been officially reported by governments to the World Health Organization (WHO) in Geneva.
- Because of defective record keeping, because of under-recognition and faulty diagnosis of the condition, because of under-reporting, inaccurate reporting and even false reporting, the WHO estimates that since the start of the pandemic a total of 1.3 million cases of AIDS may have occurred worldwide.

"A Measure of Our Humanity: The Church's Response to the AIDS Pandemic," *Catholic International,* November 15-30, 1991, pp. 961-968. Julian Filochowski is chair of the Caritas Internationalis Working Group on AIDS. This text is based on his address to the Caritas Consultation on AIDS, Hong Kong, 1991.

• The WHO estimates that between 8 and 10 million people have been infected with the Human Immunodeficiency Virus (HIV) which causes AIDS.

• The WHO estimates that by the year 2000 there may be a cumulative total of 15 to 20 million adults plus 10 million infants and children infected with HIV.

From these figures it is self-evident that the AIDS crisis is not simply an outbreak or a localized epidemic of a killer disease: it is a truly global pandemic.

This global pandemic is unprecedented in human history but, by its virulence, it reminds us of the plague of the fourteenth century, which wiped out half the population of Europe. The origin of that plague was a mystery. It was surrounded by shame and fear, and society needed to create scapegoats to cope with it, so the blame fell upon Jews and then upon women, who were persecuted as witches.

AIDS has similar characteristics today. It could be said that people with AIDS (PWAs), by the way they are treated and regarded, have become the equivalent of the lepers of former times. In the gospels, Jesus not only physically cured the ten lepers and the paralytic, and the woman with the hemorrhage, but he also restored to them their human dignity, and their rightful place in the community. Saint Francis of Assisi and Saint Catherine of Sienna kissed the lepers' sores, not simply because they were sores but because they were the living wounds of the suffering Christ. They were still sores, however, and in the lepers the saints recognized their brothers and sisters as themselves.

For those of us who are dedicated to service within the Christian community it is especially important not to become paralyzed by fear in the face of this disease, nor polarized in sterile debate. We should instead perceive the pandemic as a crucial moment in the world's history, when the church can once again respond to fresh challenges and opportunities with unselfish love and without prejudice, in the tradition of our brother and savior Jesus Christ.

In his Christmas message of 1988, Pope John Paul II drew the attention of the whole world to the plight of people with AIDS: "People with AIDS are brought face to face with the challenge not only of the sickness, but also the mistrust of a fearful society that instinctively turns away from them. I invite everyone to take up the tragic burden of these brethren of ours and I assure them of my deep affection. May the concerted efforts of science and love soon find the hoped-for remedy. This is the hope I lay at the crib of the new-born savior."

He had taken up the issue a year earlier in Arizona, during his visit to the United States, when he had encouraged the representatives of the Catholic Health Association with these words: "Today you are faced with new challenges, new needs. One of these is the present crisis of immense proportions which is that of AIDS. Besides your professional contribution and your human sensitivities towards all affected by this disease, you are called to show the love and compassion of Christ and his Church."

To respond with love and compassion, with commitment and determination, with integrity and humility to people with AIDS must be an intrinsic element of our preferential option for the poor today. The church has embraced the cause of the poor and often expressed explicitly its option for the poor. To live authentically an option for the poor is never easy. It is far more than sympathy with the poor and the suffering from a distance. In many of our societies PWAs are the excluded poor, the poorest of the poor; they are the marginalized. To share, and truly share the concerns of the marginalized always requires both courage and great discernment.

First we must banish fear and popular prejudice and understand that AIDS is not Africa's disease, but a human tragedy affecting people of every gender, race, age group, sexual orientation, marital status or state of life. Babies, high-school students, army colonels, married women and men, Catholic priests and religious, Protestant pastors and even grandparents too, have all died and are dying today of AIDS and AIDS-related conditions. Whether they contracted it from blood transfusions, from sexual intercourse, from mother to child in the womb, from sharing syringes, or from dirty hospital equipment, they are all to be loved and embraced unconditionally and nonjudgmentally as sons and daughters of our God: each one is precious and cherished. There is no division between 'innocent' victims of AIDS and 'guilty' victims of AIDS. Indeed we should avoid 'victim' language altogether. They are all people—temples of the Holy Spirit—who have to live with AIDS. Those who pretend that AIDS is God's punishment on a sinful section of our society have a vengeful God, a clumsy God and certainly not our Christian God of forgiveness, life and love.

AIDS and the Church

The Church as Provider of Services

PWAs have a condition with no cure. And despite massive global research investment, none is expected to be available for five years at least, and no vaccine for at least ten years. But even when such drugs become available it is unlikely that third-world countries will be able to pay the colossal prices to import them in significant quantities for them to be made available to ordinary men and women who have AIDS or carry the HIV virus.

The services needed by PWAs today, and for many years into the future, can be divided into three categories:
• Medical/therapeutic services,
• Social/support services,
• Pastoral/spiritual services.

The church is being called to offer all these to people affected by AIDS, especially where they are not being provided by governments or by other private institutions.

Medical and Therapeutic Services

These include:
- sympathetic referral points and specialized clinics for the proper diagnosis of AIDS and AIDS-related conditions;
- the treatment of opportunistic infections, including medication, hospitalization when necessary and careful monitoring of the progress of the condition, in order to enable people to live with AIDS;
- terminal care for the dying and hospice care, if and when the disease finally takes its toll.

The wealthy can purchase this medical care, the poor usually go without. Throughout Africa the Catholic medical services, mission hospitals and clinics are beginning to offer specialized services to PWAs. Doctors, nurses, paramedical workers and social workers are all being trained and educated to deal with AIDS. In putting themselves alongside people with AIDS, just as their predecessors had done with those suffering from leprosy, many religious orders have been able to identify in a new way with the charism of their founders. In every one of our countries we must, sooner or later, bring together those who have responsibility for a health pastoral and those who run our church social welfare institutions to define clearly our Catholic response to the pandemic and draw up an agenda for action.

Social and Support Services

The medical services required by PWAs must be backed up by a multitude of support/social services. In seeking to live with AIDS, PWAs need supportive counselling as well as advice (on diet and exercise for example), home visits to help them cope in their day-to-day survival, sometimes transport to clinics, sometimes special care for their children. Pastoral workers, parish sisters and members of Christian movements are trying to provide such services in many parts of the world. In fact, ordinary volunteers from the Catholic parishes and base communities have been mobilized in increasing numbers in the United States, Europe, Brazil and Africa, to befriend and to support PWAs, and thus take on part of this healing, caring ministry.

It is particularly important to attempt to provide the services to people with AIDS in response to the needs they themselves articulate, and not simply in accordance with what we feel they ought to need. Self-help groups of PWAs and associations of HIV-positive people have sprung up all over the world; their mutual care schemes, their determination and their achievements are a magnificent testimony for all of us, and they should make us very humble indeed. These groups need support, and church facilities and infrastructure should be put at their disposal.

The counselling needed goes beyond those who are sick and includes the 'worried well,' in other words, those HIV-positive persons who have not developed AIDS and the families, friends and loved ones of those with AIDS. Furthermore, the establishment of support groups for carers is now seen as crucially important because so many people are burning themselves out in fidelity to the demands of caring for the terminally sick.

Spiritual and Pastoral Services

Intimately linked to the provision of social services is pastoral care — the giving of sacramental and spiritual support to people with AIDS, their families and friends. These services cannot be offered by any other organization; they are unique to the church's mission. To present just one example, there is an annual anointing service in London for people with AIDS, their friends and carers, which provides enormous sustenance and affirmation to those involved.

All these different services to PWAs are essential and exceedingly difficult to separate one from another. Last September [1990], in Burundi, Pope John Paul II exhorted us all to participate in this caring work.

> It is our duty to help people with AIDS. . . . May the disciples of Christ crucified stand with love at the foot of the cross which is borne by these poor, with whom our savior also wanted to identify. And Christian communities will need to be very generous in their support of the families who have been broken by the illness of one of their members and in caring for children deprived of parents. We hope that the day is drawing near when this scourge of AIDS will be eliminated. But as we face our current ordeal, let us be living witnesses of God's merciful love. Let us be the bearers of hope, in the faith of Christ who gave his life for the salvation of all.

The Church as Educator

Education is a much debated topic when we consider AIDS. One is tempted immediately to think only of the debate about the prevention of AIDS by advocating the use of condoms. Education, however, involves a much broader range of topics. Let us consider some of them.

We can educate people about the basic facts concerning AIDS. Even in countries where the mass media is highly developed, many people are still very ignorant about AIDS. They really do not know what the disease is or how one can contract it, and they thus respond with irrational fear and discrimination toward those who have been infected by the HIV virus, who have contracted full-blown AIDS or belong to groups whose behavior is considered to put them at risk of contracting the disease. The twin disease of AIDS is "AFRAIDS," or "Acute Fear Regarding AIDS."

Government information campaigns which rely a great deal on magazine advertisements and television commercials do not, unfortunately, reach a great proportion of the urban poor. The illiterate shanty-town dwellers do not buy glossy magazines or see television. But the church's channels to inform and educate (through the parishes, base communities, radio schools and popular organizations) are ideal means through which the crucial facts about AIDS can be passed on to the poor. Who else will reach the children who sleep on the city streets of the Third World? In Uganda, for example, the church is one of the principal mechanisms for grassroots education. Alongside the government education campaign, entitled "Love Carefully," the church has developed its own "Love Faithfully" campaign, with posters, leaflets and stickers. It has been very effective.

Education to prevent the spread of AIDS is fundamentally important if we are to arrest the frightening growth of the pandemic, given that young people's sexual experimentation usually starts before the age of 12. In schools, among children in the 5-15 age range, the information about AIDS and its spread can be placed in the proper context of education about wholesome and healthy human relationships. But whether in schools, youth groups or Christian communities, the church's message will always hold up the ideal of life-long relationships of fidelity, and not simply suggest that promiscuity should be made a little safer.

While we consider this theme of education, we should not forget the need to educate ourselves. In this respect it is of vital and urgent importance that the clergy, the religious, seminarians and pastoral agents are instructed about AIDS. In many parts of the world we hear that people who contract the disease often turn to their spiritual leaders for advice, support and spiritual healing in order to make their heavy burdens more bearable. In other places, sadly, the local church is the last place that people with AIDS would go for help and guidance, and this should give us food for thought. Either way, we cannot presume that such religious leaders are automatically prepared or able to handle the emotions, the complicated issues and especially the deep mysteries which present themselves as a result of this new pandemic.

We must here underline the special educational role which can be assumed by those people who are already HIV-positive or who have contracted full-blown AIDS. Who can better teach us about AIDS than those who struggle each day with the physical, psychological and spiritual pain of this disease? It is essential that church leaders take the small step to learn from PWAs, so that they can look at the pandemic from their perspective.

After our clergy and religious are properly formed in this area, we must then rely on them to assist in the education and instruction of the wider Christian community. Basic facts about AIDS and how it is contracted must once again be presented, but also to be presented is the mandate that all

Christians have to be of service to those who are marginalized from the rest of society.

It seems that, on this latter point, the Church can assume a unique role. Many of the other educational efforts in society which focus on the prevention of AIDS seem to deny that this disease can touch the healthy, strong and good people in our population. By challenging the whole Christian community to be of service to those with AIDS, we remind them that PWAs are indeed part of the whole community and must never be cast out or shunned by others.

Official public statements from the church can have an important educational impact. Pastoral letters from church leaders and bishops' conferences which speak the truth about AIDS clearly and proclaim the church's concern and commitment to PWAs, have greatly comforted those who are suffering, have reduced fear and worry in the populace at large and encouraged cautious Catholics to play some small part in their parish, neighborhood or workplace in supporting PWAs.

The visible and active witness of our bishops and church leaders speaks louder than any number of official statements. When our pastors and bishops themselves visit and spend time talking with PWAs they bring not only direct comfort and moral support, but they are also examples to the whole Christian community.

The Church as Advocate

Because of fear and prejudice, the basic rights of PWAs and those who are HIV-positive are being eroded and violated all over the world. Many have found themselves thrown out of their jobs, some have been evicted from their homes and others have found themselves refused treatment at health centers. On frequent occasions they have been denied a proper and dignified burial by funeral parlors. PWAs have been too often blocked from receiving other necessary public services and they continually face discrimination because they carry the virus. In Africa, some priests are refusing to bury PWAs if they have not had the sacrament of the sick or paid their church dues.

Enforced blood tests are being introduced in many places. These prevent freedom of travel to HIV-positive people, block their chances to study and can be used by others as a means of discrimination when they attempt to secure employment, insurance or social services. It is tragic that certain religious orders and dioceses are now introducing mandatory testing of candidates as a criterion for selection to the seminary or novitiate. Blood tests without guaranteeing the confidentiality of the results are a violation of a person's human rights. Unfortunately this is a widespread problem. Blood tests without advice and counselling are unprofessional and damaging, and are all too frequent. So the whole ethics of testing is a major concern. The totalitarian tendencies in this respect for many governments are causing much suffering. In the Third World, Cuba's quarantine policies for all people with AIDS or HIV are deeply disturbing.

Intolerable pressures are sometimes brought to bear on women diagnosed HIV-positive to undergo sterilization. For those women who are pregnant, similar and improper pressure is exerted upon them to abort. These issues, whenever and wherever they become visible, should be on the agenda of all church agencies and commissions which struggle for justice, peace and human rights—and we must make sure that they are! It is important to plan and focus our advocacy efforts carefully, so that they will have real and positive effects. We must press government leaders to provide adequate medical and social support services to PWAs. We must push and persuade our own congregations to include PWAs within the community of parish life. Finally, we must speak out against the exploitation of PWAs by unscrupulous and professionally questionable scientists, physicians and pharmaceutical companies who use this pandemic to increase their own wealth and fame. Pope John Paul II's words of warning in this sphere give us a lead to follow; in Tanzania last year, in an address to diplomats, he said:

> The AIDS epidemic calls for a supreme effort of international co-operation on the part of governments, the world medical and scientific community and all those who exercise influence in developing a sense of moral responsibility in society. The threat is so great that indifference on the part of public authorities, condemnatory or discriminatory practices towards those affected by the Acquired Immunodeficiency Virus, or self-interested rivalries in the search for a medical answer to this syndrome, should be considered forms of collaboration with this terrible evil which has come upon humanity. . . . Those members of the Church will continue to play their part in caring for those who are suffering with AIDS, as Jesus taught his followers to do (Mt 25:36). . . . Our individual and collective concern for them is a definite measure of our humanity, taken in the loftiest sense of the word.

Opportunities for Networking

A Question of Values

It is almost surprising that so many people want to hear the church's view and witness the church's action in responding to the AIDS pandemic. By our participation in networks which are attempting to strategize and coordinate appropriate action with regard to AIDS, we can take the opportunity to emphasize our basic value system as well as the gospel mandate of unconditional love which was given to us by Jesus Christ. Some church leaders have expressed caution about entering into networks with governments and other organizations which advocate AIDS prevention techniques which may be contrary to the church's moral teachings. If we do not enter such networks, however, we then lose the possibility of bringing our own values and influence into the dialogue and debate which continue to take place within the field of AIDS services. We should consider participating in some of the following networks:

1. WHO global program on AIDS

The World Health Organization has been charged with stimulating and coordinating the worldwide response to the pandemic. WHO has invited Caritas Internationalis to participate in special meetings and seminars on AIDS. It has actively sought our views and opinions on such topics as community-based services, educational efforts and the role of non-governmental activity.

2. National AIDS committees

Most of the world's nations have already established national AIDS committees and are developing both short-term and medium-term national AIDS plans. In many countries, church leaders have been included as members on such committees and have been able to exert a positive influence on the formulation of appropriate action plans. We must find out about, and get copies of, the plans for each country.

3. Local community networks

In some countries and regions, local non-governmental groups have taken a very active role in developing services and advocacy efforts for PWAs. At times these groups find they need to network together in order to avoid conflicts and duplication of service efforts. Church-related organizations can often play an active role in such networks and can sometimes even serve as the principal coordinating body for the network.

Catholic Organizations Related to AIDS Services

At times we meet competition and lack of communication and coordination efforts within our own family of church-related organizations. Such a waste of energy must be avoided in the face of this pandemic. We must use every bit of our energy to fight the disease and to comfort those already affected by it.

For this reason it is very important to plan our specific services together. Let us remember further that an appropriate response must involve both assistance and development efforts as well as social justice activities. Thus the full range of socio-pastoral organizations should join together in networks of AIDS services, on an international, regional, national and local level.

In the course of such networking, we cannot forget the need to support those who are serving PWAs on a day-to-day basis. Such work is extremely difficult and can cause physical, psychological and spiritual exhaustion. In June 1988, the first National Catholic AIDS Ministry Conference was held in the United States at Notre Dame University. More than two hundred pastoral agents came together to learn more about the disease and to receive mutual support and comfort in their work. This might be a good model to be utilized in other nations as well.

The International Working Group on AIDS within Caritas reflects a priority commitment of the confederation to mutual assistance and support in facing up to the AIDS crisis.

Ecumenical Networking

While we differ widely in certain theological teachings and in other pastoral practices, let us not forget that we share many common values and a tradition of Christian service with our brothers and sisters who belong to other Christian churches. Many of these churches have also been active in responding to the AIDS pandemic. Networking with these churches can bring strength to our own Catholic efforts in this field. Thus we might find a "friendly voice" in the 1986 resolution of the Executive Committee of the World Council of Churches:

The people of God can be the family that embraces and sustains those who are sick with AIDS-related conditions, caring for the brother, sister or child without barriers, exclusion, hostility or rejection. Since AIDS is a global epidemic, effective action by churches and individual Christians must extend not only to the AIDS neighbor closest at hand, but also through effective global collaboration to the stranger on the farthest side of the world.

Conclusion

We must pledge to keep PWAs, their families, their friends and their care givers constantly present in the prayer of the church, particularly in the Prayer of the Faithful and the eucharistic prayer. Masses and special liturgies for them require creativity from us. There is a beautiful "Way of the Cross" written in East Africa, which has been used by many groups in different countries. The first day of December each year has been desig-nated "World AIDS Day," and it has been encouraging to see how many commemorative masses and special liturgies have been organized all over the world to mark the day.

For most of us, the starting point and reference point for all our work is the eucharist. As we share the body and blood of Christ as our food and drink in the eucharist, may we all affirm that it is the real body of Christ, who suffers today through HIV and AIDS. It is the real mind of Christ which is racked by fear and confusion. It is the real image of God in Christ which is blasphemed through prejudice and oppression.

May the bread and wine be a sign of our pledge to see in suffering, not punishment or death, but the place where the wonders of God are being revealed and where together, as sisters and brothers, we can lead each other on to life in all its fullness.

Conclusion

The Way of the Cross

Sister Kay Lawlor, M.M.M.

We adore you, O Christ, as you carry your cross along the dusty roads of Masaka.

We make the way of the cross in the homes and at the bedside of those with AIDS.

We bless you, because through this suffering you have redeemed the world.

1. Jesus is condemned to death. He sits shocked, unable to speak. His hands tremble. Marko has just been told he has AIDS. "I'm going to die," he says.

2. Jesus takes up his cross. He is weighed down with the knowledge that he has AIDS. How can he tell his children? He tells his brother, sells some land, makes arrangements for his children. It's hard; it's a heavy load that Vincent carries.

3. Jesus falls the first time. He cannot stand alone; the abscesses are too painful; Peter is too weak. With help, he makes it home and to bed, where he begins the difficult task of regaining strength so he can pick up the cross of living with AIDS and continue his journey.

4. Jesus meets his mother. She lies there waiting for her mother to return. Regina has just learned that she has AIDS and is dying. She wants to tell

"The Way of the Cross," *Catholic International*, November 15-30, 1991, p. 968. Sister Kay Lawlor, M.M.M., is pastoral care coordinator at Kitova Hospital, Masaka, Uganda.

her mother. As they meet a look of pain and love passes between them. "I have slim!" Her mother takes her in her arms and they weep.

5. Simon helps Jesus carry his cross. Richard has so many decisions to make. How can he go on? When his brothers come, he tells them he's too scared to go on. They comfort him; arrange to take him home; plan to help him tell his wife; promise to provide transport so he can return for treatment.

6. Veronica wipes the face of Jesus. She lies there, too weak to clean herself. Her clothes are dirty and soiled because the diarrhea is almost constant now. She's alone, pushed into the corridor so the smell won't disturb others. A young nurse comes, washes her, changes her clothes. Rose smiles.

7. Jesus falls the second time. He's begun to have diarrhea; no longer wants to eat. Sleep doesn't come and he's afraid. The illness is getting worse. Peter has to start work. It's hard to keep living with AIDS.

8. Jesus meets the women of Jerusalem. Jane has no land; Mary has no milk for her baby; Scovia's husband sent her away when he learned she had AIDS; Juliet was put out of her rented room; Betty works in a bar to support her children, providing "favors" for men to get food for the children. The plight of poor women and AIDS. Jesus weeps.

9. Jesus falls the third time. His head feels as if it's bursting; nothing brings relief. Peter lies in bed, unable even to open his eyes. As the end nears, relatives arrive to move him from his rented room where he suffered alone for many months. One more step along the way.

10. Jesus is stripped of his garments. They put her out of the house, but kept her clothes, saying they wouldn't fit her wasted body. They told her to go to her grandmother to die. Once there, she was again rejected, stripped of all, even her right to belong. Juliet was returned to the hospital like an unwanted commodity.

11. Jesus is nailed to the cross. He cannot move, finds it hard to breathe. He must wait for someone to care for him totally. An AIDS-related brain tumor has nailed James to his bed; his mother keeps watch.

12. Jesus dies on the cross. Rose, Peter, John, Elecha, Kakande, William, Joseph, George, Grace, Paulo, Goretti . . . Jesus' body dying of AIDS.

13. Jesus is taken down from the cross. The wailing begins; the car reaches the homestead. As men rush forward to carry Paulo's shrouded body, a woman comes from the house. She reaches out to touch the body of her son.

14. Jesus is placed in the tomb. A grave dug on hospital land, only staff for mourners. Her nine-month-old child cries, not understanding. The grave is filled. All go away. Rose is dead.

Selected Bibliography

The following books can enrich the discussion of the articles in this book. Several of the books in the second section, "Ethics and AIDS," may be especially helpful. As was mentioned in the Introduction, reflecting on the specific issues will be more fruitful when grounded in a sound moral methodology, that is, a clear and coherent way of making moral decisions.

Geography and AIDS

AIDS in the World, by Jonathan Mann, Daniel J. M. Tarantola and Thomas W. Netter, editors (Harvard University Press, 1992) presents the impact of the epidemic, the global response, and global vulnerability—comprehensive information basic to a new global vision for a world confronting AIDS.

AIDS: The Making of a Chronic Disease, by Elizabeth Fee and Daniel M. Fox, editors (University of California Press, 1992) analyzes politics and public policy, human rights, international perspectives, and the changing population with HIV infection.

And the Band Played On, by Randy Shilts (Penguin Books, 1988) reports on the early spread of AIDS in the United States and the responses of government, health authorities, and scientists.

The Screaming Room, by Barbara Peabody (Avon Books, 1987) presents a mother's journal of her son's struggle with AIDS. A true story of love, dedication, and courage that offers insight into the actual experience of living and dying with AIDS.

Ethics and AIDS

Reason Informed by Faith, by Richard M. Gula, S.S. (Paulist Press, 1989) presents the foundations of Catholic moral theology in a careful and comprehensive manner.

Conscience in Conflict, by Kenneth R. Overberg, S.J. (St. Anthony Messenger Press, 1991) provides a brief and readable process for coming to decisions about crucial contemporary personal and social questions.

Principles of Biomedical Ethics (Third Edition), by Tom L. Beauchamp and James F. Childress (Oxford University Press, 1989) includes discussions of autonomy, beneficence, justice, and virtue.

AIDS & Ethics, by Frederic G. Reamer, editor (Columbia University Press, 1991) includes a series of original, seminal essays offering a systematic overview of a wide range of ethical issues.

Habits of the Heart, by Robert N. Bellah, et al. (Harper & Row, 1986) studies

American mores, revealing both present limits and possible visions for dealing with individualism and the common good—with significant implications for the nation's response to AIDS. Also see both their sequels, *The Good Society* (Vintage, 1992) and *Beyond Individualism*, by Donald L. Gelpi, S.J., editor (University of Notre Dame Press, 1989).

Society and AIDS

AIDS: The Second Decade, by Heather G. Miller, Charles F. Turner, and Lincoln E. Moses, editors (National Academy Press, 1990) covers major issues such as trends in AIDS cases among male homosexuals, IV drug users, women, and minorities; also looks at discrimination and behavioral intervention strategies.

The Social Impact of AIDS in the United States, by Albert R. Jonsen and Jeff Stryker, editors (National Academy Press, 1993) explores how HIV and AIDS have affected fundamental policies and practices in some of the country's major institutions (religions, prisons, public health).

AIDS and the Health Care System, by Lawrence O. Gostin, editor (Yale University Press, 1990) presents views of prominent authorities on key issues of health policy, such as testing, confidentiality, and use of resources.

Multicultural Human Services for AIDS Treatment and Prevention: Policy, Perspectives, and Planning, by Julio Morales and Marcia Bok, editors (Harrington Park Press, 1992) presents specific suggestions for prevention, education, and behavioral change strategies that are culturally specific and sensitive.

Religion and AIDS

The Many Faces of AIDS, by the Administrative Board of the United States Catholic Conference (USCC Publications, 1987) presents a sensitive pastoral response. See also *Called to Compassion and Responsibility*, by the National Conference of Catholic Bishops (USCC Publications, 1989).

For Those We Love: A Spiritual Perspective on AIDS (Second Edition), by the AIDS Ministry Program of the Archdiocese of Saint Paul and Minneapolis (Pilgrim Press, 1991) focuses on spirituality by offering reflections from people living with AIDS; a handbook that reveals wisdom and hope.

Embracing the Mystery: Prayerful Responses to AIDS, by Sebastian Sandys, editor (Liturgical Press, 1993) a collection of prayers, readings, and meditations—for those with AIDS and for those who care for them.

Ministry to Persons with AIDS: A Family Systems Approach, by Robert J. Perelli, C.J.M. (Augsburg Press, 1991) sheds light on the thoughts and feeling of the family members whose loved ones are living with AIDS.

AIDS and the Church: The Second Decade, by Earl E. Schelp and Ronald H. Sunderland (Westminster/John Knox Press, 1992) presents a compassionate and prophetic vision of what the church's response ought to be.

Index

Women and AIDS, 64, 83-96; prevention, 189-99
Worship, 258-59
Wounded Healer (Nouwen), 241-42
Zagury, Daniel, 138
Zaire, 42, 46-47, 49-50, 87, 138-40

Zambia, 41, 45-46, 60
Zhang, Qingcai, 38
Zielinska, Wládysláwa, 29-30
Zimbabwe, 41-43, 46, 135, 139
Zion, Basil, 243-48
Zuger, Abigail, 234